curing cancer-*phobia*

curing cancer-
phobia

How Risk,
Fear, and Worry
Mislead Us

David Ropeik

Johns Hopkins University Press

BALTIMORE

© 2023 Johns Hopkins University Press
All rights reserved. Published 2023
Printed in the United States of America on acid-free paper
2   4   6   8   9   7   5   3   1

Johns Hopkins University Press
2715 North Charles Street
Baltimore, Maryland 21218
www.press.jhu.edu

Library of Congress Cataloging-in-Publication Data is available.

ISBN 978-1-4214-4740-7 (hardcover)
ISBN 978-1-4214-4741-4 (ebook)

A catalog record for this book is available from the British Library.

Special discounts are available for bulk purchases of this book.
For more information, please contact Special Sales at specialsales@jh.edu.

To Toby, for her patience, love, support,
and for her wisdom and courage

To everyone who shared their stories
about fear of cancer

To anyone who has ever faced,
or fears they might one day face,
those frightening words:
"You have cancer"

contents

curing
cancer-
phobia

introduction

As for us, we behave like a herd of deer. When they flee from
the huntsman's feathers in affright, which way do they turn?
What haven of safety do they make for? Why, they rush upon
the nets! And thus they perish by confounding what they
should fear with that wherein no danger lies.
—Epictetus

This book needs to start with an apology. How dare anyone claim
that fear of cancer is excessive or, in some cases, even a phobia? The disease is a terrible killer. Most of us have been a victim of its cruelty, either
as a patient or mourning the death of a family member, friend, colleague,
or neighbor. Certainly, medical providers know firsthand cancer's awful
impact. Fear of cancer is entirely understandable. A book that seems to
challenge that fear as irrational or excessive may seem an arrogant affront
to the pain and loss so many of us have endured. A fair reading of the evidence, however, supports the observation that, in some cases, our fear
of cancer exceeds the actual risk and does great harm all by itself. In the
name of our own health and public health in general, we must face that
difficult reality.

Critically, this book considers the evidence at the population level
only, from the general perspective of public health. I do not dare challenge
anyone's personal feelings about cancer or the individual choices we
make under its fearful shadow. I profoundly respect that, at a personal
level, our decisions about any health threat are ours alone to make in the
context of our own lives, and only we can judge whether those decisions
are right or wrong.

Rather, the pages that follow take the 30,000-foot view, considering
the impacts of our fear of cancer at the societal level. Seen through this

broad lens, and in light of all we've learned about cancer in the past couple decades, it is inescapably clear that in some ways our fear of cancer significantly exceeds the actual risk, and that fear does great harm on its own. It has, in a sense, become a phobia—"an extreme or irrational fear or dread aroused by a particular object or circumstance," per the *Oxford English Dictionary*—that imposes massive costs on our health, our economy, and our society in many ways. To reduce those costs, we need to recognize that our fear of cancer can itself cause great damage. So we need to see with greater resolution where that fear comes from—its history and its psychology—and to identify the specific harms it produces. And we need to acknowledge and support not just the work being done to understand and cure the disease itself, but also all that's being done to reduce the damage that our fear of cancer causes.

———

One of the central messages I hope this book makes clear is that, in crucial ways, our emotional relationship with the Emperor of All Maladies is out of date. Consider some basic facts that fly squarely in the face of what most people believe about cancer:

- *A diagnosis of cancer no longer inescapably means death*, yet "death" is still the first word that comes to mind for two in three people in the developed world when they hear the word "cancer."[1] As many as two-thirds of the nearly 200 types of cancer are either treatable as chronic diseases or entirely curable.[2]
- *Not all cancers inevitably grow, spread, and harm.* As population-wide screening programs have taught us, many of the cancers we can now detect at very early stages— among them types of breast, prostate, thyroid, colorectal, and lung cancer—never grow and metastasize, or they grow so slowly that, if left undiagnosed, people never know they have cancer. They die *with* the disease but not *from* it. Some cancers even regress and disappear on their own.
- *Screening has taught us that finding cancer as early as possible is not the panacea we almost religiously believe it to be.* Some cancer-screening programs have a more modest lifesaving benefit than the public commonly believes. Worse, ever

more perceptive screening technologies now identify tens of thousands of cancer cases that scare us into treatments we don't really need, treatments that cause serious harm, more than the cancer ever would have.

- *Cancer is not mostly caused by environmental substances* in our air, water, food, and other products. Some is, certainly, but we can do far more to reduce our chance of developing cancer by making wise choices about diet and exercise than by avoiding "chemicals" and "radiation" and all the other things "out there" we spend billions trying to control.
- Cancer is largely the result of natural biological processes that over time take their toll on the health of our DNA.
- *Cancer is essentially a disease of aging.* More than half of the people in the United States diagnosed with cancer are at least 65 years old; 87% of the people in the United States who *die* of cancer are 50 or older; nearly half are 70 or older.[3]

These facts conflict with accepted but outdated beliefs and fears, beliefs and fears that often lead to choices that feel right but cause serious damage to each of us as individuals and to society as a whole. That harm, not from cancer but from our fear of this most dreaded of all diseases, is what *Curing Cancerphobia* seeks to bring to wider attention, in the hope of helping us recognize and confront this threat, even as we battle the disease itself.

Nonetheless, to the extent that anything to follow offends you, I sincerely apologize.

For nearly 100 years, cancer has been the most feared disease in the developed world. Not once in all those years, however, has it been the leading cause of death. Not even close. Cardiovascular disease has held that morbid title by a substantial margin. In 2018 cardiovascular disease killed 17.9 million people worldwide. Cancer killed roughly half that, about 9.6 million. In the United States the cardiovascular death toll in 2018 was 659,000. Cancer killed 599,000.

So rationally, based strictly on the numbers, we should be more afraid of heart disease, right? It's more likely to kill us. Well, that might make sense to a coldhearted risk manager or insurance actuary. But not to you and me. Our fears are shaped much more by the nature of *how* we die than by the statistical likelihood of what may kill us. And cancer feels like a much worse way to go than heart disease, for unique historical and emotional reasons that we'll explore in part one.

Emotionally, then, our fear of cancer makes sense. But not when we look at the range of what that fear leads to, the subject of part two. We've been taught that the best way to fight cancer is to catch it as early as possible, so worry about cancer leads millions of us to screen for the disease. But screening is not recommended for everyone, just for those that research has found are more likely to be helped than harmed. Fear of cancer scares tens of millions of people into screening who are not in the age groups, or who don't have the medical, demographic, or family history / genetic characteristics, that indicate higher potential risk. Research shows that, for those populations, screening may catch some life-threatening cancers, but it's more likely to cause harm. This is referred to as *overscreening*, the initiating step in a cascade of harms that follow.

Overscreening can lead to frightening false positives, false alarms when people hear the dreaded words "You have, or might have, cancer" only to find out days or weeks later that they don't. Worse, more screening increases the discovery of cancers that are *over*diagnosed; these are cancers diagnosed based on what their cells look like under a microscope but that are tiny and discovered in their early and isolated stages, cancers that doctors can predict with a high degree of confidence will never spread or cause any symptoms in the lifetime of the patient.

We fear these low-risk cancers more than the clinical evidence suggests we need to, and because the fearful C-word is in the diagnosis, we often choose more aggressive and riskier treatment than our medical condition requires. This is referred to as *over*treatment, which includes procedures such as these:

- Mastectomies for pre-invasive ductal carcinoma in situ: breast cancers that haven't spread and often never will.
- Prostatectomies and radiation treatments for asymptomatic and slow-growing prostate cancers.
- Thyroidectomies for tiny papillary thyroid cancer tumors, which are almost never fatal and almost always slow- or *non*-growing. This type of indolent cancer is so common that you and many other people reading this book may have it and will never know.

- High-risk surgeries to remove lung cancers that biopsies have identified as so slow growing that they would probably never harm the patient during his or her lifetime.

These procedures all cause serious side effects: mastectomy leaves many women with long-term pain, early menopause, or psychological and sexual intimacy problems; prostate cancer treatments cause the loss of erectile function or urinary incontinence in roughly one-third of the men who undergo them; thyroidectomies leave some patients with damaged or destroyed vocal cords, as well as weight gain and fatigue; and lung cancer surgeries can cause stroke, heart attack, or infection in elderly patients. Tragically, surgeries to remove nonthreatening cancers sometimes kill the patient, even though the cancer itself almost certainly never would have.

Our fear of cancer also causes harm by keeping people *away* from screening and treatment. For tens of thousands of people who *do* have characteristics that put them at higher risk and who *should* screen, the fear of being told "You have cancer" *scares them away from* screening. Many women who are told their mammogram found something suspicious never come back for follow-up screening. Fear helps explain why. It also causes many people to delay going to see a doctor even after early symptoms develop for fear of hearing the frightening news that they do indeed have cancer. This fear-driven *under*screening and "delayed presentation" causes many truly threatening cancers to go undiagnosed until the disease has grown and spread, at which point treatment is less effective.

Beyond the health effects on individuals, excessive fear of cancer has broad consequences for society, explored in part three. At least $5.3 billion is spent per year on surgeries and other treatments of essentially nonthreatening cancer that doesn't require such aggressive intervention. That's roughly 3% of all money spent on cancer care in the United States. Another $9.2 billion is spent each year screening people for cancer who are worried about the disease but, based on their age and lack of other risk factors, are outside the groups for whom screening is recommended and are more likely to be harmed than helped. Consumers spend billions on all sorts of products that falsely claim to provide protection from cancer. Governments invest huge amounts of money and effort protecting us from environmental carcinogens that are in many cases far less of a threat than we fear, resources that are then not available to protect us from greater environmental dangers. We oppose all sorts of useful technologies—cell phone towers, power lines, clean nuclear energy—on the basis of a cancer risk that is either tiny or nonexistent.

So at both the individual and the population levels, the fear of cancer in many ways exceeds the threat and leads to choices that cause unnecessary harm. Fortunately, the medical and public health communities are starting to recognize this problem and reduce those harms, which is explored in part four.

- For some types of less-threatening cancers, new treatment standards have been adopted that offer patients the option to wait and monitor the disease rather than have surgery immediately. An increasing number of men are choosing this option for slow-growing low-risk prostate cancer.
- For some types of cancer (thyroid and uterine), the frightening C-word has been removed from the diagnosis, and in these cases the number of people choosing more aggressive treatment than their medical condition requires is dropping. Similar changes have been proposed for the nomenclature of low-risk breast and prostate cancer diagnoses.
- National screening programs, some physicians' organizations, and a few cancer advocacy groups are beginning to warn people that common types of cancer screening—mammography, PSA testing (for the prostate), and thyroid screening—have limited benefit and do widespread harm. Proposals are being studied to limit screening to only those truly at risk.
- Work is being done to make doctors, who swear to "do no harm," more aware of the problems of overscreening, overdiagnosis, and overtreatment. Decision aids have been developed to help people think through their choices about cancer screening and treatment for low-risk disease, when critical thinking can so easily be overwhelmed by fear.

Caveats

The choices we make about cancer run from whether to screen in the first place to how far to go with treatment at the end of life. This book deals only with the early choices: whether to screen, whether to go to the doctor when symptoms arise, and what to do about a diagnosis of a low-risk type of cancer. The choices we make once we've been diagnosed with a more threatening type of cancer or when we are undergoing treatment are vastly more complex than this book dares to consider.

And to reiterate, even the initial choices considered here are not for anyone else to judge as right or wrong, intelligent or "irrational." Every choice a person makes is the right choice for them in the context of their own lives. This book analyzes things at the population and policy level only, an abstract, impersonal perspective irrelevant to an individual facing a diagnosis. And of course the analysis is with the objectivity of hindsight, which we also don't enjoy as we make choices about our future. As Danish philosopher Søren Kierkegaard observed, "Life can only be understood backwards; but it must be lived forwards."

Furthermore, this book respects that "rational" is an imprecise word for describing people's decisions about their health and safety. Nobody makes such choices based solely on a dispassionate, objective analysis of the evidence alone. Emotions are a valid part of any holistically rational decision about staying safe, staying alive. Risky surgery to remove a nonthreatening prostate, thyroid, or breast may in fact be more of what I call a "fear-ectomy" than a clinically necessary removal of life-threatening tissue, but removing the fear of living with cancer in your body, even if you've been told it's a nonthreatening or a slow-growing type of cancer, is entirely reasonable. Avoiding screening or a doctor's visit out of fear of being told you have what could be a fatal disease makes emotional sense too. As long as we are fully informed about the pros and cons of each option, that choice is ours to make, and only we can decide for ourselves whether that choice is right.

In addition, this book respects that what might seem like harm to an outsider might not feel like harm to the person experiencing that outcome. Consider a mother of two young kids who, diagnosed with a nonthreatening type of breast cancer, nonetheless opts to have both her breasts removed. To a stranger, and even her doctor, that may seem excessive and harmful. But to her that may be a cost she is willing to pay for the assurance that she'll be there to raise her kids. Or consider a 50-year-old man who learns he has a nonaggressive, asymptomatic prostate cancer, highly unlikely to ever do him any harm, but he chooses a radical prostatectomy rather than "watchful waiting." The diapers he has to wear for the rest of his life and his erectile dysfunction may be costs he's willing to pay to avoid the fear of knowing he has cancer growing in his body. The definition of harm is, in the end, up to each person and not for anyone but the person facing the risk to judge.

And one final caveat: I am a journalist, former Harvard instructor in risk communication, and consultant in the psychology of risk perception. My expertise is in carefully researching subjects and summarizing that research in, I hope, useful ways. I am not a doctor. This book does not claim or intend to be a thorough medical guide to any of the conditions discussed. To ensure the accuracy of the information provided, the book was reviewed by several respected experts, including oncologists, a public health policy expert, and four health care cost analysts. I asked several sources to review how I had described their input to ensure its accuracy. If there was something in a scientific paper I read that I didn't understand, I contacted the author for clarification. But nothing written here should be taken as medical advice that you should act on without getting professional guidance.

＝＝

I may take a population perspective and present a lot of big-picture information, but cancer is ultimately a personal experience, so this book is woven through with personal stories. They are stories of real people, with their names changed. The stories contain quoted or paraphrased conversations or summaries of what people have written. The one exception is Mark's story about lung cancer in chapter 7, which is fictional but based on what patients commonly experience when they have frightening but slow-growing lung cancers.

I have avoided the most dramatic stories, the ones from angry people who regret their decisions to have more aggressive treatment than their clinical conditions required and suffered grave harm as a result. Such dramatic stories are common in the news media, but they are surprisingly rare. Most people who choose to undergo a fear-ectomy remain content with their choice, no matter how harmful the outcome. Some of this may be what cognitive scientists call regret aversion, the tendency to avoid the inner conflict of admitting that the choice you made was wrong. Mostly, though, people take comfort knowing they have done all they could to deal with the fearsome threat of cancer, even if they did more than was clinically necessary and caused themselves serious harm. The fear of cancer is that powerful. So in the spirit of fairness and accuracy, the personal stories you'll read reflect that more common reality.

Two other small things: There are extensive citations for the sources of information in the book, should you want to explore them for yourself. Where those citations include a URL, the full source was available online as of March 2023. Also, I sought out the most recent data available, but frustratingly, given the way medical research is done and the lengthy process involved in getting it published, some of those data are many years old.

A few words on the origins of this book. Several inspirations led me here. I share them in the hope that they may help you appreciate why I wrote it and what I hope it accomplishes. The first was my experience as a street reporter for a TV station in Boston. Over 22 years, I did countless stories about situations involving some sort of risk, in which people were more afraid, or less afraid, than the experts I talked to said they needed to be. That led me to research what had been learned about the psychology of risk perception, a body of knowledge pioneered by Paul Slovic and others that explains such seemingly irrational behavior. That in turn helped me recognize countless examples of what I came to call the "risk perception gap," the gap between our fears and the facts that leads to choices about personal safety that *feel* right but sometimes cause harm all by themselves. I've written about those examples elsewhere.

The second inspiration was a TEDMED talk by Otis Brawley, then chief scientific officer of the American Cancer Society, entitled "War on Cancer, Year 40: Who's Winning?"[4] He described how we are still diagnosing cancer the same way we have for more than 150 years, based on what cells collected in biopsies (and now, their genes) look like—what they *are*—but not what those cells are *going to do*, which science and medicine are still unable to predict with certainty. Dr. Brawley's talk introduced me to the ideas of overdiagnosis and the overtreatment it sometimes leads to. It helped me recognize that fear of cancer is, in some cases, a clarion instance of a risk perception gap.

A third inspiration was my brain tumor. It had been surgically removed years earlier, with no ill effects, but remembering how terrifying it was to be diagnosed with a tumor—which my doctor reassured me was a benign growth (a hemangioblastoma, which would have killed me if it wasn't removed)—made it sharply clear how fear of cancer could overwhelm reassuring information that what a patient has, even if it is cancer, is not dangerous.

Finally, as I was doing preliminary research, I came across the October 31, 1955, edition of *Life* magazine, which featured an article by oncologist George Crile Jr., who would later be Rachel Carson's oncologist. In "A Plea against Blind Fear of Cancer," with the tagline "An experienced surgeon says that excessive worry leads to costly tests, undue suffering and unnecessary operations," and in a book that came out at the same time, *Cancer and Common Sense*, Dr. Crile wrote, "Already doctors are seeing increasing numbers of healthy patients who suffer only because they are afraid of getting cancer. This fear leads both doctors and patients to do unreasonable and therefore dangerous things." He concluded, "It is possible that today, in terms of the total number of people affected, fear of cancer is causing more suffering than cancer itself." He described this as "a new disease," which he named "cancerphobia."[5]

Dr. Crile's warning about cancerphobia was made a long time ago, the year the first McDonald's opened, the Mickey Mouse Club debuted, and Rosa Parks refused to give up her seat on a Montgomery, Alabama, bus. We have come a long way since then. We know a lot more about cancer and how to treat it. Adjusted for age shifts in the population, mortality from cancer is down 32% in the United States since the early 1990s, 15% to 20% globally.

Yet more than 60 years after Dr. Crile's warning, cancer remains the emperor of our fears, and both the disease itself and the condition Dr. Crile called cancerphobia continue to take a terrible toll. Cancer kills close to 600,000 Americans a year and nearly nine million people worldwide. But millions more fall victim to excessive fear of cancer in various ways, some fatal. Just as we can't yet entirely cure the physical disease, nor can we cure our deep fear of it. Both are woven into us, the disease largely a natural part of our biology, our fear the product of deep survival instincts. But the more we understand each, the better we can treat them and reduce their harms. It is my hope that what you are about to read might in some small way build on the foundations Dr. Crile laid and help you, and society in general, think about cancer in new and healthier ways.

Part One

the
origins
of
our fear
of cancer

the historical roots

Death is life's change agent. It clears out the old to make way
for the young.
                                            —Steve Jobs

Nasty, Brutish, and Short

Around 1.7 million years ago, an adolescent boy, probably of the species *Homo erectus*, awoke one day with a sore foot. He hobbled around
for a while, but over a few weeks, his foot grew too inflamed and painful
to walk on. He lost weight and developed trouble breathing. He gradu-
ally grew weaker, and several months after that first painful step, the boy
died. Most likely from cancer.

In the 1960s a fossilized metatarsal bone from his foot was found in
a cave in South Africa. In 2016, after analyzing an odd round-shaped lump
on the bone where there shouldn't have been one, scientists reported that
they had found the oldest case of cancer in a hominin: osteosarcoma, cancer of the bone. Cancer killed this boy 1.7 million years ago, before our
species, *Homo sapiens*, even arose.[1]

Cancer has almost certainly always been a part of human existence,
a product of our biology far longer than there has been plutonium, plastic, or pesticides. The disease is natural cell growth run amok, the result
of genetic mutations that allow for uncontrolled cellular reproduction. In
some cases, mutations in those wantonly multiplying cells give them the
additional ability to escape their organ of origin and spread into the rest
of the body. Most of these mutations occur naturally as our cells and their
DNA replicate and errors occur, or as they undergo constant dynamic
changes as a result of biological processes as simple as breathing or digestion. External agents can cause these mutations too, but the common

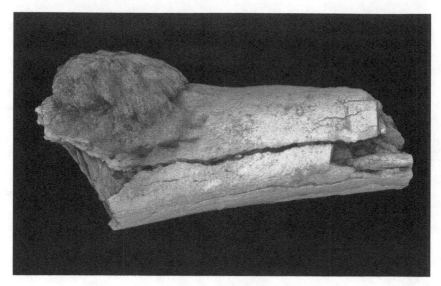

FIGURE 1.1
Bone cancer on a fossilized metatarsal bone, 1.7 million years old.
Courtesy of Patrick Randolph-Quinney, Northumbria University, United Kingdom

belief that *most* carcinogenic mutations are caused by external substances
is not supported by the evidence. The ratio of mutations that arise naturally to those caused by an external agent is debated, but recent research
suggests it may be roughly 2 to 1.[2] Long before there were carcinogens like
cigarettes, coal tar, or humanmade chemicals, there was cancer.

The scourge of cancer shows up in the earliest histories. The Edwin
Smith papyrus records observations of "ball-like tumors" on the chests
of eight Egyptian men in 3000 BCE. The ancient Sumerians, Chinese, In-
dians, and Persians all recorded diseases that seem to have been cancer,
dating as far back as 2000 BCE. Hippocrates, the Greek "father of modern
medicine," described a range of diseases whose characteristics fit cancer. But it was cancer on the surface of the breast that inspired him to
give this disfiguring growth its name: *karkinos*, a crab, or cancer in Latin.

Cancer was surely terrifying back then. Hippocrates's description of
breast cancer is chilling: a raised mass of dark tissue with a cold, hard-
as-a-rock surface with spreading claw-like extensions that bit into the
flesh. That visual description of breast cancer, for which the entire family
of roughly 200 types of these diseases is named, does not in fact fit most
other solid cancers, and it doesn't apply to nonsolid diseases like leukemia,

cancer of the blood. But another aspect of the way Hippocrates described cancer has, until recently, applied to most types. It was "too strong for the means at the disposal of medicine." Cancer was incurable.

Greek physician Galen, 500 years after Hippocrates, tried to understand and treat cancer based on the Hippocratic theory that four fluid "humors" controlled our health, and that cancer was the result of imbalance among them, a theory that would hold until the mid-1800s. But Galen too had a bleak view about what a diagnosis of cancer meant. "Only the beginning of a cancer admits of a cure," he wrote, "but when 'tis settled and confirmed, 'tis incurable and must die under a cold sweat."

Medieval physician Paul of Aegina wrote in the seventh century: "I for one could never cure a single case nor do I know anybody else who succeeded in doing so." Islamic scholar and physician Ibn Sina (commonly known as Avicenna, 980–1037) wrote in his famous *Canon of Medicine*: "It may happen sometimes that the starting cancer may be cured. But when it is advanced, verily will not."[3] Ambroise Paré (1510–1590), a French physician who attended four kings and whose battlefield techniques helped modernize the butchery of surgery, called cancer "Noli me tangere" (do not touch me), declaring, "Any kind of cancer is almost incurable and . . . [if operated on] . . . heals with great difficulty."

So we know that cancer has existed since prehistoric times, and it was surely greatly feared because it meant suffering and almost certain death. But we also know that fear of cancer was not as widespread as it is now. There just wasn't much of it around. For most cancers, it takes decades for the same long strand of DNA to suffer the several genetic mutations that allow a single cell to replicate with no controls and spread to other parts of the body (this spreading, or metastasis, causes most cancer deaths). Back then, most people simply didn't live long enough for cancer to develop.

Until the late 1800s, life for most was, in the words of English philosopher Thomas Hobbes (1588-1679), "solitary, poore, nasty, brutish, and short." From the Stone Age to the turn of the twentieth century, the average human life lasted from 20 to 35 years. If you made it to age 21 in late medieval England—and 40% of the population didn't—you had a shot at living to age 64, but only if you were among the wealthiest class. And few were. Cancer wasn't prevalent because older people weren't.

The Enlightenment, and the scientific revolution it spawned, eventually led to longer lives. We came to realize that we were not merely consigned to fate. We could figure things out. We could understand nature itself. We began to make the discoveries that have led to the longer life spans we enjoy today. Those longer lives, in turn, allowed cancer to become a far more common killer.

Some of those discoveries were about cancer itself. The disease might not have been common back then, but it was certainly feared enough to draw the attention of early researchers. In the middle 1500s Italian anatomist Gabriel Fallopius (1523–1562), for whom fallopian tubes are named, identified the difference between malignant and benign tumors. (Malignant tumors grow fast and spread. Benign tumors grow slowly and don't.) In 1713 Italian physician Bernardino Ramazzini (1633–1714) observed that, compared with the public in his hometown of Padua, celibate nuns didn't get cervical cancer (which we have learned is most commonly caused by the sexually transmitted human papillomavirus). But he also realized nuns had higher-than-average rates of breast cancer (which we now know is more common in women who haven't given birth, since the nine months of pregnancy slows the normal regeneration of breast cells—and the DNA in them—reducing the number of times DNA reproduction can make a mistake and natural mutations can occur). "You seldom find a convent that does not harbor this accursed pest, cancer, within its walls," he wrote.

In 1775 English physician Sir Percivall Pott (1714–1788) identified the first external environmental agent to cause cancer—soot—after documenting elevated rates of scrotal cancer in chimney sweeps. (The medical literature still sometimes refers to this condition as "chimney sweeps' carcinoma.") The connection between tobacco and cancer was first made in 1761 by John Hill (1714?–1775), who, in *Cautions against the Immoderate Use of Snuff*, documented elevated rates of cancer of the nose in heavy snuff sniffers.[4]

Other scientific milestones, though not directly connected to cancer, contributed even more to our longer life spans. In the early 1700s Italian anatomist Giovanni Morgagni (1682–1771) made autopsy a modern science, establishing that many diseases, including cancer, were not initially spread throughout the body but began at just one site (which is why today different cancers are identified by the organ in which they arise). In the late 1600s the advanced microscopes of Dutchman Antonie van Leeuwenhoek (1632–1723) enabled contemporary Englishman Robert Hooke (1635–1703) to discover cells, which in turn allowed mid-1800s German scientist Rudolf Virchow (1821–1902) to identify and draw detailed images of the pathology in diseased cells, including cancer cells. Virchow's images still provide a basis for cancer diagnoses today.

Far more than the work on cancer itself, progress in medicine and public health laid the foundations for life spans that, in the developed world, are nearly double what they were little more than a century ago. Hungarian obstetrician Ignaz Semmelweis (1818–1865) recognized that the unwashed hands of nurses who came in from surgical wards to deliver newborns raised the risk of infant mortality. In 1854 John Snow (1813–1858) tracked the cause of a London cholera outbreak to contaminated well water from one neighborhood pump, finally disproving the Galen-inspired theory that disease was caused by "miasma," or foul air. (More on foul air to come shortly.) In the middle and late 1800s biologists Louis Pasteur (1822–1895) and Robert Koch (1843–1910) identified the germs responsible for several diseases, and Joseph Lister (1827–1912) built on Semmelweis's observations when he developed antiseptic techniques for medical settings, including for surgery.

Surgery itself advanced. Across the millennia it had always been a barbarous last resort against cancer. (The Egyptians used "fire sticks" to burn tumors off the body.) Because surgery before the advent of anesthetic was so brutal and excruciating, it had to be done quickly, so it was mostly limited to external parts of the body. Despite all the suffering it caused, cancer surgery provided little benefit. That changed in a dim and crowded medical amphitheater in Boston in 1846, when William T. G. Morton (1819–1868) placed a glass inhaler over Edward Gilbert Abbott's face and administered anesthetizing ether before sawing and slicing a tumor from Abbott's jaw, an unthinkably barbaric surgery without such relief. Of the invisible gas that revolutionized surgery, John Collins Warren (1778–1856), Harvard's distinguished professor of surgery, declared at the time, with solid New England understatement: "Gentlemen, this is no humbug."

More extensive surgeries quickly proliferated. Invasive surgery attacking cancer of internal organs became more common. Anesthesia opened the way for radical mastectomy, a procedure that William Halsted (1852–1922) developed in the late 1800s, which stood as the default approach to breast cancer treatment until the 1960s. Such longer and more invasive operations would not have been possible without relief from the pain.

These discoveries were all critical for the development of modern medicine, which has helped lengthen the human life span. They were part of the larger scientific revolution in the 1600s through the 1800s, which figuratively took the medieval blinders off the human ability to understand the world in which we lived. And that, in turn, contributed to an age of unprecedented general optimism. The insights of Hooke and Virchow, of Semmelweis and Snow, of Koch, Pasteur, Lister, Morton and many others, contributed to a growing faith that we could figure anything out, an empowering sense that human intelligence could conquer any threat, that we could take control of our own fate. As Marie Curie (1867–1934) reportedly said when she learned she had cancer, "Nothing in life is to be feared, it is only to be understood. Now is the time to understand more, so that we may fear less."

But if the scientific revolution created hope, it still provided only a faint hope for curing cancer. Toward the end of the nineteenth century, the pervasive view of cancer was captured in the way one leading doctor described it in 1853:

> For centuries, it has been the dread of the human race. Its distinctive character has rendered its very name significant of malignancy; the ancient leprosy could scarcely have been regarded with more terror. Sad is the reflection that, even at this advanced stage of medical science, the inability to cure this disease is still one of those opprobria from which the science cannot rid itself. The physician is still obliged to look on as a bystander, unable to arrest the malady, literally eating into the very vitals of his patient.[5]

Even as science advanced, cancer remained a stubborn and terrifying opponent, and every hint of hope proved false.

Cancer Moves to Center Stage

What is to be done about cancer? No other question is so insistently demanding of medical science for a definite reply. For some unascertained reason this dread scourge seems to be increasing in a startling ration.

—*Ladies' Home Journal*, 1913

June and July 1858 in London were exceptionally hot and dry. There was no escape from oppressive heat that on some days exceeded 100 degrees. Nor from the stench. The Thames was at record low levels, exposing slimy river banks thick with miles of human waste several feet deep, rotting under a baking summer sun. The Thames had always been an open sewer, but with rising population and the invention of flush toilets, billions more gallons of filth poured into the Thames and now turned the baking London air into what became known as the Great Stink.

Dickens wrote in a letter to a friend, "I can certify that the offensive smells, even in that short whiff, have been of a most head-and-stomach-distending nature." Reporters described the river as "a pestiferous and typhus breeding abomination."[6] One wrote, "Gentility of speech is at an end—it stinks, and whoso once inhales the stink can never forget it and can count himself lucky if he lives to remember it."[7]

That last observation might have been the most telling of all, because much more was in the air of London in 1858 than just the gut-turning reek. There was deep gnawing fear. The third of three recent cholera outbreaks to sweep through the city had abated just four years earlier, after killing more than 10,000 people. Though John Snow's remarkable detective work in the second outbreak had conclusively identified contaminated water as the cause, the common belief remained that cholera and other infectious diseases were the result of "miasma," or foul air. And the air in London during those horrible two months was as foul—and as frightening—as it could get.

That fear, more than the gag-inducing stink, prompted the British government to immediately begin emergency construction of an advanced sewer and water treatment system, which began full operation only eight years later (remarkably, much of that system still operates today), probably saving more lives than any of the brilliant medical advances of nineteenth-century Europe.

The new London sewers, and similar systems built in many major cities, were part of one of the most overlooked but consequential advances in world history, the public health movement. No other program has extended the length and quality of human existence nearly as much. By the turn of the twentieth century, new sanitation systems, chlorination of drinking water, vaccines against several major infectious diseases, programs to isolate contagious tuberculosis patients in special clinics and sanatoriums, and the establishment of government public health departments (all predicated on the acceptance—finally—that germs, not miasma, caused disease) had begun reducing many major illnesses, principal players in the drama of human life and death. That, in turn, cleared the stage for cancer to emerge in the twentieth century in its starring role as the Emperor of All Maladies, the most feared disease in the modern developed world.

In 1900, cancer was at the bottom of the list of major causes of death in the United States (table 1.1).[8] Tuberculosis (TB) was the number two killer but by far the most feared cause of death. TB carried the dubious distinction of the Great Destroyer, the White Plague, and the Captain of the Men of Death. It bore those ominous labels and led the list of most feared diseases for one of the same reasons that cancer bears such titles now. Unlike the more common killers of pneumonia and influenza, tuberculosis was incurable. A diagnosis felt like a death sentence, as a diagnosis of cancer still feels for many today, despite the progress that has made many forms of cancer treatable or even curable.

In 1896 the *American Journal of Psychology* reported that when people were asked which diseases they feared, only 5% named cancer. Smallpox, lockjaw, consumption, rabies, diphtheria, leprosy, pneumonia—even being crushed in a rail accident or during an earthquake, drowning, being burned alive, or being hit by lightning—were more feared than cancer.[9]

TABLE 1.1.
Causes of Death in the United States in 1900

RANK	CAUSE	NUMBER OF DEATHS	RATE PER 100,000
1	Pneumonia and influenza	40,362	202
2	Tuberculosis	38,820	194
3	Diarrhea, enteritis, and ulceration of the intestines	28,491	143
4	Diseases of the heart	24,497	137
5	Intracranial lesions of vascular origin (stroke)	21,353	107
6	Nephritis (kidney disease)	17,699	89
7	Accidents (excluding motor vehicles)	14,429	72
8	*Cancer*	12,769	64

But thanks to rapidly increasing life spans, cancer would soon top the list. In 1890 the average white woman in the United States lived 44 years, the average white male 43. In 1900, just ten years later, the averages had risen to 48 and 46. (Statistics were not kept for people of color.) Similar shifts were under way in England, Germany, France, and Japan. By 1910 life expectancy was up to 52 for women and 48 for men. People were living longer, and as they did, cancer crept up the list of killers.

By 1910, though it was still in eighth place, cancer was killing 71 people per 100,000, a 10% increase in just ten years, while tuberculosis deaths had declined 25%. And by 1920, when life expectancy had risen to 55 for women and 54 for men (a critical threshold; roughly three out of every four cancers today occur in people 55 and older), cancer had moved up to sixth and was killing 83 per 100,000, while the mortality rate for tuberculosis had dropped dramatically, from 194 to 113 per 100,000 people. In just two decades, the death toll from America's most feared killer had dropped by 40%, while the annual death toll from cancer had risen by roughly a third.

Few people were aware of these population-level statistics, but they knew what was happening in their own lives, and increasingly people either had cancer themselves or knew someone who did. Growing awareness of the disease was magnified by increasing attention from the news media. In 1900, 90 articles in the *New York Times* mentioned cancer, a word newspapers were reluctant to use because it triggered disgust and shame: 20 obituaries, 3 about new cancer hospitals or clinics, 1 about an x-ray cancer cure, and 1 about the hopeful discovery of a "cancer bacillus." By

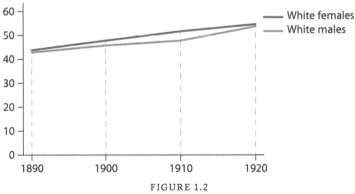

FIGURE 1.2
US life expectancy at birth, 1890–1920.

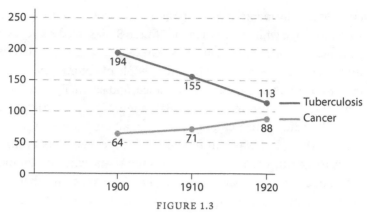

FIGURE 1.3

US tuberculosis and cancer mortality (per 100,000), 1900–1920.

1910 there were 137 mentions of cancer in the *New York Times*: 32 obitu-aries, 13 reports of potential cures, 2 reports about possible causes of cancer, and, capturing the trend of the day, 1 story reporting that in New York, "Compared with October last year there were fifty less deaths from tuberculosis. Cancer has an increase of 13."

A *New York Times* editorial in 1910 reflects the rising fear of cancer. "A Cancer Campaign" told of the new George Crocker Institute of Can-cer Research at Columbia University. George Crocker (1856–1909) was a wealthy western rancher who had lost his wife to cancer and donated $1.5 million ($41 million today) to create a research center to find a cure. And Crocker wasn't alone. As the prevalence and fear of cancer rose, philan-thropic donations in the first decade of the twentieth century established the New York State Institute for the Study of Malignant Disease, the Can-cer Commission at Harvard University, and the American Association for Cancer Research. Hospitals focusing on cancer treatment opened, as the St. Louis Skin and Cancer Hospital did in 1905, or expanded, as did the New York Cancer Hospital, opened in 1884, when it became the General Memorial Hospital for the Treatment of Cancer and Allied Diseases.

But most Americans had no access to modern medical care, nor trust in doctors, who were still largely seen as incompetent mechanics and profiteers more than reliable medical experts. People did have access to quacks, however, and the darkening cloud of cancer fed the proliferation of snake oil salesmen who feasted on, and fueled, society's growing cancerphobia.

An 11-part series, *The Great American Fraud*, in popular *McClure's Magazine* in 1905–1906 attacked the massive fake cure industry that preyed on the "ignorance and credulous hope" of a frightened public.[10] Investigative journalist Samuel Hopkins Adams (1871–1958) revealed such fake cancer cures as Dr. D. M. Bye's "Combination Oil Cure for the Treatment of Cancer, Tumor, Catarrh, Piles, Fistula, and all forms of Skin and Womb Diseases," which, Adams reported, turned out to be "a sort of paste of clay, glycerin, salicylic acid and oil of wintergreen; a mixture of cathartics for internal use; a Vaseline preparation; and the oil itself, which is ordinary commercial cotton seed oil with an infusion of vegetable matter. And with this combination [Bye] proposes to remove cancer and cure the condition that causes it! His treatment wouldn't remove a wart or a mosquito bite."[11]

Adams outed S. Andral Kilmer, proprietor of the CanCertorium in Binghamton, New York, who claimed to be "cancer's first conqueror." He revealed the fraud of a man who called himself Isham, whose "Humanity Baking Powder" and "Waters of Life" were promised not only to cure cancer but to restore hair to bald heads. And Adams uncovered the scam of the Dr. Warner Remedy Company, which was advertising its "Mineral Radium Water (which) has more miraculous and wonderful cures to its credit than any other known agency." Adams reported that the water contained no radium at all.[12]

Adams's exposé contributed to passage of the Pure Food and Drug Act in 1906, and ultimately to the creation of the Food and Drug Administration, which continues to fight precisely the same phenomenon today, fake cancer remedies that their purveyors peddle to profit from people's fears. At the turn of the twentieth century those fears had become so strong that the quack medicine industry was estimated to be worth $2 billion per year (in today's value), and exposés like the *McClure's* series did little to dampen those sales. That the popularity of quack cures and products falsely promising protection from cancer persists to this day is testimony to how the fear of a cancer death easily clouds the reasoning mind.

Fear also compels the mind to look for patterns, to find answers, to try to understand whatever threatens us so we can protect ourselves. As the prevalence and fear of cancer rose in the early 1900s, so did the breadth of suggestions about what was causing that rise. Many believed that all cancer was hereditary (as some cancers indeed are), or contagious (as a few cancers are), or the result of excessive consumption of various foods (obesity and poor diet also increase cancer risk). Some believed that cancer was caused by living in damp or dirty environments and that it was principally a disease of the poor. There was even the suggestion that since one cluster of cancer cases occurred near a popular fishing lake, that living near lakes and streams filled with trout might cause cancer. (President Grover Cleveland, who had had a secret operation to remove a tumor from the top of his mouth, bought that explanation and gave up trout fishing.)

Some of our current beliefs about what causes cancer trace their beginnings back to this search for answers in the early 1900s, as cancer incidence and fear both climbed. In the smoke and whirr and electric glow of the Industrial Revolution arose the hypothesis that modern civilization itself was causing this ever more feared menace, precursor to the widely held belief today that cancer is mostly or entirely caused by external environmental agents, products of modern industry and technology. In a 1915 *New York Times* essay, "Civilization Has Created a Long List of New Diseases; Medical Science Forced to Grapple with Ills that the Flesh of Long Ago Knew Nothing Of," E. H. Lewinski-Corwin, executive secretary of the Public Health Committee of the New York Academy of Medicine, wrote: "The ever-growing speed and tension of our life, the unsanitary conditions under which we live, work, and play, the unwholesome tendency of extreme specialization and standardization, the constantly occurring industrial changes and displacements which, in connection with internal migrations, rural exodus, and foreign immigration, produce appallingly large numbers of misfits, ignorance, intemperance, and immorality—all and every one of them contribute toward health decadence and life waste." In 1934 Henry Miller (1891–1980) named his controversial book *Tropic of Cancer* not for the latitude but because, he wrote, "to me, cancer symbolizes the disease of civilization, the endpoint of the wrong path, the necessity to change course radically, to start completely over from scratch."

Medical experts fought back against such unsupported speculation. In the 1907 book *The Control of a Scourge: Or, How Cancer is Curable*, English surgeon Charles Childe (1858–1926) wrote: "[Cancer] has been ascribed to influences of civilisation, yet closer acquaintance with savage races has demonstrated that it is present among them . . . The patent fact, indeed, is its universality, its prevalence under apparently almost every conceivable condition, whether of soil, climate, diet, race, occupation, or animal life." Childe did acknowledge, though, that part of the cancer threat was new. Not the disease, but society's growing fear. It was this fear, he claimed, that gave rise to the unsubstantiated claims about its causes, the popularity of quacks and the harm from their phony products, and the fact that people weren't coming in for diagnosis and treatment until it was too late, a problem that persists today (as discussed in depth in chapter 10).

To Childe and a few of his colleagues, the solution to this threat was education. Information. Childe dedicated his book to fighting rising cancer fear: "It is hoped that its publication may give rise generally to a less dismal feeling with regard to this disease than exists to-day." While Childe fully understood that talking openly about cancer could fuel the fear he was trying to dispel, he thought it worth taking that risk: "It may be urged that such a book and the spread of such information as it contains will alarm the public. Let that for the moment be granted. I hold that it is better even to alarm the public then to stand idly by and see the public commit involuntary suicide."[13] From fear of cancer.

A small group of doctors in the United States thought the same thing. The result of their response to the rise of cancerphobia in the beginning of the twentieth century is the army of advocacy groups offering patient support and promoting cancer education, treatment, and research today. These groups have achieved a great deal in the effort to bring cancer under control. But to achieve their goals, these advocacy organizations have played on and fueled our fear. As George Crile wrote in *Cancer and Common Sense*, "Those responsible for telling the public about cancer have chosen to use the weapon of fear. They have portrayed cancer as an insidious, dreadful, relentless invader. With religious fervor they have fashioned a devil out of cancer. They have bred in a sensitive public a fear that is approaching hysteria."[14]

The "C-word" Comes out of the Closet

At the top of the front page of the *New York Times* on April 23, 1913, next to a headline that read,

WOMEN IN SUBWAY FLEE BEFORE MICE
Then Three Small Boys Easily Obtained Seats in a Crowded Car

was this unassuming headline and story:

RICH WOMEN BEGIN A WAR ON CANCER
Mrs. Sage, Mrs. F.W. Vanderbilt and Mrs. Speyer
Helping to Plan National Campaign.
Steps were taken at a meeting of Physicians and laymen called yesterday
afternoon by Dr. Clement Cleveland to organize a National Anti-Cancer
Association and to begin a campaign of education on the prevention of
cancer similar to that which has been carried on against tuberculosis.

It would be 24 more years before Congress passed the first National
Cancer Act in 1937, establishing the National Cancer Institute, and another 34 after that before President Richard Nixon signed the second National Cancer Act in 1971, the moment generally considered to be the
start of the modern US so-called war on cancer. But if you share the understanding of that "war" as the programmatic government-funded
effort to enhance cancer diagnosis and treatment, research its causes,
and—holy grail of medical holy grails—find a cure, then April 23, 1913, is
probably a more accurate date for when that focused fight began. Much
that has come about since had its beginnings in that gathering of New
York society women and prominent East Coast medical leaders.

A month later the group announced the creation of the American Society for the Control of Cancer (ASCC) with the motto "Fight Cancer
with Knowledge." The group published leaflets and posters and offered
public lectures, mostly aimed at women, with messages like

- "Most cancer, discovered early, is curable."
- "The only cure is the knife."
- "Medicines [at that time, this meant quack remedies] are
  worse than useless."
- "Delay is more than dangerous; it is deadly."
- "The fatalism which says 'If it's cancer I might as well give
  up' is foolish, cowardly, and suicidal."

But the ASCC motto of "Fight Cancer with Knowledge" might as well
have read "Fight Fear of Cancer with Knowledge." Like Charles Childe,
the ASCC recognized even then the harm of both cancer and cancerphobia.
"There is no gainsaying the fact," the ASCC wrote, "that many women

have an instinctive dread of cancer. They believe that it is inherited and therefore unavoidable. They have known so many cases which terminated fatally that they think the diseases always incurable, and if they must die anyway, they will at least live in blissful ignorance as long as possible, and hide the truth, even from themselves."[15]

But as the ASCC tried to fight fear with the facts, it struggled to educate the public without fueling those worries. At a meeting in 1914, a senior ASCC official said, "We need to do away with this word 'cancer' and bring into use instead a number of expressions that will rightfully describe the various kinds of growths that occur among rebellious cells."[16] That's exactly what the medical community today has either already done or is considering; the diagnoses for some types of uterine and thyroid cancer have removed "the C-word," a change also being considered for some types of prostate and breast cancer. (Much more on that in part four.)

The ASCC's pamphlets, public talks, and events like National Cancer Week began to open up public conversation of and news reporting about cancer. Newspapers reached almost everybody in the early twentieth century, and the headlines from back then reflect the prevailing schizophrenia about the disease. Editors knew that the prevalence and fear of the disease were rising, but they also knew that the word "cancer" was literally offensive to most people. So they focused on the positive edge of the emotional sword of hope and fear. *New York Times* headlines between 1910 and 1916 included:

HOPE FOR CURE FOR CANCER, Doctor Tells How Cancer Vanished
CANCER: CAUSED BY BAD FOOD, CURED BY GOOD FOOD
CANCER CURES BY RADIUM
NEW BLOOD REMEDY MAY CURE CANCER
USES ELECTRICITY IN CURE FOR CANCER
CAUSE OF CANCER FOUND AT LAST BY BOSTON SCIENTIST

But along with positive news stories, a growing number of obituaries confirmed the darker truth everyone knew; hope rang false against the spreading toll of death touching more and more lives. Rarely did obituaries list cancer as the cause of death for anyone famous. But one early article that did, perhaps the first "celebrity cancer" story of modern times, played an important part in shaping rising public awareness—and fear—of cancer.

New Jersey congressman Robert Bremner (1874–1914), a friend of President Woodrow Wilson, chose to make his battle with cancer public, particularly his choice to rely on radium in the later stages of that battle. At the time radium was a controversial cancer treatment that had received extensive coverage. The headlines about "the radium cure" that ran in the *New York Times* within a few months of Bremner's illness capture the same mixed messages of hope and doubt about potential cancer cures we still get today:

WONDERFUL EFFECTS OF THE RADIUM TREATMENT
RADIUM FAILS AGAIN. Twice Employed, It Gave No Relief to Boy Cancer Victim
RADIUM IS APPARENTLY CURING CANCER
DOUBT RADIUM CURES
RADIUM CAUSE OF CANCER?

Bremner's case is important because it shaped public attitudes about cancer in two ways. The first was his openness and emotional frankness, which set a precedent. But Bremner was also leading an effort in Congress to fund a national stockpile of radium, then both rare and costly. That effort failed, but it was an early step in pressuring Congress to fight cancer. As the death toll and the fear mounted, so did that pressure. Some in Congress shamelessly responded with cancerphobic alarmism. In 1928 Senator Matthew Neely voiced the fears of millions when he described cancer as

> a monster more insatiable than the guillotine, more destructive to life and health than the mightiest army that ever marched to battle, more terrifying than any scourge that has ever threatened the existence of the human race. [It] . . . has fed and feasted and fattened . . . on the flesh and blood and brains and bones of men and children in every land. The sighs and sobs and shrieks that it has exhorted from perishing humanity would, if they were tangible things, make a mountain. The tears it has wrung from weeping women's eyes would make an ocean. The blood it has shed would redden every wave that rolls on every sea.[17]

Cancer was, Neely said, a "loathsome, deadly, insatiate monster," a growing menace that "would in a few centuries depopulate the earth."

Despite his dramatic oratory, however, in the context of the "life is good" optimism America was enjoying in the Roaring Twenties, Neely's efforts to pry more money out of Congress failed. By 1929, the ASCC, still run by cautious doctors and East Coast society women, hadn't had much success educating the public either. It was short of funds and struggling. But a new director that year expanded the group's reach, and its goals, which now included pressing Congress for federal spending. Clarence Cook Little (1888–1971) was a blueblood with a family tree that went back to Paul Revere. He would eventually become president of the University of Michigan. He took over the ASCC just as cancer had become the second leading cause of death in America, killing 108 people per 100,000. It had also become the country's most feared disease according to one of the nation's leading doctors, Charles Mayo (1865–1939), who said in a 1925 speech: "While there are several chronic diseases more destructive to life than cancer, none is more feared."[18]

In 1935 Little partnered the ASCC with the General Federation of Women's Clubs, a women's rights advocacy group. Marjorie Illig, chair of the federation's Public Health Committee, was a radiologist who had seen plenty of cancer suffering and death. It didn't take much to convince her that educating the public about cancer could help. Within a year, she and Little had created the Women's Field Army (WFA), complete with uniforms, ribbons denoting military-like rank, and ornamental swords, with "battalions" operating in every state. It was the first of many applications of the war metaphor in the struggle against cancer.

At its peak, the WFA had two million members, organizing public events and going door to door handing out pamphlets and collecting donations. But Little knew he still needed more. In 1937 he persuaded the editors of *Fortune* magazine to publish a "panoramic survey" of cancer medicine, titled "Cancer: The Great Darkness." The lengthy essay, ultimately published as a book, moved cancer further into the open with its detailed discussion of what was still a taboo topic, and by making an overt plea for federal investment in cancer research. The authors noted that while about $5 million a year was being spent on cancer research, "the public willingly spends a third of that sum in an afternoon to watch a major football game." Calling cancer "one of the most tabooed subjects in the modern scientific world," the editors observed the cancerphobia that existed back then, a description that still applies:

Public ignorance has led to strenuous campaigns to "educate" the public with well-intentioned pamphlets and utterances; which, however, reinforced by sensational and unofficial press items horrific in their implications, have stirred the public to fear. This fear, together with a vague notion that most cancer diagnoses are simply death warrants, sheds upon the whole subject a pale light of hysteria, for which the only rectification would be facts, hard and bitter perhaps, but solid and indisputable. But the unfortunate physician cannot allay fear with facts because the ultimate key Fact is missing. In the end no one knows what cancer is.[19]

That same year, 1937, *Life* magazine ran a major report on cancer, and the *New York Times* published 490 stories (including "War on Cancer Pressed" and "Cancer Research Found Seriously Handicapped"). Momentum was building for federal government action. Now, nearly a decade into the Great Depression, with the country looking to the federal government more than ever for help on all sorts of issues, and with the death toll from cancer still growing and touching almost every family or neighborhood, passionate new advocates picked up the fight in Congress. They too unapologetically used—and fueled—fear to advance their cause.

Representative Maury Maverick of Texas said on the floor of the House: "One out of every eight persons over 40 who die, die of cancer. As most of us are over 40, I have figured that there will be around 60 of us who thus meet death." Washington senator Homer Bone said, "If 140,000 persons in this country were burned over slow fires every year it would stagger the moral conscience of the world; and yet here, we, a body with our fingers on the purse strings, have it in our power to do something to stamp out a disease which not only takes 140,000 lives a year but which claims them in such a hideous fashion."

The purse strings loosened. Congress passed the first National Cancer Act of 1937, creating the National Cancer Institute (NCI) and devoting $700,000 a year (a paltry $12 million today) to cancer research.[20] The funding was a response to public fear and political pressure as much as to the medical threat of disease. At that time cancer was only the *third* leading cause of death in the country (pneumonia having overtaken cancer in second place amid the poor health conditions of the Depression). Heart disease was the leading killer, taking 269 lives per 100,000, while cancer was killing 112/100,000. Yet the National Heart, Lung, and Blood Institute, which does research on heart disease, wasn't created for another 11 years. Cancerphobia helps explain why. As *Time* magazine put it, in covering the debate over the National Cancer Act, "More than any other disease, cancer has horrified the imagination of mankind. It kills slowly, painfully, and science does not yet know its causes or mechanism." From the start, federal investment in research on public health was disproportionately skewed toward the disease people were more afraid of, not the one that posed the greatest threat to life. This too remains true today.

With the rising prevalence and fear of the disease, it surprised no one that the law creating the NCI passed Congress unanimously, or that Clarence Cook Little was named its first director. But it certainly surprised Little, who was still head of the ASCC when, in 1943, a visitor came by to find out what his organization was doing to support cancer research. As a result of that meeting, American society's relationship to cancer would change dramatically.

Mary Woodward was a successful New York businesswoman in 1940 when she married Albert Lasker, a pioneer of the modern advertising industry. As a child, Mary had been horrified after the family laundress had had both breasts removed to successfully treat breast cancer. Forty years later, when Mary's cook developed cancer and died, she was heartsick. But more than that, Mary Lasker was angry.

So when she met with Clarence Little in the Manhattan offices of the ASCC, Lasker got right to the point. What was the ASCC doing to support cancer research? she asked. Nothing, Little replied, explaining that the organization was dedicated to public education, not research. Moreover, the doctors on his board, mostly surgeons who thought surgery was the way to fight cancer, didn't think investing in research was worthwhile. Lasker gave the ASCC $5,000 to write up an overview of the state of cancer research in America and left, barely stifling her frustration.

Within two years she had engineered a coup at the ASCC. Most of the old directors, medical men, were gone, replaced by executives from the advertising, pharmaceutical, and film industries. Clarence Little was gone. The name itself was gone too, replaced by the American Cancer Society (ACS). The mission of education only was also replaced. The objective of the new ACS, captured in their slogan "Beating cancer," was nothing short of the end of the disease itself.

One dollar out of every four raised would go to research. Mary Lasker and her business-world board of directors were phenomenally successful fundraisers. The relatively sleepy ASCC was replaced with the advertising juggernaut the ACS, raising $12.45 million in 1947 ($132 million in current value), just four years after Lasker took over. And all of this was occurring on the threshold of a remarkable confluence of other events that would turn the growing fear of cancer into the modern version of cancerphobia that grips us today.

The Rise of Modern Cancerphobia

Fear is contagious. You can catch it.
—Neil Gaiman

It happened more than half a century ago, and yet David Nathan's voice tightens, and he grimaces as he recalls: "I remember the smell, how awful the smell was. People were moving away from this poor woman as she walked into my office. And the look on her face, of shame and of embarrassment . . . and . . . ," he gropes for the right word, "fear."

It was 1956 and young Dr. Nathan was just starting what would be a career of exceptional accomplishment in oncology, capped by five years as president of the prestigious Dana-Farber Cancer Institute. "The open sores on her breast . . . open leaking wounds. Her condition had deteriorated so badly. Yet when I asked her why she had waited so long to come in . . . and our care was free then and she seemed to me to be a poor woman . . . she said it was because she was afraid to learn that it might be cancer. She was so afraid of cancer, the idea of cancer . . . she said 'I couldn't face it. I couldn't allow myself to think that I had cancer,' . . . that she had let things deteriorate so badly that there was nothing we could do for her except ease her pain."

By the 1950s fear of cancer had reached unprecedented levels. The number of cancer deaths in the United States, and much of Western Europe, was skyrocketing. The promises from doctors and surgeons of effective treatment and potential cures were all proving empty. And all of it was happening under the chilling Cold War threat of nuclear annihilation.

On the other hand, by the end of the 1950s our ever more modern world had fluoride and antibiotics, soda in cans and satellites, a birth control pill and microwave ovens, Jello and frozen food and an understanding of DNA. Sir Edmund Hillary and Tenzing Norgay had climbed the world's highest mountain. Roger Bannister had run a supposedly unachievable sub-4 minute mile. It was also a decade of optimism and hope, of faith in government, in science, in modern medicine, a time when many Americans believed that anything could be achieved.

Hope and fear. Those extremes set the emotional context in which several events and trends over the next two decades would come together to frame our modern emotional relationship with cancer. As important as fear of the disease might have been in the past, that was only prologue.

The American Cancer Society's Emotional Campaign

After World War II, Mary Lasker and the new ASC really went to work. Gone was the more measured tone and purely educational content of the ASCC. Now the message was a direct appeal for donations for nothing less than the end of cancer itself. And that message was more overtly emotional. In two decades the ASCC had produced only eight films, with titles like *Reward of Courage*, which avoided direct appeals to fear.[21] Now, with executives from the advertising and entertainment industries on its board, the new ACS dropped all hesitancy about tapping public anxiety about cancer, releasing a film per year starting in 1946. Their first was a ten-minute animation called *The Traitor Within*.[22] It opens with a silent image of a ticking clock in front of a brooding dark sky. Then a graveyard cross appears on the screen, then another, then another, and as the clock ticks ominously on, more and more crosses progressively fill the screen as the narrator soberly intones: "Every three minutes someone dies of cancer. Day after day, week after week, month after month. Cancer kills close to 200,000 of our people each year."

Tick. Tick. Tick.

That frightening theme was the core of most early ACS communications. A poster claimed, "Every Three Minutes Someone Dies of Cancer. Guard Those You Love. Give to Conquer Cancer." Another warned, "Cancer, Our Number Two Killer." To drive the fear home, the ACS often put

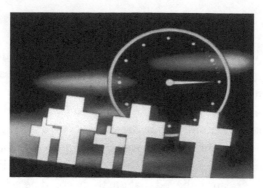

FIGURE 1.4
Still from the American Cancer Society's film *The Traitor Within*
(Atlanta, GA: John Sutherland Productions, 1946).
Courtesy of the American Cancer Society

the threat in personal terms. "One in five of *us* here," said one ACS leader at a public talk, "every fifth person in *this* audience—will die of cancer."

Perhaps the most overt ACS appeal to emotion was the boy America got to know as Jimmy. One evening in 1948, Ralph Edwards, host of the nationally popular radio show *Truth or Consequences*, said his California-based program was being linked to Boston "to take you to a little fellow named Jimmy. Jimmy is suffering from cancer, but he doesn't know he has it," Edwards said. "He's a swell little guy, and although he cannot figure out why he isn't out with the other kids, he does love his baseball and follows every move of his favorite team, the Boston Braves. Now, by the magic of radio, we're going to span the breadth of the United States and take you right up to the bedside of Jimmy. Up to now, Jimmy has not heard us. Now we tune in a speaker in a room in his hospital. Okay, engineers, give us Jimmy, please."

In a hospital bed lay Jimmy, a 12-year-old Maine boy being treated for intestinal lymphoma. He had been chosen to be the face of a fund-raising campaign envisioned by the show-business people on the board of the ACS, who wanted to start a charity campaign like the successful March of Dimes for polio or the Christmas Seals program for tuberculosis. Jimmy was chosen as the face of the campaign because he was one of the few children under cancer care who was not so ill he couldn't speak. He was also chosen because he was one of very few who had an outside chance of survival.

As millions of Americans listened in, Jimmy named his favorite Boston Braves players, and one by one each of those stars crowded in to the dazzled boy's room; gave the boy autographed balls and T-shirts, a Braves uniform in his size, tickets behind home plate for the game the next day; and together sang "Take Me Out to the Ballgame" with him. The audience in Edwards's California studio sobbed. Across the country thousands of his listeners sobbed. Edwards wrapped it up a few minutes later with "Now listen, folks. Jimmy can't hear this, can he? Let's make Jimmy and thousands of boys and girls who are suffering from cancer happy by aiding the research to help find a cure for cancer in children . . . Give from the heart for a cause so worthy it's impossible to describe." (You can listen to the Jimmy broadcast here.[23])

Before the players had even left the hospital, people were lined up at the front entrance, not to see the baseball stars but to donate. Within days the post office in Boston was flooded with letters, some addressed simply to "Jimmy, Boston, Massachusetts." Red and white cans were passed around in Boston movie theaters and placed outside baseball stadiums in America to collect donations. They filled quickly. Edwards had asked his audience for $20,000 to get Jimmy a television set in his hospital room so he could watch Braves games. Within two weeks the fund had raised a quarter of a million dollars. As of 2016 the Jimmy Fund had raised more than a billion dollars, raising $86 million in 2016 alone.

(The world finally met Jimmy, actually Einar Gustafson, after his sister called the Jimmy Fund offices a month before the fiftieth anniversary of the radio program and stunned everyone by telling them that Jimmy was alive and well and living in Maine. I had the good fortune during my broadcast reporting career in Boston to interview Einar during pregame festivities for him at Fenway Park. He was a retired long-distance truck driver and small business owner, as well as a grandfather. He was warm, smiling, excited, and a little overwhelmed at all the attention he was getting. On May 22, 1998, Einar stood on the mound at Fenway Park, and with his family standing behind him and kids with cancer standing behind home plate, scarves or hats on ther bald heads, a grinning Einar threw out the first pitch at the Red Sox / Yankees game. Thirty-six thousand fans stood and roared, more than a few of whom, including me, were weeping. Einar passed away in 2001.)

The ACS's emotional fund-raising campaign was wildly successful. But its appeal to emotion and fear was so overt that in 1948, the American

Psychiatric Association complained that ACS "propaganda" was fomenting fear of cancer, suggesting that the ACS adopt a visual icon less frightening than its sword (of hope) and more cheerful, like a helping hand. Edna Kaehele, who had become famous for publishing one of the earliest first-person books about battling cancer, *Triumph Over Cancer*, in 1952 called the ACS approach "extraordinarily inept" fearmongering that would drive cancer patients into hiding rather than into treatment.

But the public relations effort of the ACS was only one part of Mary Lasker's campaign. She knew that not even the most successful fundraising could raise the kind of money necessary to entirely cure cancer. That would take the federal government, which meant a sustained political campaign, a crusade. And a crusade had to be led by a white knight. Lasker found hers in Sidney Farber.

Stiff and formal (his medical school colleagues called him Four Button Sid for the suits he always wore to class), Farber was head pathologist at Children's Hospital in Boston in 1947, where he was trying to understand cancer by focusing on childhood leukemia. In 1948 he published a paper describing how injections of a drug that inhibited cellular reproduction, aminopterin, had produced remissions of leukemia in 10 of the 16 children he had tried it on.[24] This was revolutionary: treatment of cancer with drugs, not surgery, and treatment that appeared to work, the first glimmer of real hope. Farber was Jimmy/Einar's doctor at Boston's Children's Hospital. Lasker learned of Farber's groundbreaking chemotherapy work, and by the mid-1950s the two were working as partners in Washington, DC, lobbying for what culminated in the National Cancer Act of 1971—Lasker tapping her social and business connections, and Farber adding the authority of his doctor's coat, his fastidious bearing, and his passion for saving the lives of children.

Lasker waged a full-scale modern political lobbying campaign. She brought Farber and other famous doctors to hearings and meetings with congressional leaders and federal officials. She directed huge campaign donations from the ACS to the heads of key congressional committees. She got her wealthy friends to make private donations and tapped their political connections. A lobbyist Lasker worked with called her impact "probably unparalleled in the influence that a small group of private citizens has over such a major area of national policy."[25]

Lasker's lobbying prompted a lot of news coverage and far greater public discussion of cancer, as well as growing pressure on Congress. By the end of the 1950s the NCI budget had risen to $118 million (nearly $1 billion in today's dollars). But the Lasker-Farber campaign did not take place in isolation, and it might not have succeeded but for several additional developments in post–World War II America, a mix of events, shifting attitudes, social movements, and scientific developments through the fifties and sixties that together contributed significantly to the fears and beliefs we have about cancer today.

The Rise of Modern Environmentalism

In 1962, life expectancy had reached 73 for women and 67 for men, cancer was now killing 370 people per 100,000, and the bestselling book at the end of October was Rachel Carson's *Silent Spring.* The October 12, 1962, edition of *Life* magazine featured a profile of Carson and some photos in which Carson looked haggard and tired. The story called her appearance "gentle." It was anything but.

Earlier that year, as she was polishing up chapters on the link between pesticides and cancer, Carson had discovered two lumps in her left breast, from which she'd had a cyst removed years before. By the time *Silent Spring* and the *Life* interview were published, Carson had had a radical mastectomy, but not until she discovered that her doctors had misled her by not telling her she had cancer and only calling her tumors "suspicious," at which point she fired them and found a new oncologist, George Crile Jr., who told her with respectful honesty that it was unlikely he could save her life. As she smiled for *Life*'s cameras, Rachel Carson knew she was dying. Of cancer.

That same month, hundreds of millions of people around the world were also worried—deeply, viscerally worried—about the imminent prospect of a horrific death, not from cancer, but from nuclear war. Just ten days after Carson's profile ran in *Life*, President John F. Kennedy revealed that the United States had detected Soviet offensive missiles under construction in Cuba that could reach targets across the United States within minutes. He told a stunned global TV audience that US naval vessels were preparing to confront Soviet ships in a quarantine of Cuba. On the evening of October 22, 1962, a somber president of the United States said that the world was facing "the abyss of destruction."

The existential fear of global nuclear war that had gripped the world since the atomic bombings of Japan was suddenly terrifyingly plausible. And that fear, it turns out, had indirectly inspired *Silent Spring.* It spawned the first global protest movement, to "ban the bomb," which campaigned against the atmospheric testing of nuclear weapons and the cancer threat from the radioactive fallout from those tests raining down around the world. Isotopes of cesium and strontium from these explosions were found in the soil in western states (several tests were detonated in Nevada), in milk from cows that grazed along the East Coast, and in fish around the globe. Ban the Bomb protestors warned that the world was being poisoned, blanketed by radioactive material . . . *that caused cancer*.

By the mid-1950s, the campaign against radioactive fallout blossomed into the beginnings of the modern environmental movement, which only later added fears of industrial chemicals to its initial focus on radioactive fallout. *Silent Spring* brought those fears together. Carson wrote:

> Chemicals are the sinister and little recognized partners of radiation in changing the very nature of the world—the very nature of its life. Strontium 90, released through nuclear explosions into the air, comes to earth in rain or drifts down as fallout, lodges in soil, enters into the grass or corn or wheat grown there, and in time takes up its abode in the bones of the human being, there to remain until his death. Similarly, chemicals sprayed on croplands or forests or gardens lie long in soil, entering into living organisms, passing from one another in a chain of poisoning and death.[26]

Death from cancer. From its very beginning, the environmentalism Carson helped champion focused on cancer as the penultimate peril posed by the human products and processes of modern progress. These are the roots of our modern fear that cancer is principally the result of exposure to environmental substances. Carson wrote: "With the dawn of the industrial era the world became a place of continuing, ever-accelerating change. Instead of the natural environment there was rapidly substituted an artificial one composed of new chemical and physical agents, many of them possessing powerful capacities for inducing biological change. Against these carcinogens which his own activities had created man had no protection."[27] But the rise of environmentalism was still just one of several developments in the years following World War II that set up how we feel about cancer today. Another was the controversy about smoking and cancer.

Smoking and Lung Cancer

On January 11, 1964, Surgeon General Luther Terry spoke to a packed room of 200 reporters in Washington, DC. The doors had been locked so no one could rush out in the middle of reading the 384-page report they had just been given. The event was held on a Saturday, when the stock market was closed and couldn't be affected, so momentous was Terry's news. The reporters were given an hour and a half to read before the uniformed surgeon general, holding a copy of the report, pronounced the findings from an exhaustive review of all relevant research by the country's top experts: smoking *causes* lung cancer.

The announcement made front page news around the world. But it was less fresh news than the culmination of a controversy that had been building for years. Science had been tracking the connection between tobacco and cancer since John Hill's 1791 *Cautions against the Immoderate Use of Snuff*. Smoking specifically had been a focus since the early 1800s, when a succession of European scientists established a correlation between pipe smoking and cancer of the lip and tongue. In 1929, German Fritz Linckint provided the first statistical link between lung cancer and tobacco. Linckint coined the term *passivrauchen*, passive smoking, in 1936. The momentum grew as more studies came out of Germany in the thirties and even during the war years in the forties, and two major studies were published a month apart in 1950, one by Sir Bradford Hill and Richard Doll in England and one by Ernest Wynder and Evarts Graham in the United States, that found a strong statistical association between smoking and lung cancer deaths.

The public had been tracking the connection between smoking and cancer as well. In burials. In 1930 lung cancer was the cause of just 5% of all cancer deaths in America. By 1955 it was leading the pack at 18%, tripling in 20 years as most other forms of cancer mortality dropped or stayed basically the same. And a majority of the bodies were male. In 1930 overall cancer mortality for men (about 170/100,000) was slightly lower than for women (about 190/100,000). But by the mid-1950s, cancer was killing far more men (roughly 210/100,000) than women (about 180/100,000).[28]

Small wonder. World War II, in which cigarettes were handed out to America's soldiers with their rations (to keep them calm during battle and to avoid boredom during noncombat time), had helped turn the country into a chimney. In 1952 Americans smoked a stunning *11 cigarettes a day per person!* Half of men and one-third of women smoked. Lung cancer deaths among men—3,000 in 1930—had risen to 18,000 in 1950 and soared to 41,000 in 1962 as the postwar smoking toll began to hit home. By 1960 lung cancer alone was the ninth leading cause of death in the country. The connection between smoking and cancer touched a lot of Americans personally.

Headlines magnified public concern. *New York Times* headlines from 1952 and '53 mirror what newspapers around the country, and the world, were reporting.

CANCER DEATH RISE OVER WORLD FOUND
LUNG CANCER HELD RISING
LUNG CANCER RISE IS LAID TO SMOKING

The tobacco industry had been fighting these headwinds for decades, with ads like one in 1930 saying, "20,679 physicians say 'Luckies are less irritating,'" one in 1947 saying, "More doctors smoke Camels than any other cigarette," and one in 1949, "As your dentist I would recommend Viceroys." So by the early fifties the industry was in full defense mode. In early 1954 the *New York Times* reported:

INDUSTRY CONFERS TO AID CIGARETTES
Secret Meetings Here Weigh Drive to End Fears Caused
by Lung Cancer Charges

This marked the start of an insidious program of corporate deceit, which an industry memo said was designed to create "doubt about the health charge without actually denying it."[29] The tobacco industry poured money into challenging the science connecting smoking and lung cancer (and other diseases), in part by hiring their own scientists to reach more favorable findings.

On January 4, 1954, the industry placed full-page ads in 400 newspapers across the country:

A FRANK STATEMENT
Distinguished authorities point out . . .

1. That medical research of recent years indicates many possible causes of lung cancer.

2. That there is no agreement among the authorities regarding what
   the cause is.
3. That there is no proof that cigarette smoking is one of the causes.

The ad stated, "We believe the products we make are not injurious
to health." It announced, "We are establishing the TOBACCO INDUSTRY
RESEARCH COMMITTEE," and "in charge of the research activities will
be a scientist of unimpeachable integrity and national repute." Remarkably, that scientist was Clarence Little, the same Clarence Little who had
led the ASCC and, just before joining the tobacco industry, the NCI.

Little was a devout eugenicist who believed that inferior humans
should be bred out of the population. He believed that cancer was hereditary—a genetic defect. So to Little, lung cancer was just nature's way of
weeding genetically defective people out of the gene pool, and smoking
merely helped that defect do its work. As forceful an advocate for cancer
education as he had been, Little was equally adamant in leading the
industry-funded fight against the mounting evidence that smoking *causes*
cancer. The *New York Times* reported in February 1954:

EXPERT ON CANCER GIVES KINDLY
NOD TO CIGARETTE

Dr. Clarence Cook Little, director of the Roscoe B. Jackson Memorial
Laboratory at Bar Harbor, Me., and an internationally known investigator in the field of cancer, said here yesterday that he doubted there
existed a direct relationship between cigarette smoking and cancer
of the lung.[30]

On the other side of the public relations battle was Mary Lasker and
the ACS. Rising concern about smoking and cancer fit perfectly into the
society's campaign to raise concern about the disease generally. The ACS
funded its own research, which the *New York Times* reported on regularly,
including this article in June 1954.[31]

CIGARETTES FOUND TO RAISE DEATH RATE IN MEN 50 TO 70;
DEATH RATE RISE LINKED TO SMOKING

Cigarette smokers from 50 to 70 years of age have a death rate from
all diseases as much as 75 percent higher than that of nonsmokers, the
ACS reported today . . . Deaths among smokers in the age group were
mainly from cancer and heart attacks, the study showed.

The public pressure mounted on the government to act. In 1962 the ACS, the American Public Health Association, the American Heart Association, and the National Tuberculosis Association wrote to President Kennedy, who tossed the political hot potato to Surgeon General Terry. The result was that seminal 1964 report, which, in dry language buried on page 31, said, "Cigarette smoking is causally related to lung cancer in men; the magnitude of the effect of cigarette smoking far outweighs all other factors. The data for women, though less extensive, point in the same direction."[32]

The 1964 surgeon general's report on smoking and cancer capped a decade of news that had added to public cancer fears. "Few medical questions," Terry said as he announced the findings, "have stirred such public interest or created more scientific debate than the tobacco-health controversy."[33] But as historic as his 1964 report was, it too was just one among several developments that helped shape society's evolving emotional relationship to cancer.

The Coining of "Cancerphobia"

George Crile Jr., Rachel Carson's final oncologist, was one of the few doctors in the 1950s unafraid to use the C-word. Indeed Crile's whole attitude toward cancer and cancer medicine was unique.

Crile had royal blood in the world of American medicine. His father, George Sr., had been called the most important man in surgery since Lister for his work preventing shock in surgical patients (by applying anesthesia not just to the patient but directly to the organ being operated on). George Jr., known as Barney, served in World War II and saw a lot of injured and sick soldiers who did just fine without immediate and extensive surgery. "I came home from World War II convinced that operations in many fields of surgery were either too radical, or not even necessary," he once said, according to his obituary in the New York Times. He would lead the challenge to the orthodoxy of the brutal Halsted radical mastectomy, the unquestioned standard of care for breast cancer for 50 years. "Universal acceptance of a procedure," he wrote, "does not necessarily make it right."

Crile Jr. was a pioneer in other ways as well. He championed the attitude just starting to take hold among a few doctors that cancer patients deserve honesty, even if the diagnosis means death. He also helped lead a new approach to more flexible patient-centric cancer treatment, writing, "Every cancer is a separate problem that should be dealt with in an individual way and no generalization as to treatment should be made." Moderate surgery or even no surgery, rather than automatic radical surgery for every patient, started to become more acceptable options. Ultimately that shift would reframe how many people feel about cancer today, since the prospect of radical surgery, now uncommon, scared many patients away from screening and treatment altogether.

These challenges to the accepted practices of mainstream medicine made Crile plenty of enemies. So did his criticism that doctors and organizations promoting cancer education were playing on fear and making things worse. Perhaps the most profound of his insights was the alarm he sounded that public fear of cancer was excessive and dangerous all by itself.

The October 31, 1955, edition of *Life* magazine features a cover photo of a glamorously dressed society woman attending a function in Washington, DC. A box at the upper right corner of the cover teases an article inside: "A Surgeon Deplores Blind Fear of Cancer." In the article, "A Plea against Blind Fear of Cancer," Crile wrote:

> Those responsible for telling the public about cancer have chosen to use the weapon of fear, believing that only through fear can the public be educated. Newspapers and magazines have magnified and spread this fear, knowing that the public is always interested in the melodramatic and the frightening. This has fostered a disease, fear of cancer, a contagious disease that spreads from mouth to ear. It is possible that today, in terms of the total number of people affected, fear of cancer is causing more suffering than cancer itself. Already doctors are seeing increasing numbers of healthy patients who suffer only because they are afraid of getting cancer. This fear leads both doctors and patients to do unreasonable and therefore dangerous things.[34]

"No one," Crile wrote, "need be afraid of the word cancer."

His article set off shock waves, prompting a defensive reply that ran as an insert in Crile's article from the heads of the American Medical Association, the NCI director, and the medical director of the ACS, which dripped with professional arrogance and conservativism: "His thesis is contrary to the teaching of the country's 81 medical schools and to the experience of physicians and surgeons . . . Dr. Crile . . . raises technical questions that can only be resolved by physicians in scientific publications and sessions."

Crile counter-attacked by revealing that fee-for-service doctors had an incentive to do surgery, and radical surgery at that, since they were literally paid by the pound; the more of the body they cut away, the more they earned. He also reported his horror witnessing colleagues perform extensive surgery on patients far too sick for it to do them any good, referring to those patients as they lay asleep being cut up by the surgeon's scalpels as "teaching material." This controversy among doctors, who by this time had become elite and high-profile members of society, got huge media attention, which brought Crile's ideas to a wide national audience.

So did his book *Cancer and Common Sense*, which came out at the same time, in which he wrote: "Fear of cancer has been beaten into (people) until this fear has become almost as great an enemy as cancer itself . . . Those responsible for telling the public about cancer . . . have portrayed cancer as an insidious, dreadful, relentless invader. With religious fervor they have fashioned a devil out of cancer. They have bred in a sensitive public a fear that is approaching hysteria. They have created a new disease, cancer phobia."[35]

It would take a few decades, but by the eighties Crile's more respectful and open approach to patient communication had become the norm. So had his rejection of radical surgery for breast and other cancers. But his provocative and prescient call to recognize the dangers of what he called cancerphobia was soon forgotten. (The term "cancerphobia" was first used in 1948 by John Ryle in a lecture to other doctors in a London psychiatric hospital. See chapter 14.) These warnings are only just now, two decades into the twenty-first century, starting to prompt reflection in the medical community. But as was true for Crile, the suggestion that fear of cancer is in some cases excessive and harmful all by itself is still rejected by many medical leaders. Several experts interviewed for this book resist the very idea of "cancerphobia" and only with reluctance acknowledge that excessive fear of the disease does sometimes lead to a range of harms, including death.

Chemotherapy, the First Rays of Hope, and Broken Promises

When Carson contacted Crile, looking for "a new evaluation of the whole thing by someone else," he informed her of the work at the NCI that was having some success. It involved human-made chemicals, so Carson chose not to avail herself of that progress, in part because she feared that relying on industrial chemicals to save her life while campaigning about the danger of such substances might undermine her credibility and cause.

But the development of those cancer drugs was the final development in the fifties, sixties, and early seventies that shaped how we feel about cancer today. From antiquity it had been simply accepted that there was no cure for cancer, no hope, that having cancer meant only suffering and death. That's why doctors rarely told their patients they had cancer. It would be cruel, these physicians argued, to tell people that they had an incurably fatal disease. As Susan Sontag wrote in 1978 in *Illness as Metaphor*, "No one thinks of concealing the truth from a cardiac patient: there is nothing shameful about a heart attack. Cancer patients are lied to, not just because the disease is (or is thought to be) a death sentence, but because it is felt to be obscene—in the original meaning of that word: ill-omened, abominable, repugnant to the senses."[36] But now, with the work of Sidney Farber and a few more pioneering researchers willing to use powerfully toxic substances to attack cancer, the first cracks were appearing in the foundational assumption that there was no hope. Now, for the first time in human history, the promise of a cure for cancer, made and broken so often in the past, started to seem like it might actually come true.

History pivots greatly on fear. When we are afraid, our leaders do difficult, expensive things they could never do when we aren't. Fear sent America into the war in Vietnam. Cold War fear sent people to the moon. And fear of cancer led to the second National Cancer Act, in 1971, and its Declaration of Purpose, which begins:

(a) The Congress finds and declares:
(1) that the incidence of cancer is increasing and cancer is the disease *which is the major health concern of Americans today.* (my emphasis)

It would be unfair to suggest that the National Cancer Act of 1971 passed only because of fear. But it is fair to suggest that fear, more than anything else, got that momentous piece of legislation through Congress with nearly unanimous votes in both House and Senate at a time when America was torn apart politically over the war in Vietnam. It is also fair to call Americans' fear of cancer at that time excessive, at least statistically. When President Nixon called the National Cancer Act a declaration of war on cancer, the mortality rate for cancer was 163 per 100,000, a new high. But the rate of mortality from heart disease was more than twice as high, at 359/100,000. There was not then nor has there even been a commensurate war on heart disease. History pivots most on fear.

But remember, as the ACS symbol captures, the other edge of the Sword of Fear is hope, and hope too helped pass that law, as noted in the second line in the "Purpose" section of the National Cancer Act:

> (2) that new scientific leads, if comprehensively and energetically exploited, may significantly advance the time when more adequate preventive and therapeutic capabilities are available to cope with cancer.

Hope had been inspired in part by the soaring achievement of landing a human on the moon a few years prior, fueling immense public faith in science. After all, if we could put people on the moon, then science could achieve anything, even cure cancer. The lunar landing prompted Solomon Garb to suggest something similar in his widely read book *Cure for Cancer: A National Goal.*[37] That book inspired Lasker and Farber to further intensify their political campaign and to relabel their goal a "moon shot" for cancer, language still used today.

The hope was not just the result of blind faith in science. Advances in chemotherapy and other treatments had been made in the years since Sidney Farber first used aminopterin to treat childhood leukemia. Now, childhood leukemia could be treated with more effective multidrug regimens, like VAMP, an acronym for a stew of ordinarily toxic drugs whose success (albeit in a small minority of patients) "changed the mood among pediatric oncologists virtually overnight from one of 'compassionate fatalism' to one of aggressive optimism."[38] Multidrug treatments were also prolonging life for people with a few other types of cancer, such as MOPP for Hodgkin's disease. In 1958 researchers Anthony Epstein and Yvonne Barr discovered that a virus (which now bears their names, Epstein-Barr, more familiar as the cause of infectious mononucleosis) causes Burkitt lymphoma, a disease that had only been identified a few years earlier. If viruses could cause cancer (as suggested in research in 1910 by Francis Peyton Rous, for which he won the Nobel Prize in 1966), it meant that cancer might indeed be infectious (cervical cancer is), which was frightening, but it also made real the hope for a cancer vaccine (which now exists for cervical cancer). The NCI spent half a billion dollars in the sixties on its cancer virus program alone.

David Nathan, whom we met earlier, was a young pediatric oncologist as all this was happening. He was swept up in that hope. "The ability to treat. It changed everything. It certainly changed the doctors' attitude. That's what gave everybody encouragement . . . hope . . . a sense that finally we could do something," he recalled. From all this progress arose the belief that, as the director of the NCI said in 1963, "the next step—the complete cure—is almost sure to follow." In the context of those heady days of remarkable scientific achievement, the promise that had been made for hundreds of years of an overarching cure for all cancer now finally seemed in reach.

To be sure, some warned against the excessive optimism of a "National Program for the Conquest of Cancer," as the Senate version of the National Cancer Act was titled. The lunar landing was built on what science *knew*. Curing cancer, these experts noted, meant identifying its root causes, which were poorly understood. Some of the sciences needed to understand them didn't even exist. One cancer researcher noted, "An all-out effort at this is like trying to land a man on the moon without knowing Newton's laws of gravity." Another warned that "people have become impatient with what they take to be lack of progress," suggesting that setting the bar of expectations too high was adding to public impatience and reinforcing beliefs that cancer could not be cured.[39]

But like a tsunami that builds without being recognized as the giant wave it is until it reaches the shore and then can't be stopped, the momentum of both fear and hope about cancer that had been building in America for 70 years came ashore in 1971, setting in place the final development that shaped our modern emotional relationship with this disease.

Fear Cuts Deeper

No wave maintains its crest. As the receding waters of hope about curing cancer ebbed away in the post-Vietnam seventies and eighties, the limited effectiveness of the first few cancer drugs became clear, and mistrust of promises made but not kept began to erode some of that optimism. One study found that chemotherapy was now saving 35,000 to 40,000 lives per year, but cancer was still killing roughly 500,000 per year. Another report found that, adjusting the numbers for age, the overall cancer mortality rate had actually risen, by nearly 9% per year. You didn't have to be a statistician to know that we were losing more battles than we were winning in the war on cancer. Hope was still vastly outweighed by fear, as a 1975 editorial in the *New England Journal of Medicine* observed: "When it comes to cancer, American society is far from rational. We are possessed with fear ... cancerphobia has expanded into a demonism in which the evil spirit is ever present ... American cancerphobia, in brief, is a disease as serious to society as cancer is to the individual."[40]

American society was also in social and political turmoil. The final years of the Vietnam War, public outrage over President Nixon's Watergate attempt to subvert democracy itself, the discontent of Age of Aquarius baby boomers fueling the rise of feminism and "back to the Garden of Eden" environmentalism, social tension around issues of abortion and race, and rampant inflation all contributed to a continuing erosion of the general optimism the country had enjoyed throughout the fifties. The seventies were a hard time to be hopeful in general.

The explosive growth of the modern environmental movement in particular, coming hard on the heels of the National Cancer Act, played a significant part in dimming the glow of hope about progress against cancer. There were dire cancer alarms about events like the meltdown of the Three Mile Island nuclear reactor in Pennsylvania; toxic waste dumps at Love Canal, New York, and Times Beach, Missouri; and "cancer clusters" in Woburn, Massachusetts, and Toms River, New Jersey. These alarms were also raised about Agent Orange, PCBs, vinyl chloride, pesticides, and a constantly growing list of potentially carcinogenic industrial chemicals. We could get cancer from air pollution, water pollution, and even food dyes. Cancer was *the* threat that modern environmentalism relied on to raise public concern about the harms caused by the material progress humankind was making. Harkening back to a similar response to the Industrial Revolution in the late 1800s and early 1900s, some in the sixties and seventies saw environmental contamination as evidence that modern life itself was bad for health; rivers caught fire, acid rain damaged forests and sterilized lakes, thick urban smog choked people living in increasingly crowded cities and leading increasingly stressed "rat race" lives. The postwar "population bomb" was said to threaten the very future existence of humanity.[41] Social critics who argued that industrial and technological progress were an inherent threat to the natural world cited the rising cancer death toll as proof. The organic movement, the "pesticide-free" food industry, "natural" medicines, advocacy campaigns warning about too much salt or fat or sugar or processed ingredients in food, all blossomed based on the promise of protection from modern ills, and all of them promised protection from cancer specifically, prompting Joe Jackson's satirical response to what he felt was excessive fear, in his song "Cancer" in 1982.[42]

> Everything,
> Everything gives you cancer.
> Everything,
> Everything gives you cancer.
> There's no cure, there's no answer.
> Everything gives you cancer.

Changes in the news media that began in the seventies, especially the growth and influence of local and network television news, were gasoline on the fire of these fears. Stories emphasizing the danger of cancer frequently led network newscasts in that decade. The major broadcast networks all did documentaries about cancer risk, dramatizing the threat. CBS aired *The American Way of Death* in 1975 and *The Politics of Cancer* in 1976. Local TV news was proliferating as the public's main source of information, and almost any story about cancer was featured prominently. (I did my fair share of scary "it could cause cancer" stories as the environmental reporter for a TV station in Boston from the late seventies through the nineties.) Newspapers and magazines competed for the "cancer" audience. The NCI counted almost 1,500 articles about cancer in one 40-day period at the end of 1981.[43]

As it became more acceptable to talk openly about cancer, movies like *Love Story* and *Brian's Song*; books like Betty Rollin's first-person *First You Cry* and Doris Lund's bestselling tearjerker novel *Eric* (about a boy with leukemia); the cancer deaths of Duke Ellington, Betty Grable, Vince Lombardi, Shirley Temple Black, and NBC anchorman Chet Huntley; and the much-publicized breast cancer ordeals of First Lady Betty Ford and Margaretta "Happy" Rockefeller, wife of the vice president, all kept awareness of the threat of cancer high in popular culture.

All these trends have rapidly accelerated in the past few decades. Environmental advocates have continued to sound alarms about suspected new carcinogens. The topic of cancer has exploded onto movie and TV screens. (Most of those stories involve sickness and death.) Google Ngram, which tracks the use of words in books over time, reports that the number of books containing the word "cancer" has quintupled since 1970.[44] A search of the word "cancer" in Google News in February 2021 yielded 429 million entries.[45] There are endless stories about potential cures, personal cancer stories about everyone from international celebrities to local citizens, controversies about suspected cancer clusters, and constant public campaigns by cancer advocacy groups promoting early screening, treatment, and research. The modern 24/7 media world, both information and social media, magnifies all this awareness, dramatizing the fear and exacerbating its harms.

Fortunately, the trends that began in the twentieth century, accelerated by key events in the decades following World War II, have made a word that could scarcely be spoken in public 100 years ago commonplace. The stigma, disgust, and shame once associated with cancer have greatly diminished. But not the fear. Why?

We have made extraordinary progress. Since 1991 the cancer mortality rate in the United States has dropped a remarkable 33%.[46] Mortality rates for lung, prostate, breast, uterine, colon, stomach, leukemia, and thyroid cancers are all down. These advances are so dramatic that one expert, Vincent DeVita Jr., former NCI director, asserted in his optimistically titled 2015 book *The Death of Cancer*, "We can now cure more than 68% of all cancers—more if you count the easily curable skin cancers, which are very common."[47]

Why then are we still so afraid? Why, with such remarkable progress, progress that is only accelerating as one new discovery provides the foundation for others, did President Barack Obama feel the need, in his final State of the Union address, to promise "a new moonshot. America can cure cancer." A *new* "moonshot," promised again by President Joe Biden, uses the same metaphor first invoked by Mary Lasker half a century before, offering the same sweeping promise used to encourage passage of the first National Cancer Act, in 1937, and the second version 34 years later. Why, with mortality rates dropping everywhere, does cancer remain the disease that frightens us the most?

There are several likely reasons. Partial progress does not change the frightening nature of the disease. Some cancers cause great suffering, and some are still incurable. Mortality rates are down, yes, but cancer is still killing roughly 600,000 Americans per year and reducing the quality of life of millions of others, who now survive but live with cancer as a chronic disease, many suffering side effects from the treatments that keep them alive. These are people we know and care for: our loved ones, our family, our friends . . . ourselves. The frightening realities of cancer still loom in all our lives, progress notwithstanding.

Also, the progress is recent, some of it coming in only the past few years. Not everyone is aware of it all, and it has been incremental, a small step here and there. There has been no single "cure for cancer," the penultimate "moon shot" goal we've been promised, the ultimate victory in the war on cancer all those advocacy campaigns and federal spending programs have used to tap our fears and hopes—and bank accounts. We feel we're not "there" yet, and unfulfilled promises dull the hope offered by the extensive but incremental progress we've made.

Still, you might think that an objective consideration of the evidence would counteract at least some of that fear. But that's not how the psychology of risk perception works. All our perceptions, especially of anything that might portend danger, are *affective*, a subjective mix of the facts we have and how we feel about those facts.[48] This is probably the biggest reason that our excessive fear of cancer resists the evidence of progress, and it explains why intense fear of this disease will be harder to eradicate than even that last lurking cancerous cell.

Even the optimistic Dr. DeVita, one of the most informed people on the planet about all the progress we've made, has personally experienced how readily fear of cancer can become a phobia and overwhelm reason. In his book he tells of suffering from an enlarged prostate but putting off going to a doctor, "because the symptoms and signs of an enlarged prostate gland and prostate cancer are similar. My deepest fear was that I had prostate cancer." Two years later, when he learned that he did in fact have a fast-growing and dangerous type of prostate cancer, but it was a type that he knew could be successfully treated, this pioneer in cancer medicine recalled: "For close to a week, I lived in a daze. What ran repetitively through my head were the various scenarios that would take place leading to my death. I knew them all; I had seen them happen."

In a fundamental way, Dr. DeVita was not unlike that poor woman suffering from advanced breast cancer who had come to see Dr. Nathan back in 1956. Fear overwhelmed reason in both of them. So the history of how we've come to fear this disease is only one strand of cancerphobia's DNA that we need to understand. The other is the psychology of risk perception, the specific emotional characteristics that explain *why* cancer feels so much more frightening than any other disease.

---

Chapter 2

the psychological roots

No passion so effectually robs the mind of all its powers of act-
ing and reasoning as fear.
                    —Edmund Burke

The 75-year-old woman was paralyzed and unable to speak. After
a thorough examination, the family physician told her children that he
had found a lump in their mother's thyroid and suspected that cancer may
have started there and spread to her brain. He referred them to an oncologist, suggesting as a last hope that treatment with radioactive iodine
might destroy the cancer and help their mother recover.

This is how the oncologist described the family's surprising reaction
when he delivered what seemed to be dire news:

> The old lady lay paralyzed and stuporous in her bed. At last the
> tests were completed. There was no evidence of cancer.
> "There is nothing that can be done," the family was told.
> "Your mother has suffered a stroke from a broken blood vessel;
> the brain is irreparably damaged. There is no operation or
> treatment that can help."
> The oldest daughter leaned forward, tense, and with a qua-
> ver in her voice, asked, "did you find cancer?"
> "There was no cancer," I replied.
> "Thank God," the family exclaimed.[1]

For decades, around the world, cancer has been the disease people
fear most. Why? Based on the likelihood it will kill us, cardiovascular disease should frighten us more. The World Health Organization reports
that it killed 17.9 million people worldwide in 2018. Cancer *only* killed

9.6 million.[2] In the United States in 2018, cardiovascular disease killed roughly 9% more people than cancer did. Given these facts, doesn't our fear of cancer seem, well, irrational?

Sure, if you use only the facts to gauge risk. But we don't. We use our feelings too. You can hear this in the comments of men in a study of why they chose aggressive and risky treatment for nonthreatening types of prostate cancer that were almost surely never going to harm them. Based purely on the medical facts, that seems an irrational choice. But as the men said, "It's *cancer*, man!"; "It's a time bomb and you don't know if your time is going to be short or time is going to be long"; and "Yeah, a train doesn't look dangerous when it's going 5 mph but if it runs you over you'll be just as dead." The researchers summed up their interviews more dryly: "Patient treatment preferences were not based on careful assessments of numerical risks for various clinical outcomes."[3]

You can also hear the reality of risk perception psychology in what women say about choosing aggressive and risky surgery for treatment of low-grade ductal carcinoma in situ (DCIS), a type of breast cancer that their doctors told them was unlikely to ever cause them any symptoms at all, much less kill them. Respondents to one survey said: "I thought if I ever had DCIS, I would wait. But when faced with DCIS, all I could think was, 'Get it out, get it out, get it out.'" "I had two little kids and was so afraid for them. I couldn't stop crying." "My emotions definitely drove my decision. Doctors will never be able to tell you what will happen to you; they can only give you statistics."

Research has established that we perceive and respond to potential danger with both a rational analysis and an emotional interpretation of the facts, as we try to make sense of those facts in the context of our lives. And cognitive psychologists and neuroscientists have learned that, between the facts and the feelings, feelings have the upper hand. Down at the most basic biological level, the wiring of the brain's danger detection system guarantees that in the initial millisecond when we detect a potentially threatening stimulus, before we're even conscious of it, we react with an instinctive fight, flight, or freeze response. We are hardwired to fear first and think second. Then, over time, even as we think things over, feelings have a stronger influence on our perceptions. As neuroscientist Joseph LeDoux puts it, "The wiring of the brain at this point in our evolutionary history is such that the connections from the emotional systems to the cognitive systems are stronger than the connections from the cognitive systems to the emotional systems."[4]

Cognitive psychologists Melissa Finucane and Paul Slovic call this "the affect heuristic," an academic name for the suite of subconscious mental shortcuts we use to make emotional judgments about the facts in the context of our life circumstances, education, experiences, and values.[5] A key part of that cognitive toolkit is a set of psychological characteristics that give those facts emotional valence and make some things *feel* scarier than others.

The result of this is that "risk is a feeling," as pioneering risk perception researcher George Lowenstein and colleagues have put it.[6] And that feelings-based risk perception system creates what I call the risk perception gap—when fears that don't match the level of danger (sometimes we're too worried, and sometimes we're not worried enough) lead to choices that feel right but put us at greater risk. Our sometimes excessive fear of cancer is a profound example.

This, in essence, is why the number two cause of death reigns as our most feared disease. This is why millions of people for whom cancer screening is not recommended choose such screening anyway, and why millions who *should* be screened *avoid* tests that could help save their lives. This is why tens of thousands of people opt for more aggressive and risky cancer treatments than their clinical condition requires, and why many who have symptoms that may be early signs of cancer avoid going to the doctor, afraid to learn they have this terrifying disease, though that knowledge could save their lives. Our *affective* system of risk assessment is why we so readily believe that cancer is caused by everything "out there," despite the evidence that most cancer is the result of natural biological processes. The emotional nature of our feel-and-think risk perception psychology is why reasonable fear of cancer so often turns into the excessive and seemingly irrational fear this book examines.

But that word "irrational" is dangerous. It sounds judgmental, smugly implying that people who make choices based more on their feelings than on the facts are less educated, less intelligent, or just plain wrong. That implication denies all that we have learned about human psychology, which has established that we're not the "just the facts" rational decision makers we pretend to be. All our choices are the product of a mix of information and how we *feel* about that information in the context of our circumstances. So if people choose to have themselves screened for cancer despite having no risk factors that warrant such exams, or if people who do have those risk factors are so afraid of finding out they have cancer that they *avoid* screening, those choices are right for them, even though those choices increase the risk that they'll die. A double mastectomy to remove precancerous DCIS in only one breast is right for any woman who makes that choice, despite the risk of long-term pain, body image issues, and the low but real risk of death from a surgery she does not clinically need. Surgery to remove a slow-growing prostate cancer highly unlikely to ever cause any symptoms is right for any man who makes that choice, despite the high risk of erectile dysfunction and urinary incontinence from such surgery. A thyroidectomy to remove a tiny nonthreatening papillary cancer is the right choice for anyone who makes it, even though that surgery will leave them dependent on medication for the rest of their life to control their hormone levels.

On the medical evidence alone, those choices don't seem to make sense. But to the people who make them, such choices *do* make sense, and it is not for anyone to second-guess them or judge them derisively as irrational. Nonetheless we have to understand *why* people make such choices: Why do we subject ourselves to more risk than our clinical conditions alone require, screen when we shouldn't, or don't screen when we should? Understanding the psychological roots of our sometimes excessive fear of cancer is the critical first step toward reducing the vast harm that fear can cause. We can use our general understanding of the emotional nature of our risk perception psychology as a warning light to guide us toward healthier choices.

But that's not enough. We need a better awareness of the specific psychological factors that make some things feel scarier than the evidence says they are. If we're aware of the emotional tripwires that shape our fears about cancer—the specific components of the overall affect heuristic—we can step over those tripwires and give reason more of a voice in shaping our judgments.

We're all afraid of the same things. All you have to do is ask yourself what frightens you and you'll know what frightens me.

—John Carpenter, horror film director

In Edna Kaehele's 1953 book *Living with Cancer*, one of the first to openly describe the personal experience of having cancer, she describes the shock of hearing her diagnosis: "It is an unclean word to our minds. A horror beyond which there is no reasoning . . . Cancer! The word filled the universe. I could feel it start from some place too deep for conscious thought, whirring to slow life, swelling to immense proportions, bursting at last with the force of an atomic explosion somewhere in the top of my head. Cancer! CANCER! CANCER!"[7]

We are each unique in so many ways: in our gender and age, our experiences and life circumstances, our health status, our cultures, values, and beliefs. Yet it is true for nearly all of us that few words would be more frightening to hear than "You have cancer." Why is that? Why does this group of diseases so universally frighten so many different people around the world? Why has cancer become, practically everywhere, the emotional Emperor of All Maladies? The synonyms for what cancer has come to mean include malignancy, blight, scourge, poison, pestilence, plague, rot, corruption. Why has cancer come to mean malevolence itself?

In 1977, as society was beginning to talk more openly about cancer, and as doctors were finally being more open and honest about it with their patients, psychiatrist Jimmie Holland pioneered treatment for cancer patients' mental and emotional health. (She had been moved by the stories that her oncologist husband, James Holland, told about his patients. Dr. Jimmie Holland graciously contributed to the research for this book and was eager for its publication. She passed away as it was being written.)

Thousands now work in the field she helped create, known as psycho-oncology, focused on the psychological, social, behavioral, and ethical aspects of cancer. Most of that work understandably focuses on patients undergoing cancer care or recovering from such treatment. But a bit of research has investigated how people feel as they decide whether to undergo cancer screening, as well as the psychology behind their choices about how to respond to diagnoses—the choices we're exploring.

Most of that research merely asks people how they feel, not specifically why they feel that way. But the broader study of risk perception psychology has explained that "why," identifying several discrete psychological characteristics—fear factors, if you will—that we subconsciously use to assess how worried to be.[8] While doctors usually present risk in statistical terms, some numeric version of the likelihood that we'll die, research has found that what matters most to how we *feel* about a risk is not the statistical likelihood that we will die but the specific nature of *how*. Australian journalist Pamela Bone put it perfectly while in remission from multiple myeloma: "I'm not afraid of being dead. I'm just afraid of what you might have to go through to get there."[9]

Risk perception "fear factors" can be thought of as the psychological filters by which we subconsciously assess the nature of how it would feel to experience a risk. Several of these characteristics regularly appear in the way people describe their fear of cancer. They are the psychological keys to decoding the harmful phobia that otherwise reasonable concern about cancer can become. (These fear factors, while common in most people in most cultures, affect people differently depending on their unique circumstances, experiences, and personalities.)

Pain and Suffering

The greater the pain and suffering an experience involves, the more afraid of it we are, regardless of the odds. We are more afraid of burning to death than of dying in our sleep, for example, or of death by shark attack rather than by sudden drop-dead cardiac arrest. Many types of cancer cause severe physical suffering. So do treatments for many cancers. And death from many forms of cancer often entails the agony of slowly withering away. Although not true of all cancers, many types of the disease unquestionably involve a great deal of physical suffering.

In the 2018 national survey conducted by the American Society of Clinical Oncology (ASCO), in which cancer retained its title as the most feared disease, the biggest reason people gave for their fear of a cancer diagnosis, tied with fear of death itself, was pain and suffering.[10]

You can hear this factor in the comments of psycho-oncology researchers, patients, and other sources talking about why cancer is so frightening.

> Perceptions of "quick" deaths following heart attacks or trauma were contrasted with images of protracted and painful cancer deaths. Participants recalled friends and relatives "fighting for every breath, wanting an extra day all the while" and ending up in a "pitiful state."[11]

Cancer is associated not only with death, but with death in its worst form—a lingering, slow, miserable death.[12]

More than any other disease, cancer has horrified the imagination of mankind. It kills slowly, painfully.[13]

In the end it isn't dying that scares me but pain. The ending of life is expected, we all live in this mortal plane. What I resent is that death being longer and more painful than it needs to be. My body will self-destruct, day by day. The tumour will grow, spread, consume, squash the very organs that work to sustain it.[14]

Control

The less control we feel we have over a potential threat—the less we feel we can do something to protect ourselves—the more afraid we are likely to be. Even though many forms of cancer are now treatable as chronic conditions, or curable outright, most people around the world still believe cancer is invariably fatal, something they ultimately can't do anything about. In 2017 the Health Information National Trends Survey (HINTS) asked respondents to rate how much they agreed or disagreed with this statement: "When I think of cancer, I automatically think of death." Sixty-one percent agreed.[15] Fundamental to our fear of cancer, both the reasonable concern and the sometimes excessive version of that fear, is that we don't think we can do anything about cancer.

Cancer is still a word that strikes fear into people's hearts, producing a deep sense of powerlessness. (Angelina Jolie in an opinion essay announcing she'd had a double mastectomy)[16]

"Scared, death, feeling that you can't control it, it's out of your control."
"As soon as you hear cancer you think of the ultimate. There's nothing more then, but for this person to die."
"My basic image I grew up with is cancer: dead!" (Patients cited in a study of fear of cancer)[17]

The powerful need for control helps explain many of the behaviors our fear of cancer leads to. Probably the clearest example is overscreening, when people choose to undergo cancer screening even though they have none of the risk factors that make such screening likely to benefit them. Screening, researchers report, offers a sense of control.

> It is not surprising then that many women under 50 with no family history of breast cancer get screening mammograms, and some doctors advocate it, despite evidence that they are either ineffective at saving lives or have some minimal impact but incur substantial physical and financial costs. Many women and their doctors feel that a screening mammogram is the only positive action they can take to allay their fears.[18]

> These early detection and screening programs largely "worked" by giving individuals a way to assert some control over their fears of cancer.[19]

But the fear of not having control works both ways. It also drives many people *away* from screening. They take control of their fear by avoiding it.

> "I'd rather not go [for screening], that way the doctor can't tell me that I have cancer, because just by knowing, that I will die, . . . I would die . . . From knowing. From the fear."
>   "I don't want to know it before my time."
>   "Just finding out that something may be wrong is definitely the biggest fear of all." (Patients in a meta-analysis of several surveys of cancer fears)[20]

Our need for control also helps explain why the majority of people diagnosed with a slow-growing, nonthreatening type of cancer that can be treated with no more than ongoing surveillance choose far more aggressive and risky treatments than their clinical conditions require. Just watching and monitoring things doesn't feel like doing as much—taking as much control—as having surgery.

Uncertainty

Uncertainty—not knowing what we need to know to protect ourselves— leaves us feeling powerless. It's a corollary to not having control. Three basic types of uncertainty play a role in why cancer is so frightening.

First is the uncertainty about any threat we can't see, smell, hear, or detect with any of our senses. This factor helps explain why appeals to fear about undetectable environmental carcinogens have so much impact. Most of those suspected carcinogens are invisible, odorless, and tasteless. Environmental alarms about these substances play on this fear factor. This type of uncertainty also helps explain the appeal of screening, which makes the invisible visible, reducing uncertainty.

> In addition to whatever impact [screenings] have on the probabilities of suffering disease and ill health, they also provide a means to control the uncertainty and fear associated with disease.[21]

> Beliefs were expressed that risk of cancer was reduced by participation in screening. This may be a coping strategy to gain protection from the risk and uncertainty of the threat of cancer. (Survey of South Asian breast cancer patients)[22]

The second form of uncertainty can be thought of as "It's complicated and hard to understand." The science and medical details of cancer, and the numbers, odds, and other probability statistics that doctors use to explain risk, are complex. Not understanding is the same as not knowing, a form of powerlessness that turns many of us into personal Google doc(tor)s, as we go online or to other sources to learn more and give ourselves a sense of control.

Then there is the final and perhaps most frightening type of uncertainty. Screening biopsies and blood tests can give doctors a precise idea of what kind of cancer we have, and a *reasonable* idea of what those cancers are likely to do, but they can't provide absolutely certainty about the future. This element of uncertainty lies at the heart of how we respond to "overdiagnosed" types of breast, prostate, thyroid, and lung cancer that are highly unlikely to ever harm us—unlikely . . . but doctors can't say for sure. Even if there is only a one in a million chance that your cancer might be lethal, you could be that one, and that tiny remaining uncertainty creates fear that vastly exceeds the statistical odds.

Is the Risk Human-Made or Natural?

We are more afraid of risks that are human-made than those that arise naturally. When the HINTS survey in 2001 asked people what they thought increased their risk of getting cancer, 80% believed that pesticides and food additives raised their risk, and 88% said pollution.[23] In a 2019 version of the survey, 79% agreed a lot or somewhat that "everything causes cancer."[24]

The widespread fear that many modern products and processes cause cancer arose amid the smog, burning rivers, and hazardous waste dumps that spurred our awareness of and concern about environmental problems in the sixties and seventies. In chapter 14 of *Silent Spring* (ominously titled "One in Four," as in, one in four of us will get cancer), Rachel Carson wrote: "With the dawn of the industrial era the world became a place of continuous, ever-accelerating change. Instead of the natural environment there was rapidly substituted an artificial one composed of new chemicals and physical agents, many of them possessing powerful capacities for inducing biologic change. Against these carcinogens which his own activities had created man had no protection."

Stunningly for a scientist (a marine biologist), Carson instinctively played on the psychological tendency to fear the human-made over the natural when she wrote, "Man, alone of all forms of life, can create cancer-producing substances." That isn't close to true. Nature "creates" all sorts of carcinogens too.

Though we now know that most cancers are the result of natural processes that cause DNA mutations leading to uncontrolled cell growth, and that diet, exercise, and other lifestyle choices can reduce the risk of cancer by as much as 40%, the myth remains embedded in common belief, reinforced by environmental advocates and the general news media, that cancer is largely the result of modern human-made products and processes.[25]

Consider this example: In 2010 the *Telegraph* (a British newspaper) reported that a study of mummies had found very few cancers. According to the study's authors, that meant, as the headline read,

CANCER CAUSED BY MODERN MAN
as it was virtually non-existent in ancient world. Cancer is a modern man-made disease caused by the excesses of modern life, a new study suggests.

The newspaper's *science* reporter, who surely should have known better, repeated the huge leap the study authors had made to reach their biased conclusions: "The findings suggest that it is modern lifestyles and pollu-tion levels caused by industry that are the main cause of the disease and that it is not a naturally occurring condition."[26] The study would have made Rachel Carson proud. The authors wrote, "A striking rarity of ma-lignancies in ancient physical remains might indicate that cancer was rare in antiquity, and so poses questions about the role of carcinogenic envi-ronmental factors in modern societies."[27] Neither the study nor the news report made any mention of the fact that people in "antiquity" usually didn't live long, and that the modern rise in cancer prevalence corre-sponds with our longer life spans. Or that cancer in soft tissues wouldn't show up in fossils.

Fighting the entrenched misbelief that "everything causes cancer" is hard. The highly respected Cancer Research UK tried, calling the study factually incorrect and misleading, as well as directly addressing the psy-chological factors of control and less fear of what is natural than what is human-made, saying, "It can be tempting to worry about our cancer risk from external things like pollution and chemicals more than from things we can control, like our lifestyles. But decades of research have shown that lifestyle factors—such as not smoking, keeping a healthy weight, lim-iting alcohol, getting enough exercise, and avoiding sunburn—have an important effect on cancer risk. In contrast, the evidence that pollution and industrialisation has a widespread role in UK cancer rates is weak."[28]

The belief that cancer is mostly caused by human-made substances explains why any mention of the word "chemicals" or "radiation" sets off alarms. (Magnetic resonance imaging was originally called nuclear mag-netic resonance imaging. The "nuclear" was dropped to avoid the fright-ening allusion to weapons and radiation.) And it explains why scientists frustrated by "chemophobia" and "radiophobia," corollaries of cancer-phobia, try to reduce those fears by arguing, "All of nature is made out of chemicals," and, "If we're worried about nuclear power we should also worry about natural sources of radiation like the sun and bananas." Those arguments fail to convince, however, because of the next risk perception characteristic.

Is the Risk Imposed or Voluntary?

We are more afraid of risks that feel imposed on us—radiation from a nuclear power plant accident—and less afraid of those that we engage in voluntarily, like radiation from the sun. Unlabeled ingredients that manufacturers have put in our food worry us more than what we *choose* to eat and drink. We readily blame plastics and pesticides for imposing cancer risk on us but absolve ourselves of responsibility for the dietary and lifestyle choices that increase our cancer risk far more than those imposed bogeymen.

Consider the 2015 survey by the American Institute for Cancer Research (AICR) ranking how many people ascribed cancer to which causes. Of the top 16, 10 are imposed on us:

   3. Radiation (not including the natural kind from the sun)—89%
   4. Industrial pollution—88%
   6. Asbestos—83%
   7. Pesticides on produce—74%
   8. Nuclear power—68%
   9. Food additives—62%
   10. Radon—59%
   11. Genetically modified food—56%
   16. Artificial sweeteners—51%

The voluntary lifestyle and diet choices that elevate our cancer risk far more showed up far down the list.

   15. Being overweight or obese—52%
   19. Alcohol use—43%
   20. Lack of exercise—42%
   21. Diet low in fruits and vegetables—42%
   24. Diets high in red meats—35%[29]

Consider a regular wine drinker who avoids the (disproved) cancer risk of artificial sweeteners. That is a risk perception gap.

Personification

A risk we know about only as a concept doesn't worry us as much as one with which we have some personal experience. Unlike the abstract idea of climate change, for example, most of us have experienced cancer's cruelty firsthand, either ourselves or through the experience of a relative, a friend, a colleague, a neighbor, or maybe just in the public story of a celebrity. Someone real. Someone with a face and a name, not just a number. A person, someone who could be *us*. That personification makes cancer more frightening.

Many people who notice a "suspicious" symptom have encountered cancer before through the illness of a loved one, such as a parent or grandparent. If a symptom suggests that you might have the same type of cancer as your loved one did, you may become terrified. Fear that you might go through the same vividly recalled cancer experience as someone close to you did can be overwhelming.[30]

"I was shocked when a friend of mine died from the disease. That incident made me realize how dangerous breast cancer can be if not detected at an early stage. So, after that I said to myself that anything you like it or not but you are now going to have mammograms on a regular basis."

"I saw a woman who had a large scar on her left chest in a public sauna in Korea. Her scar was on her left chest from shoulder to middle of the chest. I felt so bad for that woman. Cancer is so fearful for me since I saw her." (Two women in a survey about breast cancer fear)[31]

So many people I know have died of cancer. I'm afraid. (Patient in a survey regarding fear of cancer)[32]

The role of personification affects doctors and health care providers as well as patients. As one physician told researchers in a study of what doctors tell their patients about ovarian cancer screening, "We're physicians, but we also have life experiences . . . for better and for worse, our personal experience may affect our practice."[33] Their personal experiences can't help but shape how doctors talk to us about cancer and what they recommend. A study found that doctors in the United States who had personal experience with cancer themselves or in their families were 17% more likely to ignore the expert recommendations against ovarian cancer screening and recommend that screening anyway, compared to doctors who had no personal experience with the disease.[34]

Just as personification raises fear, the same psychological factor tends to diminish our concern if we have little or no personal experience with a risk. The literature review of studies into why we fear cancer, Vrinten et al., found, "A dozen studies described people who were not afraid of cancer at all, because they . . . had never experienced it in anyone close to them."[35]

Even More Cognitive Impediments to Critical Thinking about Cancer

The powerful influence of these subjective psychological filters—pain and suffering, control, uncertainty, human-made versus natural, imposed versus voluntary, personification—goes a long way toward explaining why our fear of cancer in some cases exceeds the evidence. But they are not the whole story. Research on human cognition has identified all sorts of unconscious biases and mental shortcuts that interfere with our ability to see information objectively. Many also shape how we feel about cancer.

Availability/Awareness

When we experience anything with emotional power, like something frightening, the brain encodes that memory in a way that makes it more readily "available" to come quickly back into consciousness if we are in a similar situation again. Because of that speed, recalling these important memories carries extra emotional impact. Many of us have had emotionally powerful experiences with cancer. "Availability" gives those experiences extra influence whenever we think about the disease.

Connected to "availability" is "awareness." The more aware of a threat we are, the bigger and brighter that blip is on our mind's radar screen, and the greater the emotional weight it carries. Through personal experiences, stories in the news, the constant barrage of education and fund-raising messages from the cancer advocacy community, and seemingly ceaseless warnings about external carcinogens from environmental advocates, cancer is an ever-present bright blip on our risk radar. As one person put it to researchers on cancer and emotion, "I don't know; I feel like it is so, so common, and it's just kind of like a constant scare."

Loss Aversion

Loss aversion is the tendency to place undue emotional weight on the side of a choice that involves a loss, in this case, the loss of our health or lives. To illustrate the influence of loss aversion, researchers presented women 40 or older who had not yet had mammograms with two differ-ent messages describing mammography. Half the women saw a message describing screening and its benefits. Half saw a message describing screening and all the harms suffered by women who don't screen. Only half of the women who got the optimistic information describing screen-ing's benefits started coming in for mammograms, but two-thirds of the women presented with the loss-framed message did. The message framed in terms of loss was more motivating.[36]

Regret Aversion

Another kind of aversion shapes our choices about cancer: regret aver-sion. No woman wants to look back and regret her decision to have both breasts removed in response to a diagnosis of cancer in one breast that was unlikely to spread and cause harm. No man wants to look back at the decision to have prostate surgery or irradiation for slow-growing localized prostate cancer and regret that the side effects of erectile dysfunction and urinary incontinence weren't worth it, as some men do—16% in one study.[37]

Regret aversion isn't about hindsight. It's looking ahead to think about how you'll feel about a choice later, after you've made it. It shapes our choices as we make them. Researchers describe it this way: "When assessing the risks associated with a given decision, people often weigh the risk of regretting that decision—a risk that may be as important as any of the other risks."[38]

The dramatic case of Susanna Dillwyn Emlen, relayed in Robert Aronowitz's book *Unnatural History: Breast Cancer and American Society*, makes the power of regret aversion poignantly real. It happened a long time ago but remains relevant to the choices considered in this book. In 1817, at age 50, Susanna had struggled with breast cancer for six years. Wasting away and in pain, she was given the choice of doing no more or having her diseased breast amputated. There was no anesthesia back then. Surgery meant unimaginable pain. And her doctor told her bluntly that surgery was unlikely to save her life. But Susanna did not want to re-gret in her final dying moments not having done all she could. "It ap-peared best to me to endeavor to submit to an operation believing that if it should prove unsuccessful I should suffer with more patience from be-lieving I had availed myself of those means of relief placed providentially within my power."

Susanna died two years after willingly enduring the excruciating brutality of the operation, in peace and with no regrets.

Innumeracy

Risk information is frequently presented in statistical terms, but many of us struggle to understand numbers, especially when described with percentages. Consider this quiz (from my book *How Risky Is It Really? Why Our Fears Don't Always Match the Facts*):

1. Which risk is greater, one in 100, 1 in 1,000, or 1 in 10?

2. Let's say you buy an "I'm Feeling Lucky!" lottery scratch ticket. One player in 1,000 wins. So if 1,000 people (including you) buy that ticket, what percentage of those folks are going to feel lucky after they scratch off the ticket?

3. Let's say you buy an "I Am Going To Be Filthy Stinking Rich!" ticket. One percent of the "investors" in this game win the big prize. If 1,000 people play this game, how many people end up filthy stinking rich?

4. If you take one die from a set and roll it 1,000 times, about how many times would it come up on an even number?

The answers are at the end of the chapter. If you want to peek now, take a look.

How did you do? Don't feel bad if you got less than a perfect score. Regardless of education, people have trouble with numbers, a cognitive limitation that impairs our ability to be objective about the risk of cancer or the risk of side effects from various treatments, because doctors usually provide their information in numeric form. The seeming rationality of numbers is appealing to doctors, which is part of why they rely on them to explain risks to their patients objectively. But because of innumeracy, it's often like they are speaking in a foreign language, even as they think they're helping us make an informed choice.

To illustrate how common this problem is, in one study of people with a greater-than-high-school education who took the quiz above, about one

in five got the first question wrong.[39] Question 2 stumped eight in ten participants. Question 3 stumped four in ten. Question 4 was the easy one.
Still, stunningly, only half got it right.

Besides struggling to understand what numbers actually say, we have
additional problems understanding risk in quantitative form. One is our
confusion about the difference between the *relative* risk—how much more
or less likely one outcome is compared to (relative to) another—and the
absolute risk, the actual number of people in a given population who suffer that outcome. An increase from one victim to two out of a million is a
frightening relative increase of 100%, but it raises the absolute risk to just
two in a million. Very often, journalists, environmentalists, cancer advocacy groups, and medical providers—anybody who wants to play up the
drama of a cancer risk—offer *either* the relative *or* the absolute risk, but
not both, highlighting the one that is more dramatic.

Then there is the difference between statistics about incidence—the
number of people who *get* cancer—and mortality, the number of people
who die. Many alarming stories report that cancer incidence is rising.
Fewer report that the mortality rate is steady or declining. And finally,
statistics—like many of those in this book—report population-wide averages or totals, without cautioning the reader that each person and each
case of disease is unique.

Some aspects of innumeracy are just struggling with math, basic addition and subtraction, multiplication and division. But some are due to
the heuristics our brain uses to assess numbers, even the numbers we
understand:

- *Denominator neglect.* When we consider a risk of 1 in 100,
  represented mathematically as the fraction $\frac{1}{100}$, we disregard the denominator because all we care about is the
  numerator, if that one might be us.
- *Probability neglect.* The probability that something might
  cause cancer only means it *might* cause cancer to *some* people
  at *some* ages who are exposed to *some* doses of some substance depending on the route by which they're exposed (did
  they get it on their skin, breathe it in, or swallow it?) and for
  how long they were exposed (every day for their whole lives
  like rodents in toxicology tests, or only once or twice?).

Probability lumps all those critical variables together, and it only means there is a *chance* something might happen, not a *guarantee*. But when we hear that something *might* cause cancer, we often leap to the conclusion that it *always does*, in everybody. Journalists, including good science journalists, generally fail to make this important point about risks, using the frightening but not very informative phrase "[this substance] *has been linked to* cancer." (This is a huge failure in the risk reporting about the class of industrial chemicals generally referred to as PFAS, the latest in a long series of human-made substances found to be *associated* with *some* cancers and other health risks.) There is a huge difference between association and causation that, with cancer, we often ignore.

- *Base rate neglect.* This is a fancy way of saying that we tend to look at one simple risk number and fail to consider all the other numbers that would paint a more complete and accurate picture. One in two American men and one in three women will develop cancer in their lifetimes. Scary, right? But that is just one part of the overall picture. Three cases in four occur in people over 55 years old. So the thinking of a 35-year-old woman who considers only the first number and neglects the second—which adds critical information about the overall picture—is influenced by "neglect" of the actual base rate *for her.*

Several more cognitive instincts shape our perceptions and help explain why cancer is so uniquely frightening. We are exquisitely sensitive to anything that triggers a feeling of *disgust*: smells, tastes, sounds, ideas, or diseases that warn us against something that might be dangerous. For a long time, cancer was thought of as a disgusting disease. For some, it still is. Disgust affects whether we screen for and how we choose to treat colorectal cancer, cancers related to sexual activity, and cancers of the breast or genitals.

Cancer also still carries a fearful *stigma*, defined as "a permanent mark of shame, disgrace, dishonor, ignominy, opprobrium, humiliation." (This is particularly true of certain cancers, like lung and cervical cancer.) It's hard to overcome that permanence. As Jimmie Holland wrote,

For many years, cancer carried a stigma for the patient and the family . . . Cancer was called the big C, because the word itself was still so scary. A taxi driver once refused to drive me to Memorial Hospital saying, 'No ma'am, that place is for the big C. I drive all the way around it.' And many patients felt guilty for bringing the shame of cancer on the family. This cultural silence and stigma limited the opportunity for people even to talk with one another about their illness.

Holland was describing experiences in the fifties and sixties, but the stigma attached to cancers associated with personal behaviors, like lung cancer in smokers or sexually transmitted cervical cancer, remains, particularly for some populations, including African Americans and Asian women (particularly for breast cancer). In research on Asia-born women living in the UK, the authors note, "Perceptions of cancer and health behaviour were influenced by cultural beliefs. Common themes were cancer is a taboo subject and cancer is a stigma."[40]

Part of this stigma includes the persistent fear among some that a worrisome personality, a stressful lifestyle, or even fear of cancer can cause the disease, a controversial theory in the medical literature but certainly a burned-in belief among some, contributing to an exaggerated stigmatization of cancer in the public's mind.

"Just by worrying can we become sick . . . I always worry and that I might get cancer."
    "Just uttering the word [cancer] would result in getting the disease." (Patients from a survey of cancer fear)[41]

Trust also contributes to our emotional relationship to cancer and to the choices we make about screening and treatment options. Personal physicians are the single most trusted professionals. We follow their recommendations in large part because we trust them. But as we'll see, our health care providers often don't provide balanced and complete information about cancer screening or choices for handling a low-risk diagnosis. People of lower socioeconomic status have less trust in the entire health care system, doctors included, which contributes to higher overall rates of poor health outcomes in these groups.

Finally, on top of all those general truths about the way human cognition works, there are all sorts of differences in how we feel about cancer based on our gender, race, ethnicity, educational status, and how worried we are about things in general. As just one example, a study of more than 13,000 British residents between 55 and 64 years old found, "All cancer fear indicators were significantly higher in women, respondents with lower education, and those with higher general anxiety. Ethnic minority respondents reported more worry."[42]

———

Cancer involves so many different choices that it would be impossible to tease apart the psychology that shapes each choice, even just the few choices this book considers. And it would be pointless because each of us is unique, and those choices are for us alone to make in the context of our personal lives.

But as we prepare to move into the following sections detailing the ways that an excessive fear of cancer does great harm, it's vital to keep in mind the specific psychological and cognitive factors described above, because they offer insights into how we make our own choices. Being aware of the emotional factors that color how we feel about cancer will hopefully help us make those choices more carefully, producing outcomes that will do us the most good.

Quiz answers
1. 1 in 10
2. 0.1% (or 0.001)
3. 10
4. 500

Part Two

the costs
to
individuals

overscreening, overdiagnosis, overtreatment

An Overview

Seek and ye shall find
—Jesus of Nazareth

Erwin Schrödinger had a cat named Milton. Milton never became famous, at least not by name. The Austrian scientist Schrödinger did, for his discoveries in physics. But the anonymous Milton also made his mark on history, as the cat in an oft-cited thought experiment named for his owner. Though Schrödinger conceived his conceptual conundrum to describe his puzzling over quantum mechanics (which puzzles most of us), it speaks directly to the central question we're about to explore: What harm might we be causing, just by looking for cancer?

What is known as the puzzle of Schrödinger's cat goes like this. A cat (presumably Milton) is inside a closed box. Quantum theory suggests that the cat can be both alive and dead at the same moment, something called superposition, and only the act of observing the cat triggers it into one state or another. *Leave it unobserved and nothing happens.*

3-D mammography. Prostate-specific antigen (PSA) analysis. Low-dose computed tomography. Colonoscopy. Genetic testing. The development of ever more perceptive cancer-screening technologies is driven by a core belief about cancer—find it as early as possible. "Cancer is curable if treated early" has been preached by doctors, public health officials, and cancer advocacy groups for as long as we've battled this disease. That blind belief urgently needs updating.

It may sound heretical, but several kinds of cancer don't need to be treated as aggressively as we assume, cancers that fit the standard characteristics of the disease when examined under a microscope but that would never harm the patient over their remaining lifetime. (Eighty percent of cancers are diagnosed in people 55 or older; 50% in people 65 and older.)[1] While it remains true in general that finding cancer as early as possible increases the chances for successful treatment, finding certain common cancers early often does more harm than good. Cancer screening itself has taught us that *early detection is not always beneficial.*

As with Schrödinger's cat, the very act of observation triggers the harm, not from cancer itself, but from fear of the disease. That fear drives millions of people to look inside the box—to screen for various kinds of cancer even though they have none of the risk factors (age, genetics, etc.) that warrant such exams. That is *overscreening.* Then, if anything is found that meets the cellular characteristics of cancer, the patient receives a frightening diagnosis that includes some version of the C-word, even if it's the low-grade, low-risk, slow- or non-growing kind highly unlikely to cause the patient any harm. That is *overdiagnosis.* Fear then drives many people to choose more aggressive treatments than these less-threatening types of disease clinically require, and those tests and treatments often cause serious side effects, including death. That is *overtreatment.* For tens of thousands of people each year, this fear-driven cascade causes more harm than the cancer itself ever would have.

Overscreening

It's hard to imagine how there can be too much screening for a disease as insidious as cancer, an affliction described by Philadelphia surgeon David Hayes Agnew in 1883 as "a monstrous and aimless accumulation of tissue elements which observe neither order or form." That's not far from how cancer is described today, albeit without the reference to monsters.

Cancer is a condition where cells in a specific part of the body grow and reproduce uncontrollably. The cancerous cells can invade and destroy surrounding healthy tissue, including organs. (UK National Health System)

Diseases in which abnormal cells divide without control and can invade nearby tissues. (US National Cancer Institute)

Crucially, however, those definitions miss one key qualifying element. Yes, *some* cancer cells rapidly divide and reproduce uncontrollably. Yes, *some* develop the additional ability to metastasize, to spread into the body from the organ they've started in. And yes, *some* types of cancer, certainly many, kill. *But some don't.* All cancer is not the same. Without wider appreciation of this vital distinction, we don't stand much chance of rethinking our fear of cancer. So it bears emphasis: *Some common forms of cancer pose little or no threat to our health.*

As doctors H. Gilbert Welch and William Black, pioneers in raising awareness of the problem of overdiagnosis, put it, "Although the concept of nonprogressive cancers may seem implausible, basic scientists have begun to uncover biological mechanisms that halt the progression of cancer. Some cancers outgrow their blood supply (and are starved), others may be recognized by the host's immune system or other defense mechanisms (and are successfully contained), and some are simply not that aggressive in the first place."[2] Barry Kramer, former director of the Division of Cancer Prevention at the US National Cancer Institute, shared similar thoughts: "Unfortunately the term cancer doesn't fit all sizes. It is an outdated term at least for some lesions and doesn't convey the mounting evidence that we have about the actual natural behavior of those cancers, some of which don't act like cancer at all."[3] Pediatrician Virginia Moyer, who once chaired the US Preventive Services Task Force, commented, "The public thinks once you have a cancer cell in your body, it will progress predictably and inevitably to a terrible death. That is simply not true of most cancers."[4]

Against our deep fear of cancer, it is stunning how many types aren't as threatening as we believe. According to Otis Brawley, professor at Johns Hopkins University and the former chief medical officer of the American Cancer Society, as many as "20% to 30% of cancers are not genomically programmed to grow, harm, and kill."[5]

But our beliefs about cancer have not caught up to this relatively recent realization. We're stuck with the widespread but outdated belief that if left untreated, all cancer kills, as well as the associated belief that catching any cancer as early as possible is always best. So we want all the screening we can get. Belief in cancer screening is deep, an almost religious faith, undoubtedly generated by our equally as profound fear of cancer itself. A 2004 study had these findings:

- Eighty-seven percent of adults believe that cancer screening is "almost always a good idea."
- Sixty-six percent would want to be tested for cancer *even if nothing could be done.*
- More than half (56%) would want to be tested for cancers that would never cause problems in their lifetime, even if those cancers were left untreated.
- Nearly all (98%) of those who had endured a false positive—a screening result suggesting cancer that later turned out not to be cancer at all—were still glad they'd had screening, though half of them described the experience as "the scariest time in my life."
- Of women, 58% said that they would disregard suggestions from their doctors to screen less often for breast cancer. Seventy-seven percent of men said that for prostate.[6]

Other studies have found that people still want specific types of cancer screening even after they're expressly told that the same number of people die with *or without* it.[7] And stunning research found that people want cancer screening even when they know it won't help and *might harm* them. In a study titled "A Bias for Action in Cancer Screening?," half the participants were told about a cancer-screening test (mammography for women, PSA testing for men) and were then warned that "years of research have unquestionably shown that the test does not extend life or reduce the chance of death" *and* that the test could "lead to unnecessary treatment." More than half (51%) wanted that screening anyway. The other half of participants got all that information, plus warnings about the specific harms caused by screening, including emotional suffering, physical pain, bleeding, hospitalization, or even death. Knowing all those details, and that the test would not help them and was more likely to harm them, 34% of those people still wanted the screening.[8]

Belief in screening makes psychological sense. It's one of the few things we can do to give ourselves a reassuring sense of control against our fear of cancer. Cancer screening is done by millions of people as much for its emotional value as for its clinical benefit. As the authors of "A Bias for Action in Cancer Screening?" put it: " Some people believe that there is something to be gained from screening even when the test does not save or extend lives, and that something is information. Cancer screening information may provide reassurance and reduce uncertainty."[9] Medical historian Robert Aronowitz noted how screening provides a feeling of control: "When you've oversold both the fear of cancer and the effectiveness of our prevention and treatment, even people harmed by the system will uphold it, saying, 'It's the only ritual we have, the only thing we can do to prevent ourselves from getting cancer.' "[10]

Study after study finds that the principal reason people screen for cancer, both those who meet the recommended criteria and the millions who don't, is worry, worry so ingrained that doing anything possible against the monster of cancer just seems like it must be the right thing to do. The authors of a British study of cancer-screening decisions wrote, "Our finding of experiences of fear from a number of sources in cancer screening is consistent with patients' reported experiences of seeking help for cancer symptoms. The role of fear and its link with cancer worry and perceived susceptibility in cancer screening uptake . . . [is clear]."[11] As George Crile Jr. wrote more than half a century ago in *Cancer and Common Sense*: "The demand for these tests stems from the philosophy of fear."[12]

Let me be clear. The problem isn't screening per se. Some screening methods for some types of cancer—cervical, colorectal, breast, lung—do save lives.[13] But not all screening is equally effective. Some screening technologies don't save lives at all, or save so few that the harms they cause—from the stress of worrisome false positives to the harmful side effects of overtreatment for frightening but less-threatening types of cancer—outweigh their benefits. Not all people are alike either, and even the most effective screenings, like Pap tests for cervical cancer and colorectal exams or low-dose CT scans for lung cancer, aren't right for everybody. They are only recommended for people who have some demographic characteristic (e.g., age, race) or other risk factor (family history) that makes screening more likely to help than harm. Tens of millions of people who have none of these characteristics choose cancer screening anyway. Fear of cancer is why.

Panels of experts assembled by governments or professional medical societies periodically review all the available research to compare the benefits of screening against its harms, as well as to determine whom screening is most likely to help and whom it's more likely to harm. (In the United States, the government panel is called the US Preventive Services Task Force, or USPSTF.) These expert panels publish screening recommendations designed, as the World Health Organization puts it, "to be sure that as few as possible with the disease get through undetected and as few as possible without the disease are subject to further diagnostic tests."[14]

Since screening recommendations are based on risk factors, it's worth a few paragraphs to describe the important ones. The most influential is our age. Cancer is largely a disease of aging. Mutations in our DNA occur all the time as the result of natural errors during cellular reproduction. They also occur as the natural by-product of normal biological processes (e.g., digestion) that cause inflammation. As we age, the chance increases that the several mutations necessary to allow a cell to reproduce without normal restraints and to evade controls that normally keep cells in one organ from spreading to another, will finally build up and initiate cancer in that single cell. For most cancers it takes decades for all those mutations to accumulate. This is why, though the *lifetime* risk of developing cancer (in developed countries) is roughly one in two, more than three-quarters of all new cancers occur in people 55 and older.[1]

Thus, screening guidelines identify the age prior to which cancer screening is not recommended, which only means that, although such screening might save some lives, at the population level, it will do more harm than good. Guidelines also include an age after which screening is not recommended. After a certain age, cancer incidence per age group drops. (That age varies for different types of cancer.) Doctors offer two likely reasons for this decline. First, people who have survived to older age have lived longer because they have always been generally healthier. And second, some cancers (breast, for example) that develop late in life seem to be slower growing and produce fewer symptoms.[2] So even if people in the final several years of their lives have some type of cancer, they are more likely to die of something else before the cancer can harm them.

Then there's the risk factor of genetics. Some cancers are more likely among those with close relatives who have had it: sister, mother, or daughter for breast cancer, brother or father for prostate cancer, for example. Heritable genetics (as opposed to genetic mutations that occur *after* we're born) play a significant role in 5% to 10% of all cancers. There are more than 50 of these inherited genetic cancer syndromes.[3] (Most people believe that genetic abnormalities cause much more cancer than they actually do. A survey of Americans rated "family history" as the second most common cause of cancer, after "lifestyle choices.")[4]

There are numerous other risk factors for various types of cancer. Some are well known: smoking and lung cancer, too much sun exposure and skin cancer. Some are less well recognized: only 30% of Americans realize that moderate to heavy alcohol consumption raises the risk of various cancers (esophageal, liver, breast, colon, and rectum), and that obesity is a huge risk factor for various cancers.[5] Racial and cultural characteristics are also associated with higher risk of some cancers.

The full list of cancer risk factors is too long to include and not the point here. The point is that some of us are more at risk than others. That's why screening is recommended only for people in certain subpopulations, for whom, research has established, it is likely to do the most good. For people without any risk factors (including age), screening is essentially *over*screening, because though it may still save some lives, across the entire population of people screening, it's more likely to cause harm than benefit.

But we don't worry about the safety of others as much as we worry about our own. So what can fairly be called overscreening at the population level, motivated significantly by our deep fear of cancer, doesn't feel like that to the individuals who choose to screen though they are outside the groups for whom it's recommended. They are quite reasonably making choices for themselves, in the context of their own lives.

1.   A. S. Ahmad, N. Ormiston-Smith, and P. D. Sasieni, "Trends in the Lifetime Risk of Developing Cancer in Great Britain: Comparison of Risk for Those Born from 1930 to 1960," *British Journal of Cancer* 112 (2015): 943–47, https://www.nature.com/articles/bjc2014606.
2.   P. G. M. Peer, J. A. A. M. Van Dijck, A. L. M. Verbeek, J. H. C. L. Hendriks, and R. Holland, "Age-Dependent Growth Rate of Primary Breast Cancer," *Cancer* 71, no. 11 (1993): 3547–51.
3.   "The Genetics of Cancer," National Cancer Institute, last updated Aug. 17, 2022, https://www.cancer.gov/about-cancer/causes-prevention/genetics. "The Genetics of Cancer,"
4.   American Society of Clinical Oncology, *ASCO 2018 Cancer Opinions Survey*, Oct. 2018, https://old-prod.asco.org/sites/new-www.asco.org/files/content-files/research-and-progress/documents/2018-NCOS-Results.pdf.
5.   American Society of Clinical Oncology, *National Cancer Opinions Survey*, https://www.asco.org/about-asco/press-center/news-releases/national-survey-reveals-most-americans-are-unaware-key-cancer.

Unfortunately, though they're all looking at the same research evidence, various expert review panels don't always agree about the optimal age ranges for screening or the optimal frequencies (annual, biennial, every five or ten years). The medical societies and advocacy organizations focused on a particular type of cancer usually recommend screening for a wider age range, starting at an earlier age and ending later, than the USPSTF recommends. The task force, for example, recommends that mammography begin at age 50. (Before this book went to press, the USPSTF issued a draft recommendation to change the age to 40. The discussions of mammography that follow are based on the recommendation as it stood in May 2023.) The American Cancer Society recommends that it start at 45. The National Comprehensive Cancer Network, a consortium of leading cancer hospitals that provide (and profit from) breast cancer care, recommends beginning at age 40.

A consumer trying to decide about screening has to sort out this confusion. This book relies on the recommendations from the USPSTF. It consists of 16 volunteer doctors, with a wide range of expertise, who serve four-year terms. This group chooses which medical condition to investigate (not just cancer, and the public can contribute suggestions) and then relies on extensive research done by people with expertise in that specific disease. The panel drafts suggested recommendations, and there is a period for public comment before the final recommendations are made. The USPSTF has no financial incentive for recommending more screening or less, as the medical groups do, no extra passion for maximizing treatment for specific diseases, as advocacy groups do (e.g., prostate cancer groups and the PSA test), and it works harder to fairly and thoroughly consider not only screening's benefits but also its limitations and harms. Members who have direct professional involvement or economic interest in a disease or a type of screening being reviewed are required to recuse themselves from that review, to avoid conflicts of interest (for example, a urologist making recommendations about PSA testing for prostate cancer). The USPSTF grades screening on a letter scale, with A and B being recommended: an A grade means "There is high certainty that the net benefit is substantial," and a B grade means "There is high certainty that the net benefit is moderate or there is moderate certainty that the net benefit is moderate to substantial." A C grade is essentially neutral, meaning "talk it over with your doctor," and D is essentially "Don't."

Any screening or medical procedure that gets an A or B ranking is supposed to be covered by health insurance programs.

Controversies erupt when new USPSTF recommendations leave some groups out of recommended screening (women under 50 for mammography), or don't recommend a screening test at all (PSA testing for prostate cancer). Criticism comes from the people left out of the eligibility criteria and their advocacy groups, from the medical specialties that treat the kind of cancer the guidelines cover and who profit from that treatment, and from the health care industry and screening equipment manufacturers that make more money the more people are screened. Politicians and the news media frequently misinterpret these recommendations as denying access to anyone who doesn't meet the eligibility criteria. But the USPSTF guidelines never ban anybody from screening. Though they do influence what insurers cover, they issue recommendations only, not rules, and they assess things only on a population-wide basis. They leave the final decision up to the patient and doctor, even for screenings they don't recommend.

Despite these carefully researched recommendations, however, our sometimes excessive fear of cancer drives millions of people younger or older than the recommendations specify to screen anyway. That is what we define as overscreening. An analysis conducted for this book by Ingrid Hall and colleagues of the US Centers for Disease Control and Prevention (CDC) found that in 2017:

- Despite the recommendation that only women aged 50 to 74 have an every-other-year mammogram, 15.6 million US women under 50 and 5.7 million over 74 said they'd had one sometime in the past ten years anyway.
- PSA blood tests to screen for prostate cancer had a grade of C, meaning that men from 55 to 75 should talk to their doctors about whether to have such a test. It was not recommended with an A or a B because research determined that PSA testing was more likely to cause harm than provide benefit. Yet 3.9 million US men below 50 and 6.2 million men over 75 had a PSA test anyway.
- Colorectal screening was recommended for people from 50 to 75, yet 251,000 people between 40 and 50, and 1.1 million

over 75, had a colorectal screen (either a stool sample or a colonoscopy) that year. In mid-2018 the USPSTF added a B recommendation for those 45–49.

Overscreening among the elderly is especially problematic, more likely to do harm—from tests and treatments for a frightening disease—than good by extending lives. But belief in cancer screening runs deep in this age group. A study that asked older US adults whether they intend to continue screening, and whether their doctors had advised them to stop, reported: "Among women 75–84 with <10-year life expectancy, 59% intend on future mammography and 81% recall no conversation with a doctor that mammography may no longer be necessary. Among men 75–84 with <10-year life expectancy, 54% intend on future PSA screening and 77% recall no discussions that PSA screening may be unnecessary."[15]

And in the study "Cancer Screening Rates in Individuals with Different Life Expectancies," Trevor Royce and colleagues measured the screening rates among the elderly and reported that, among those with the shortest expected remaining life spans based on age and other health factors, 40% still did some form of colorectal screening, 55% of men continued to screen with PSA tests, 38% of women continued to have mammograms, and 31% of women still had Pap smear testing for cervical cancer. The authors of that study summed up their findings: "A substantial proportion of the US population with limited life expectancy received prostate, breast, cervical, and colorectal cancer screening that is unlikely to provide net benefit. These results raise concerns about overscreening in these individuals, which not only increases health care expenditure but can lead to patient net harm."[16]

People worried about cancer hardly deserve all the blame for overscreening. Surely some falls on the health care industry, which heavily promotes screening because it turns people who screen into more lucrative patients for follow-up tests and treatment. Hospitals offer free screening for some types of cancer, and the industry that manufactures screening equipment and tests spends heavily to promote such programs. More than two years after screening levels had returned to nearly normal following a decline for a few months at the beginning of the COVID-19 pandemic, for example, many hospitals and medical associations were still sounding alarms about the initial dramatic drop as though the decline were continuing, trying to get more people (custom-ers) in for screening.[17] The money to be made by those in the cancer-screening business is enormous. The overall global market for cancer screening and other diagnostic technologies was $169.1 billion in 2020.[18]

1. The global colonoscopy equipment market alone was esti-mated to be worth $36 billion in 2020.[19]
2. The global prostate cancer diagnostic market was estimated to be worth $2.3 billion in 2019.[20]
3. The North American (mostly US) breast cancer–screening market was estimated to be worth roughly $2.1 billion in 2020, and the breast biopsy market alone was estimated at nearly $1 billion in 2020.[21]

The heavy promotion of screening is not driven only by profit. The cancer advocacy community and many government public health depart-ments firmly believe in the efficacy of early detection and do little or nothing to warn of its harms—overdiagnosis and overtreatment. As Lisa Schwartz and colleagues at Dartmouth wrote, "In the name of improved population health, many well-meaning public health agencies and dis-ease advocacy groups use powerful messages to persuade individuals to undergo screening with slogans like 'take the test not the chance' or 'don't be a victim,' or by the use of fear- and guilt-inducing images like a pic-ture of the young children who lost an unscreened parent to cancer."[22] This is the same observation George Crile Jr. offered nearly 70 years ago: "The basic error is the fault of those who . . . have exaggerated the value of early detection and treatment of disease."[23]

A degree of the responsibility for overscreening also lies with the family physicians and general practitioners whose recommendations in-fluence their patients' choices and who are strongly biased in favor of screening, playing up its benefits and mentioning little about its limitations and harms. One study of patients found: "Nearly all participants reported discussing the pros of screening with a health care provider, and the pros of screening were most likely to be discussed 'a lot.'"[24] "The proportion of participants who reported discussing the cons of screening to any extent was consistently low, ranging from just 19.5% (breast cancer screening) to 29.6% (prostate cancer screening)." Another study analyzed physician rec-ommendations about mammograms after the USPSTF recommended breast cancer screening for women starting at age 50. Looking at women outside the recommended age range, the study reported, "Overall, 81% of physicians recommended screening to women ages 40 to 44 years, 88% to women ages 45 to 49 years, and 67% for women 75 years or older."[25]

This "selling" of screening by physicians is understandable. Just as it's hard for the public to change its deep belief in cancer screening, it's hard for doctors too. "Changing culture," observed Brawley, "is never easy. It will be a difficult struggle to change, to get out of the culture of automatic early detection." And that struggle has only just begun. The problem of overscreening has only begun getting more widespread attention in the medical community in the past few years. It's also fair to suggest that some doctors recommend screening to practice defensive medicine in our über-litigious society. You can't get sued for a test you *did* recommend, but you can get sued by somebody who thinks they suffered because of the one you *didn't*. Then there is resistance in the medical community to the very idea that overscreening is a significant problem. This remains particularly strong among radiologists, who perform or interpret the results of many screening exams, professionals who want to save lives and honestly believe in screening, but who also have a personal financial interest in more screening rather than less.

On top of all these motivations in favor of screening, many doctors overestimate its benefits because of confusion over two obscure but actually rather simple concepts: "lead time bias" and "length bias," both of which make screening look more effective at extending life than it is. A common term to quantify effectiveness in cancer treatment is "survival time," the time between diagnosis and death. Treatment options for cancer patients are often described in metrics like "the 5-year survival rate" or "the 10-year survival rate." Screening increases survival time by finding cancer earlier, before symptoms appear, when it is less likely to have spread and is more treatable. That earlier detection is "lead time," and we just assume that's always good.

But now consider the example of a cancer that is overdiagnosed, a cancer so small, localized (hasn't spread), and indolent (slow growing), if it grows at all, that it would never harm the patient in their remaining lifetime. Again, screening finds it earlier, but because it's a disease that was overdiagnosed, earlier detection adds to the survival time statistic but does not change the age at which the patient dies. The extra lead time adds no mortality benefit. It just makes the survival time look better than it really is.

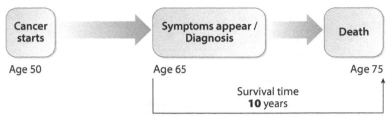

FIGURE 3.1

Timeline of cancer X (which needs treatment) with no screening.

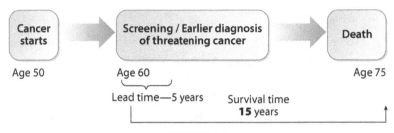

FIGURE 3.2

Timeline of cancer Y (which does *not* need treatment) with screening, providing earlier detection, or "lead time," but no increased actual survival time (i.e., the age of death remains the same).

Length time bias makes screening look better at saving lives than it actually is, because screening tends to pick up more slow-growing types of disease. The more indolent some cancers are (like some types of prostate, thyroid, and colon cancer), the longer they are in the presymptomatic phase, compared to more aggressive cancers, which go from start to symptomatic in much less time. So more of these small slow-growing cancers are out there in the pool of people being screened, and as a result, the length of time we know about screen-detected cancers is longer. But these slow-growing, less aggressive cancers are more likely to be the ones that never become symptomatic in the lifetime of the patient, so even though we know about them for a longer length of time, that doesn't add any years to how long those patients would otherwise live. They die of other causes, with the cancer but not from it.

Many doctors, trained to think that detecting cancer as early as possible is always beneficial, still think of longer lead time, length time, and survival time as signs of success. Screening advocates—manufacturers, radiologists, advocacy groups—enhance this confusion by citing survival

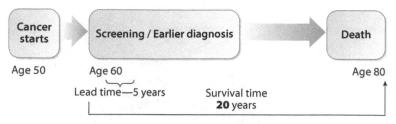

FIGURE 3.3
Timeline of cancer X (which needs treatment) with screening, providing earlier detection and longer survival time to death *from other causes*, not the detected cancer.

time, based on lead-time and length-time statistics, to argue their case. Sadly, taking advantage of misunderstanding about those measures contributes to the harm screening can cause.

One more general issue about screening is how to measure its effectiveness. Screening is recommended if it has been found to do more good than harm, but how is "good" measured? The best metric, one might think, is the change in the mortality rate—how many fewer people died of the particular cancer the screening helped catch. A more comprehensive metric, however, is known as "all-cause mortality."

Using only cancer-mortality-specific criteria, if screening found a cancer, and that led to treatment, and then something about the *treatment*—not the cancer—killed the patient, screening would nonetheless be considered a success: the screening found a cancer, and the patient didn't die of that cancer (even though the screening led to the patient's death). But if we use the metric of all-cause mortality, that patient would not count as a success. With all-cause mortality, only the *net* lifesaving fully reflects the overall benefit.

But all-cause mortality is a challenging metric to use. It simply measures how many people who were screened died a year or five or ten years later. It often doesn't consider what they died from. Maybe a person's medical treatment for a nonthreatening cancer led to their death, in which case screening should not be considered a success. But maybe screening led to treatment, and the person was truly cancer free but two years later was hit and killed by a truck. Screening may indeed have saved that person's life, but with all-cause mortality it wouldn't get the credit.

A bigger problem with using all-cause mortality in this book is that most research on the efficacy of screening provides only data on cancer-specific mortality reduction. All-cause mortality data are often not even included. So in the chapters ahead, when quantifying the effectiveness of screening, this book uses cancer-specific mortality reduction.

Overdiagnosis

In an indirect way we can blame the problem of overdiagnosis on Rudolf Virchow's weak voice. The nineteenth-century German scientist, known as the father of modern pathology, wanted to be a pastor but didn't think he had a strong enough voice for preaching. So the brilliant Virchow chose a career in medicine. Well into that career in the 1840s, as he peered through a microscope at cancer cells, Virchow saw, and drew, the unique anatomical features that pathologists still look for today when they diagnose cancer: the ragged edges and distorted shapes of the cells, the swollen nucleus and abnormal layout of the cells' inner components, the dense, uneven, packed-together arrangement of cells of various sizes, as opposed to the open, regular spatial distribution of uniform-sized cells in healthy tissue.

The visual inspection of cells by pathologists is still the principal basis for a cancer diagnosis today. The problem is that under a microscope, or even with today's additional ability to look at individual genes, we can see what cancer cells and their genes look like but not what those cells and genes are *eventually going to do*. That's what we really need to know. The gap between what we *can* see and what we *can't predict* is in essence what turns a diagnosis into overdiagnosis.

More specifically, in one of the seminal papers in the relatively new field of medical research known as overdiagnosis and overtreatment, Welch and Black describe the problem this way: "Overdiagnosis is the term used when a condition is diagnosed that would otherwise not go on to cause symptoms or death. Cancer overdiagnosis may have of one of two explanations: (1) The cancer never progresses (or, in fact, regresses) or (2) the cancer progresses slowly enough that the patient dies of other causes before the cancer becomes symptomatic."[26]

So it's not that diagnoses of slow-growing and nonthreatening cancers are wrong. They are technically correct, a finding of "abnormal cells dividing without control." But in the context of this book, they become dangerous *over*diagnoses because the word "cancer" is involved, with all

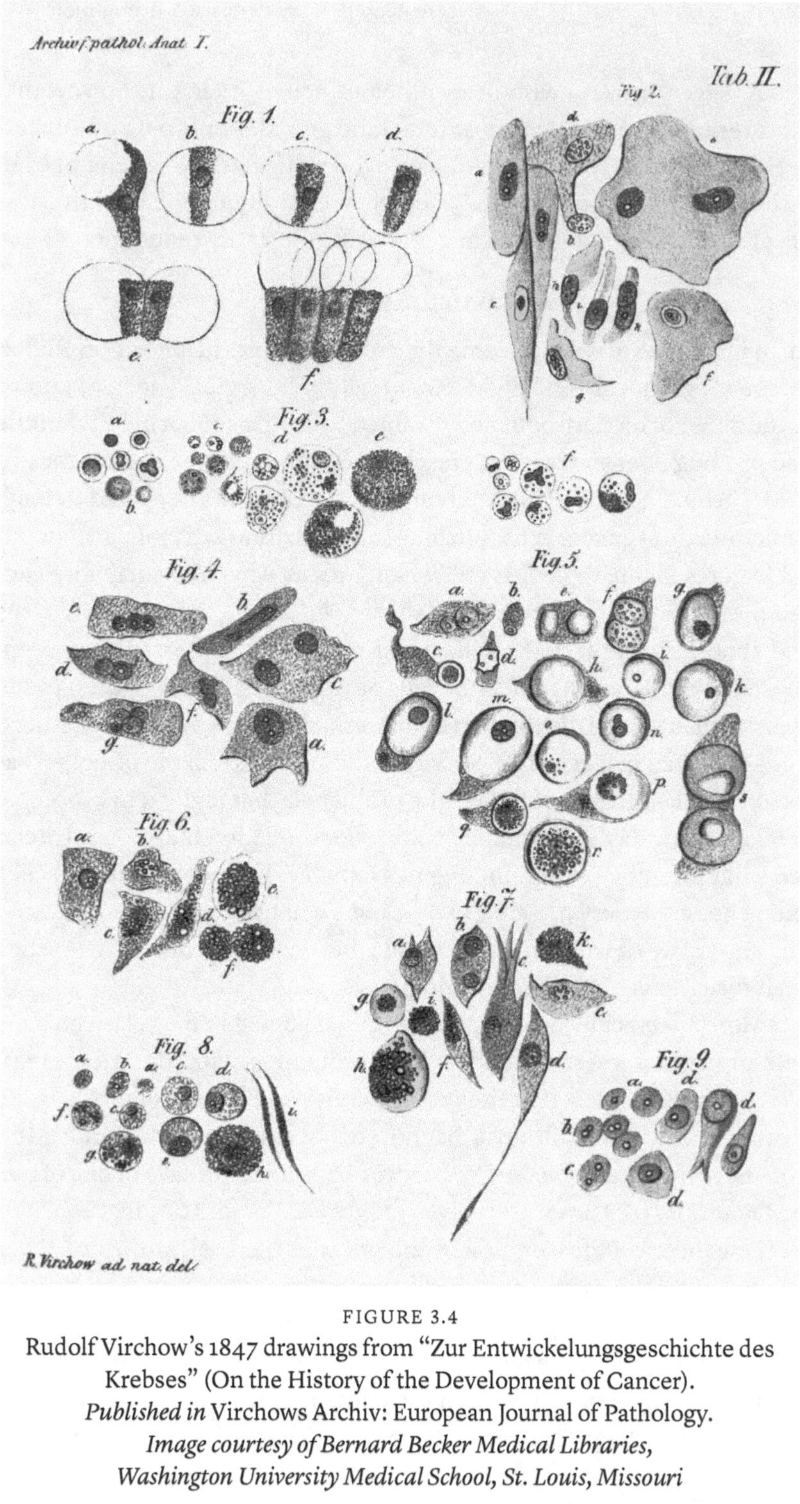

FIGURE 3.4
Rudolf Virchow's 1847 drawings from "Zur Entwickelungsgeschichte des Krebses" (On the History of the Development of Cancer).
Published in Virchows Archiv: European Journal of Pathology.
*Image courtesy of Bernard Becker Medical Libraries,
Washington University Medical School, St. Louis, Missouri*

that frightening word implies. Overdiagnosis then becomes a problem when the tripwire of the C-word triggers fear that leads people to choose more aggressive and risky treatment than their clinical conditions require.

Some resist the very idea of cancer overdiagnosis, however, and this resistance revolves around two psychological elements described in chapter 2: *uncertainty* and *loss aversion*. A great deal is known about which cancers are *almost* surely slow growing and nonthreatening. But medicine still cannot discern with *absolute certainty* which cancers will kill and which ones won't. That uncertainty raises a fair challenge to the very concept that Welch and Black and others suggest. Overdiagnosis is an abstract concept based on population-level statistics collected by looking back over years of medical and public health data. In the long run and with hindsight, we can see that many cases are overdiagnosed. But inside the personal emotional world where each of us make medical choices for ourselves, in the moment, about the future, the only relevance of a diagnosis is "What does it mean to me, now?" If we are told we have a disease that is almost certainly never going to harm us, but there remains even a slim chance that it might—and it's CANCER—there is nothing *over* about that diagnosis to any individual. Fear of the slim but real chance of a negative outcome—loss aversion—emotionally dominates our choice. Understandably.

Nonetheless, with full respect for the individual choices we make in our own lives, lived in the here-and-now and not in the future looking back, this book considers such choices and their outcomes at the big-picture population level, with the clarity only hindsight can provide. From that perspective, the problem of overdiagnosis is real, and the immense suffering it causes is a major health care problem. Millions of people endure real harm, and many die, because of this medical reality. We need to recognize it for the threat it is. But first we need a general introduction to the kinds of harm being caused.

Overtreatment

In Otis Brawley and Paul Goldberg's book *How We Do Harm*, they wrote about a patient, Ralph, who saw an ad for free prostate cancer screening and, under pressure from his wife, decided to go.[27] He had no symptoms, and his PSA level turned out to be only slightly above normal, but that worried him enough to have a biopsy, which revealed a slow-growing less-threatening type of prostate cancer for which doctors now often recommend active surveillance, a series of ongoing checks to monitor the disease, but nothing more. Nonetheless, frightened, Ralph chose surgery to remove his prostate, and four years later, after several progressively more intensive medical procedures to deal with successive side effects from the previous step, Ralph was dead.

This is what doctors James Mold and Howard Stein labeled "medical cascades," where one initial action sets in motion a chain of events, one triggering the next, leading to a drastically worse outcome than doctor and patient ever envisioned when they agreed to that first step.[28] Overscreening is the first step in such cascades. Overtreatment is the last. It's where the harm of our often excessive fear of cancer finally occurs, the harm Crile warned about when he wrote: "The thousands who die from unnecessary operations are human sacrifices to the gods of fear."[29]

A few basic types of health harm occur along the cascade of overtreatment for cancer.

1. Even before the biopsies and treatments begin, *false positive screening results* often cause psychological or physical harm. Screening designed to find any tiny sign of cancer also sometimes identifies what *might* be a cancer, and the patient gets the worrisome news that they may have cancer, but further investigation reveals that it was nothing to worry about at all. *These* results are false positives, which are frighteningly common in breast and lung cancer screening, and they trigger the fear of possibly having cancer. Though for most people this worry is brief and relieved when follow-up tests show that they are cancer free, a substantial minority of people who experience false positives endure persistent elevated worry even after the all clear. Many victims of false positives suffer elevated worry about cancer for the rest of their lives. Biologically, that worry equates to chronic stress, which does all sorts of physical and emotional harm. (The interpretation of screening sometimes misses cancers that are there. *These* results are called false negatives.)
2. False positives also trigger the next step in the cascade, the follow-up diagnostic tests to check that first suspicious finding. These tests are often invasive procedures, like painful bi-

opsies for prostate and lung cancer, which involve a low but not insignificant risk of infection and other complications.

3. The category of overtreatment that does most serious damage, however, is clinically unnecessary treatment of diseases that have been overdiagnosed. The standard of care for most low-grade, slow-growing, early stage cancers—including a common form of breast cancer known as ductal carcinoma in situ (DCIS; more on that in chapter 4), as many as half of all prostate cancers (chapter 5), more than 80% of thyroid cancers (chapter 6), and a substantial number of lung cancers (chapter 7)—is surgery. In some cases of prostate and thyroid cancer, doctors now recommend merely ongoing surveillance, known as either watchful waiting or active surveillance. But even patients given that less aggressive option, facing a frightening diagnosis of cancer, often choose surgery anyway. These surgeries are all generally safe, but at low rates they produce both physical and psychosocial side effects, which run the gamut from temporary to lifetime, mild to severe, including chronic pain, loss of sexual function, urinary incontinence, psychological costs for women who have breasts removed and for men who lose erectile function, stroke, heart attacks, and in thousands of cases, death, caused by treatment for disease that was almost certainly never going to cause any symptoms at all.

Yes, while some cancer screening saves lives, it also kills.

===

Before getting into the overscreening, overdiagnosis, and overtreatment details of specific cancers in the chapters ahead, it's important to once again emphasize that some screening programs have been found to have true net benefit for some populations. It also bears repeating that choices made about cancer screening and treatment are personal and, no matter the outcome, are not judged here as right or wrong, wise or irrational. The decisions people make to deal with fear of cancer are theirs to make and theirs alone, in the context of their own lives.

Further, it's vital to respect that fear of cancer can do psychological and physical damage all by itself. So choosing a "fear-ectomy"—more aggressive treatment than one's clinical conditions may call for—is choosing peace of mind. Eliminating the chronic stress of worrying about that cancer inside you—even if it is nonthreatening and you're constantly monitoring it—can have tangible health benefit.

Finally, from the population-level perspective, while the side effects of some cancer treatments can be labeled "harm," harm is in the eye of the beholder. What an outsider might describe as harm may feel perfectly acceptable to a woman willing to live with no breasts and chronic post-mastectomy pain syndrome, or to a man willing to endure erectile dysfunction and wearing diapers to live free from fear of this dreaded disease. Only the individual can look back at their choice months or years later and judge whether screening was the right choice, or whether the risky treatment cascade that followed turned out to be *over*treatment for them.

But from the 30,000-foot view it is undebatable that these decisions cause great harm, for tens of thousands of people, more harm than the screening or treatment prevented. We are only at the dawn of recognizing these harms. It will take time to modify the public's nearly blind belief in the benefit of cancer screening and make people fully aware of the damage screening can also cause. It will take time to make doctors, who take a professional oath to do no harm, more aware that screening can do just that. And it will take evidence from our personal experience or that of family members, friends, or colleagues that our fear of cancer sometimes does more harm than good. Sadly, tens of thousands of people are learning that painful lesson every year.

Chapter 4

$$=$$

breast cancer

$$=$$

When Worry Causes Us to Do Too Much

I wrap my fear around me like a blanket
I sailed my ship of safety 'til I sank it.
—Indigo Girls, "Closer to Fine"

Kathy is 50, an award-winning investigative TV reporter. She's happy, confident, and healthy. Her youngest child, Jake, was two and a half when she went in for her annual mammogram, something she'd been doing for years. Later that day she got a call from a nurse informing her that something suspicious had shown up and asking could she please come back in for a follow-up. "No big deal, I thought," Kathy remembered. "Plenty of my friends have had these false positives, and they usually turned out to be nothing."

But after the second mammogram the nurse who called had a different message. "She told me, 'We've found something, and it's probably nothing, but we recommend a biopsy to check it out.' " Worrying news. "I'm glad it didn't take too long. It was in my mind, sure," Kathy said. "In the background mostly. I was really busy, with work and the kids, and we were doing a big home improvement project, and our house was all ripped up, so I was kind of crazy. But in the quiet moments, with myself, it was there, sure. You try to put it out of your mind, but you can't. It's CANCER!"

The day after the biopsy, Kathy was at her desk in the newsroom when she got a call. The caller ID said it was the hospital. "My heart started pounding before I even picked it up. I could almost tell what they were going to say. I went into the conference room, where I could take the call and be alone. I had ductal carcinoma in situ,

DCIS, they said. Hearing that word . . . that's when it hits you . . . hits you at the knees. You hear the word 'cancer' . . . the word nobody ever wants to hear. I teared up. I tried to stay in control, but I basically crumbled. After we hung up I just sat there and cried and cried."

For as long as we've been aware of cancer, one type has prompted more fear than any other. Breast cancer. In part that's because it's among the leading cancer killers of women and attacks a part of the body associated with female identity. In part it's because it often causes great suffering. But breast cancer has also had a lead role in the public's cancer concern for another, surprisingly simple reason. It's one of the few types of the disease that, in some forms, we can see. The visibility of some forms of breast cancer is among the reasons it was the principal focus of cancer treatment and research right up to the early 1900s.

It is not surprising, then, given its prominence in our fears, that breast cancer was one of the first forms of the disease for which screening technology was developed. Mammography has been available for more than 40 years now, and in that time it has revealed many things. Hundreds of thousands of breast cancers, certainly. But beyond disease itself, mammography has also helped us recognize that some of our most deeply held beliefs about cancer simply aren't true. More than perhaps any other type of cancer screening, mammography has taught us that cancer does *not* always kill, and finding some cancers earlier can actually make things *worse*.

These valuable truths have been learned at a terrible cost. Driven by deep fear of cancer and the belief that early detection is always beneficial, millions of women have undergone mammography, producing life-saving benefits more modest than most people assume, and harm far greater than nearly anyone realizes.

Overscreening

The History

It seemed a macabre thing to do. For weeks in 1913, German surgeon Albert Salomon visited the Berlin morgue and harvested tissue samples from the breasts of 3,000 cancer victims. In his office he examined them with the new and exciting technology of x-ray and was able to see hazy differences between cancerous and noncancerous tissue. That was the dawn of mammography. But it would be another 50 years before the images were sharp enough to be reliable—50 years and the death in 1947 of one woman, Bertha Goldberg Strax.

New York physician Philip Strax adored his young wife, and his grief at Bertha's tragic early death at age 39 inspired him to take up the still new field of radiology, determined to help others avoid the pain that Bertha, and he, had endured. He dedicated himself to developing a reliable technology to screen for breast cancer, to catch it early enough that it might be treatable.

As Strax worked in the years immediately after World War II, cancer care was exclusively the domain of surgeons, and William Halstead's brutal radical mastectomy, pioneered decades earlier, was still the standard treatment. Even though nearly all their patients died, regardless of how extensively the surgeons carved into their bodies, with no small degree of professional arrogance, the men with the scalpels (and they were all men back then) nonetheless discounted the ability of x-rays to detect breast tumors early enough so that they might be more treatable. As one surgeon put it, "If I can't feel it, it isn't there." But surgeons hadn't been able to save Bertha, and Strax believed that by finding tumors before they were big enough to feel, x-ray screening could do what surgeons could not: actually save lives. So he organized the first randomized clinical trial to study mammography. The Health Insurance Plan (HIP) study began in 1963.

In 1971 Strax and his colleagues published a paper claiming remarkable success.[1] Mammography, they reported, was reducing the death rate from breast cancer by 40% compared to women in a control group who weren't being x-rayed. The hope this report promised was enormous, but sadly, the benefits of breast cancer screening were oversold. The actual number of women saved by x-ray screening was quite low, because the number of women being saved who weren't screened and were just being examined by their doctors was practically zero, so a relative 40% increase over that still didn't amount to many actual lives.

But the fact that screening saved *some* lives was enough for Arthur Holleb, senior vice president at the American Cancer Society (ACS). He knew of the successful Papanicolaou (Pap) test to screen for cervical cancer and passionately wanted to find one for breast cancer too. Holleb was elated by the 40% mortality improvement from mammography. Historians credit doctors Strax, Jacob Gershon-Cohen, and Robert Egan for pioneering the technology of modern mammography. But Holleb, more than anyone else, gets the credit for popularizing it, and the blame for promoting a form of cancer screening that—despite deep public faith and acceptance—provides valuable but surprisingly modest benefit, while causing significant harm.[2]

Holleb and the ACS used the flood of money from the National Cancer Act of 1971 to set up the Breast Cancer Detection Demonstration Project (BCDDP). "No longer can we ask the people of this country to tolerate a loss of life from breast cancer each year equal to the loss of life in the past ten years in Vietnam," Holleb wrote as he lobbied for federal spending. "The time has come for greater national effort. I firmly believe that time is now." The BCDDP that Holleb championed was a huge success. But it was also a sloppy experiment that turned American women, fearful of breast cancer and eager to participate, into guinea pigs.

Twenty-nine mammography centers were set up across the United States, but not as part of a careful randomized clinical trial. There was no control group of women who *weren't* screened to serve as a comparison, to truly test whether mammography saved lives, and if so, how many. Research like that would take years. Neither the ACS nor American women were willing to wait that long. The fear of cancer was just too great. So unlike the more cautious HIP study, the BCDDP rushed to bring breast cancer screening into common use as fast as possible.

Historical events set the stage for this urgency. At the time the BCDDP was being set up in the early seventies, Shirley Temple Black became one of the first celebrities to break the hush-hush taboo about breast cancer and talk openly about her personal experience. First Lady Betty Ford followed with her story. Barbara Walters, host of the popular *Today Show*, demonstrated mammography for her viewers (fully clothed). Modern feminism was empowering women, and public fear of cancer in general was reaching new heights. So by late 1974, mammography had gone from rare to so popular that waiting lists at the BCDDP screening centers were months long.

Not surprisingly, there was a sudden leap in breast cancer incidence. In just one year, from 1973 to 1974, the number of reported cases jumped a stunning 14%. Mammography seemed like a great success. The goal was to find more cancers, earlier, and that goal was being achieved. The war on cancer had a major new tool. But even while the BCDDP was still becoming established, a few cautious experts took a closer look at the earlier HIP results and discovered that mammography was not doing much of what it was actually supposed to do—save lives—and that Holleb had overstated mammography's benefits and utterly ignored its harms.

John Bailar, a senior official at the National Cancer Institute, found that only 12 to 14 lives had been saved out of 20,000 women screened in the HIP trial. And even that might not have been from mammography. The women who were screened also got rigorous full physical examinations at some of the country's leading hospitals. In "Mammography: A Contrary View," Bailar wrote, "I regretfully conclude that there seems to be a possibility that the routine use of mammography in screening asymptomatic women may eventually take almost as many lives as it saves."[3] He was warning about overscreening leading to overtreatment and serious harm. Back in 1976.

The Evidence

It's nearing 50 years since Dr. Bailar first challenged the efficacy of breast cancer screening and raised concern about its harms. His cautions sparked fierce resistance then, and they still do. A battle continues to rage between advocates of screening—especially the radiologists who perform mammography, the clinics and hospitals that perform the test and treatment that sometimes follows, the manufacturers of mammography equipment, and some breast cancer advocacy groups—and on the other side a growing number of medical experts warning about the dangers of overscreening. Bailar didn't have much evidence to go on back then. But now, nearly two generations later, after tens of millions of mammograms, the evidence is clearer, stronger, and points compellingly in one direction. Several randomized control studies, and a lot of additional observational evidence, suggest that in terms of total numbers, mammography may have actually harmed more women than it has saved.

(Several important caveats run through this chapter. Here's the first: this book discusses things in general population-level terms, but there is no "average" woman. The risks and benefits of mammography vary from person to person and depend on several factors: family history, other health issues (comorbidities), and significantly, a patient's age. For example, the US Preventive Services Task Force (USPSTF) estimates that mammography *over a 10-year period* will result in 2.1 fewer breast cancer deaths per 1,000 women screened between ages 60 and 69 years old, but only 0.8 fewer deaths per 1,000 among those aged 50–59, and only 0.4 per 1,000 among those 39–49. So the benefit from screening is lower for women under 50 and over 74. It is not zero but low enough that the harms outweigh the benefits, which is why, as of May 2023, the USPSTF did not recommend mammography for women of those ages.)

Here is some of the key research establishing the problem of over-screening for breast cancer (a brief caution: all the studies described below share similar findings, but each calculates outcomes over different lengths of time).

- A review in the UK reported in 2012 that for every 1,000 women aged 50 and up invited to screening over the next 20 years, 4.3 deaths from breast cancer would be prevented, but 13 cases of breast cancer would be overdiagnosed.[4]
- The USPSTF reported in 2016 that, considering benefits over the entire lifetime of those screened, for every 1,000 women ages 50–74 screened annually, screening would prevent 9 cancer deaths but produce 1,798 false positives (frightening false alarms like Kathy's), leading to 228 unnecessary breast biopsies and the overdiagnosis of 25 tumors.[5]

  If those women had mammograms every *other* year (the current recommendations), the benefit/harm ratio over the lifetime of these women would be 7 breast cancer deaths prevented, 953 false positives, 146 unnecessary breast biopsies, and 19 cancers overdiagnosed and treated for a type of the disease that would almost certainly never have harmed them.
- The Canadian National Breast Screening Study reported in 2014 that, after following women for 25 years, 3,250 breast cancers had been detected in those who were screened, and about the same number of cancers—3,133—had been found in women who were not screened. Among the cases found by screening, 500 lives were saved. Of the cases found *without* mammography, 505 lives were saved. Of women aged 40–49 years, 40% were overdiagnosed, along with 30% of those 50–59.[6]
- The widely respected Cochrane Review, a British nonprofit set up in the 1990s to provide neutral systematic reviews of

the evidence on various health care issues, analyzed all the randomized clinical trials on overscreening and found that if 2,000 women are screened regularly for 10 years,

- One will avoid dying from breast cancer.
- Two hundred healthy women will experience a false positive.
- Ten healthy women will be overdiagnosed, become cancer patients, and undergo unnecessary treatment.[7]

• Among the 10 studies on which the Cochrane Review based its findings was an analysis of two groups in Denmark. For 17 years women in only one area were screened. Years later, a comparison with women in other parts of the country who *weren't* screened found no difference in breast cancer mortality between the two groups.

• The same thing was found in a comparison of neighboring European countries with similar quality health care systems that introduced screening at different times (Northern Ireland / Republic of Ireland, the Netherlands / Belgium, Sweden / Norway). There was no difference in breast cancer mortality between those that started screening earlier and those that started later.[8]

It runs squarely against common belief that screening, which catches so many cancers, especially early and therefore more treatable, doesn't save many more lives than no screening at all. But it bears repeating: not all cancers are alike. Mammography does indeed catch many more breast cancers, but as noted previously, most are the less-threatening early stage, slower growing noninvasive cancers that haven't spread (and sometimes never do), not the late stage, faster growing cancers—the kinds more likely to kill. An analysis of 30 years of mammography in the United States found that the total number of cases being detected rose from 111 in 1974 to 234 cases per 100,000 women in 2004, an increase of 123/100,000. But the number of more dangerous late stage cancers being detected rose only 8 cases per 100,000. On the other hand, the incidence of lobular and ductal carcinoma in situ (small, early, and usually nonthreatening cancers) jumped from 11 per 100,000 women per year in 1975 to an astounding 91 per 100,000 women in 2002.[9] As the authors of one study put it, "The imbalance suggests that there is substantial overdiagnosis accounting for nearly a third of all newly diagnosed breast cancers, and that screening is having, at best, only a small effect on the rate of death from breast cancer."[10]

As Susan Love, a pioneer in breast cancer advocacy who has tempered her advocacy of mammography, told the *Los Angeles Times*, "Screening is really good at finding the slow, ploddy, probably-not-going-to-kill-you cancers, but it's not so good at finding the fast, aggressive ones."[11] (The "fast, aggressive ones" are referred to as "interval cancers," because they arise and spread so fast that they become lethal in the interval between even annual mammograms.)

Screening advocates argue that mammography is in fact saving many lives, noting big reductions in breast cancer mortality since it was introduced: 39% in the United States, 38% in the UK, 28% in Australia, 16% in Europe. But this is the same misleading half-truth that Arthur Holleb used to overstate the benefits from the HIP trial (and that advocates of various types of cancer screening often use, as we'll see). To fully appreciate how beneficial a risk reduction policy is, you have to know both the *relative* risk reduction—the *percentage* change compared to how things were without the policy—and the *actual* risk reduction, the number of people the policy actually saved. The 16% *relative* decrease in breast cancer deaths in Europe was an *absolute* reduction from 18 per 100,000 in 2002 to 15 per 100,000 in 2012: three fewer women per 100,000 in all of Europe, over 10 years of screening.

But even that minimal success may be only partly due to mammography. The declines in breast cancer mortality in most places started before screening did, as treatment improved. After mammography became widespread, between 1989 and 2005, breast cancer mortality in 30 European countries dropped 37% in women under age 50, *fewer* of whom received screening, but only 21% among women 50 and older who got *more* screening. As the Cochrane Review summarized, "Declines in breast cancer mortality were not caused by screening but by better treatment."[12]

The lessons from all this evidence—that cancers are not all the same, and that catching all cancers earlier is not the panacea—are still relatively new and radically contradict what nearly everyone believes, including many doctors. But most experts responsible for developing cancer-screening guidelines—recommendations for who should screen, at what age—are already convinced that overscreening is a serious problem.

COCHRANE REVIEW

It no longer seems beneficial to attend for breast cancer screening. In fact, by avoiding going to screening, a woman will lower her risk of getting a breast cancer diagnosis. However, despite this, some women might still wish to go to screening.[13]

CANADIAN TASK FORCE ON PREVENTIVE HEALTH CARE

Screening leads to overdiagnosis resulting in unnecessary treatment of cancer that would not have caused harm in a woman's lifetime, as well as physical and psychological consequences from false positives. Women less than 50 years of age are at greater risk of these harms than older women.[14]

USPSTF

In addition to false positive results and unnecessary biopsies, all women undergoing regular screening mammography are at risk for the diagnosis and treatment of noninvasive breast cancer that would otherwise not have become a threat to their health, or even apparent, during their lifetime (known as "overdiagnosis"). Beginning mammography screening at a younger age and screening more frequently may increase the risk for overdiagnosis and subsequent overtreatment.[15]

NATIONAL CANCER INSTITUTE (US)

Screening tests can have harms [that] include the following:
- False-positive results can lead to extra testing and cause anxiety.
- False-negative test results can delay diagnosis and treatment.
- Finding breast cancer may lead to breast cancer treatment and side effects, but it may not improve a woman's health or help her live longer.[16]

SWISS MEDICAL BOARD

The relative risk reduction of approximately 20% in breast-cancer mortality associated with mammography that is currently described by most expert panels came at the price of a considerable diagnostic cascade, with repeat mammography, subsequent biopsies, and overdiagnosis of breast cancers—cancers that would never have become clinically apparent.

No new systematic mammography screening programs should be introduced, and *a time limit should be placed on existing programs* (my emphasis; more on how that recommendation turned out in part four).[17]

NATIONAL BREAST CANCER COALITION (US)
NBCC has recognized for many years that the benefits of screening
mammography in reducing mortality are modest at best and that
there are significant harms associated with screening.[18]

Against all those cautions, it is crucial to acknowledge, as screening
advocates point out, that mammography for breast cancer in asymptomatic women *does* prevent some breast cancer deaths—roughly
2/1,000 screened *per ten years* of screening—and is recommended by
government guidelines in many countries as being of more benefit than
harm for certain age groups. But it's also important to spend a bit of
time looking closely at the arguments of those advocates, because they
often oversell the benefits and downplay or entirely ignore the harms,
leaving women misinformed, confused, and at risk.

The Controversy

In my 25 years of daily journalism, I often had to sort out competing in-
terpretations of the same set of facts and figures to provide the public with
what seemed to be the most honest version of the truth. The fight over
the efficacy of mammography is an example, and one aspect of it bears
out the wisdom of Mark Twain's oft-cited observation in *Chapters from
My Autobiography*: "There are three kinds of lies: lies, damned lies, and
statistics." Consider the findings of a 2019 paper touting mammography's
benefits. "Since 1989, between 384,000 and 614,500 breast cancer
deaths have been averted through the use of mammography screening
and improved treatment."[19]

In news interviews about those findings, the lead author of that paper emphasized how they contradict mammography's critics and the
claims of limited benefits. But the study doesn't specify how many lives
were saved by mammography and how many were saved because of
improvements in treatment. Lumping both together is deceiving and
makes mammography sound better than a lot of other evidence suggests
it is.

Then there is the tactic of simply dismissing research you don't like
as flawed, essentially calling findings you don't like "fake news." This is
a common tactic in many disagreements about scientific evidence and
has been frequently used by some of mammography's most ardent advocates. One example is the "40 not 50" campaign, suggesting that

screening should start at age 40.[20] The campaign simply dismisses as faulty all the evidence that the benefit of mammography is lower between 40 and 50 and the harms much higher. That campaign is funded by Rad-Net, a for-profit professional association of radiologists, which has a direct financial incentive to promote more screening, as do many advocates of mammography, from hospitals and clinics to radiologists and equipment manufacturers.[21] The research raising concerns about mammography, on the other hand, has mostly been done by governments or independent investigators.

The "science war" is another common tactic in such fights, in which advocates of one view publish their own studies to counter the studies done by the other side. One such piece of research provides an illustration. The lead author was László Tabár, a well-respected and ardent screening advocate.[22] He and his co-authors reported that "women who have participated in mammography screening (in one county in Sweden, between 1977 and 2015) [have a] 60% lower risk of dying from breast cancer within 10 years after diagnosis and a 47% lower risk of dying from breast cancer within 20 years after diagnosis." Recall the discussion of the misleading metrics of lead-time and length-time. Longer seems better, but if screening finds a cancer that would never kill, finding it earlier makes screening look better than it is at actually saving lives. Like many who argue in favor of screening, the Tabár study makes no mention of the harms caused by overscreening.

To be fair, these disagreements aren't just about money and profits. Radiologists and other medical professionals who deal with breast cancer are sincerely devoted to saving lives. They spend their careers caring for patients who are afraid, whom they want to help however possible. They believe in the tools they use, tools they've been trained to rely on, tools that some of them have even helped develop. Through their lenses, the harms of mammography, which most do in fact acknowledge, are simply outweighed by the benefits. Consider, for example, the comments of Carol Lee, a highly admired radiologist at the Memorial Sloan Kettering Cancer Center in New York and former president of the Society of Breast Imaging: "These so-called harms are hardly equal to the possible benefit of having a small, treatable breast cancer detected through screening." Or the plea of two radiologists and a breast cancer surgeon in a 2015 op-ed in the *New York Times*: "Let's stop overemphasizing the 'harms' related to mammogram callbacks and biopsies."[23]

Many radiologists at top cancer centers, as well as leading breast cancer advocacy organizations who still support mammography, have come to the more cautious conclusion: that breast cancer screening has small to modest lifesaving benefits but also causes great harm, and *patients should be honestly and fully informed about both*. The National Breast Cancer Coalition, an advocacy group, says, "From a public health perspective, the harms and public health costs of screening mammography may outweigh the modest benefits of the intervention. Therefore, a woman's decision to undergo a screening mammogram must be made on an individual level, based on quality information about her specific risk factors, and her personal preferences."[24] Eric Winer, director of the Breast Oncology Center at the Dana-Farber Cancer Institute, is also cautious. As he told me in an interview, "We have oversold mammography to the American public. People need to be aware of the potential risks, not just the benefits."

Nonetheless, belief in mammography is so entrenched in the public's mind that these cautions are falling on mostly deaf ears. Despite growing news coverage of the evidence questioning mammography's effectiveness, as well as recommendations that only some women should get screened, a study in the *Journal of the American Medical Association* (*JAMA*) reported that in the years after the USPSTF recommended biennial mammography for women aged 50-74, the advice had little effect. "Evidence from the National Health Interview Survey, which assessed patients' reports of their most recent mammogram in 2008, 2010, 2013, and 2015, showed minimal changes in rates of mammography screening."[25]

It's not just the public ignoring these carefully researched recommendations. Hospitals and medical societies are too. A review of more than 600 cancer centers in the United States reported that 80% of them recommend starting mammography at an earlier age than the USPSTF suggests, as well as urging annual screening rather than once every two years, despite the evidence that while this may save more lives, it is also likely to do more overall harm than good.[26] The American College of Radiology, Society of Breast Imaging, American Society of Breast Surgeons, and American College of Obstetricians and Gynecologists recommend that women start getting annual mammograms at age 40.

Doctors are ignoring the USPSTF recommendations as well. A 2017 survey found that 81% of general family physicians and gynecologists still recommended screening to women ages 40 to 44 years, 88% recommended it to women ages 45 to 49 years, and 67% recommended it to women 75 years or older.[27] The 2018 *JAMA* study reported, "Among primary care physicians surveyed in 2016, recommendations for screening were high across all patient age groups, with more than 80% of 871 surveyed physicians reporting they would recommend screening to women aged 40 to 44 years, for whom major guidelines recommend against routine screening."[28]

Public belief in mammography is so deep that in 2009, when the USPSTF recommended against screening for women 40–49, the response was volcanically hostile. Congress stepped in and passed the Protecting Access to Lifesaving Screenings (PALS) Act, ruling that the new USPSTF recommendations could not be used to determine whether mammograms would be covered by insurance.[29] As noted in the previous chapter, research done for this book by the Centers for Disease Control and Prevention found that in 2017, 15.6 million women under age 50 and 5.7 million over age 74 said they had ignored those expert recommendations over the past two years and had a mammogram anyway.

But screening is only where the harm cascade begins.

Overdiagnosis

Kathy sat alone in the empty conference room and sobbed, her mind spinning. After a few minutes she managed to bring her emotions under a bit of control and, collecting herself with a few deep breaths, went back to her desk in the newsroom. Nobody noticed her puffy red eyes.

Then, just as most people do when they face a threat, she tried to give herself at least some sense of control. "I got right on the phone with all my friends who I knew were breast cancer survivors. I called all my contacts, to try and get the best doctor, the best person. I went online and read and read about DCIS. I tried to learn everything I could, to give myself the sense that at least I was doing something . . . fighting back. I knew that cancer isn't always fatal, and DCIS isn't always fatal. But that's not how it felt. It's *cancer!* So it helped, felt good, just to do something."

Back in 1976, in "Mammography: A Contrary View," John Bailar, deputy associate director of cancer control at the National Cancer Institute, offered an intriguing observation. "Some (prostate cancer) lesions seem to have benign biologic behavior but malignant microscopic appearance. There seems to be no evidence for a similar situation with breast cancer, but the possibility should not be dismissed without some thought."[30]

Bailar was prescient. He foresaw precisely what screening has taught us since then about one of the most common forms of breast cancer, DCIS, in which abnormal cells are confined to the lining of the milk ducts. Under the microscope, DCIS cells have many of the sinister morphological characteristics by which cancer is clinically identified. But that only reveals what those cells look like, not what they're going to do. Most DCIS does not spread into the breast or the rest of the body.[31] Although DCIS cells have the physiological characteristics of cancer, they often lack the full suite of genetic mutations that enable those cells to metastasize. Essentially, most DCIS is trapped, and unless it changes, it poses no threat. That's why some doctors—including the doctor who first identified it—call DCIS a *precancer*, or merely a risk factor for cancer, something to be *watched*, not removed right away. It is malignant under a microscope but essentially benign in the body. As Dr. Winer of the Dana-Farber Cancer Institute put it in our conversation, "The chance of dying from DCIS is almost zero."

DCIS is a poster child for the dangers of our sometimes excessive fear of cancer and a clarion challenge to two foundational beliefs on which the edifice of that fear stands: that it's always beneficial when cancer is found as early as possible, and that if you find it, it's always safest to remove it. Prior to screening, when DCIS was found only after it had grown large enough to be felt by a physical exam, this type of cancer was practically unknown. It made up less than 5% of diagnosed breast cancers in the United States. But perceptive modern screening technologies now find many more cases, nearly all of which are tiny tumors too small to be felt by hand. In essence, the prevalence of this common type of breast cancer has been *created* by mammography. According to the ACS, 20% of all diagnosed breast cancer, one case in five, is DCIS, roughly 60,000 cases per year as of 2018.[32] The USPSTF makes the worrisome implications of that figure clear: "The best estimates from randomized, controlled trials (RCTs) evaluating the effect of mammography screening on breast cancer mortality suggest that 1 in 5 women diagnosed with breast cancer over approximately 10 years will be overdiagnosed."[33]

But has finding it earlier saved more lives? We've been able to study this type of breast cancer for a generation, largely because of mammography, and the answer is—DCIS rarely kills. A major study published in 2015 reported that, following a diagnosis of DCIS, only 3 women out of 100 had died 20 years later, *essentially the same 3-in-100 mortality odds for those women whether they had cancer or not.*[34] The problem is, while most DCIS remains in situ and never gains the ability to spread out of the milk duct where it begins, as many as 20%–30% of cases do spread.[35] And while most DCIS, once surgically removed, never recurs, a few rare cases do. Doctors can identify DCIS as low, medium, or high grade (the higher the grade, the more likely it is to spread or recur), but they can only talk to patients like Kathy in general statistics. They can't guarantee an outcome for any individual, and they still can't be absolutely certain how any given case of disease is going to behave.

That's why most patients are told what Kathy was, that the precautionary standard of care for DCIS is surgical removal of the tiny microtumor, with a simple lumpectomy (also known as breast conservation therapy, or BCT), a lumpectomy followed by radiation or drugs to reduce the chance of recurrence (that's what Kathy chose), or a mastectomy— removal of the entire breast. A few doctors informally suggest the option of active surveillance: no surgical intervention, just frequent follow-up mammograms and biopsies to see if the cancer is still only in situ—hasn't spread beyond the milk duct. Kathy was told she had that option. But like Kathy, most women diagnosed with any kind of DCIS choose some version of surgery.

And no wonder. DCIS is still formally diagnosed as breast cancer. Regardless of the low odds of mortality based on the whole population, under the ominous shadow of the C-word, exacerbated by the fearful influence of uncertainty, caution almost demands that the tumor be cut out. A fear-ectomy feels like the only reasonable choice. Women may understand the odds of both the disease and the side effects of surgery. They may factually grasp the idea of overdiagnosis and rationally understand the difference between DCIS and other types of breast cancer. But the deep fear of cancer, particularly breast cancer, erases most of the distinction. It's not surprising, then, that 97% of women diagnosed with stage 0 breast cancer—almost all of which is DCIS—choose the same treatment, surgical removal, as women diagnosed with stage 1, which is bigger and has begun to spread. Those two disease conditions have different prognoses, but both have cancer/carcinoma in the name. A study comparing the psychological and emotional reactions to a diagnosis of

DCIS versus a diagnosis of stage 1 "early invasive breast cancer" found similar rates of depression, trouble sleeping, nervousness, and anxiety in women diagnosed with either type of the disease.[36]

Few doctors even suggest active surveillance for DCIS because no reliable evidence compares the mortality outcomes of surgery versus surveillance. Clinical trials with names like COMET, LORD, and LORIS are trying to compare the outcomes for women who undergo surgery to those for women who agree to wait and watch.[37] But researchers doing these studies report difficulty getting women to sign up because many worry they might be assigned into the surveillance group. Even after these studies are finally under way, they'll have to follow the women for years. Initial results are not likely before the late 2020s.

Although no studies confirm that active surveillance is as protective as surgery, a lot of evidence supports that idea. The most revealing is the comparison between how many more slow- or non-growing DCIS cases are being found and how many of the more dangerous invasive breast cancers are being detected. While the overall incidence of breast cancer has shot up since mammography began, the incidence of invasive cancers—the kind more likely to be life-threatening—has hardly dropped at all. The huge gap, which is a way of quantifying overdiagnosis, looks like the graph on the opposite page.

Archie Bleyer and H. Gilbert Welch summarized their findings this way: "We estimated that breast cancer was overdiagnosed (i.e., tumors were detected on screening that would never have caused death) in 1.3 million U.S. women in the past 30 years. We estimated that in 2008, breast cancer was overdiagnosed in more than 70,000 women; this accounted for 31% of all breast cancers diagnosed."[38]

Findings from other research support those conclusions. A study of more than five million women who had annual mammograms in the UK between 2003 and 2007, for example, found that for every three cases of DCIS detected, only one additional invasive cancer was detected in the women after they were followed for three years.[39] The authors of that study say that screening that detects DCIS is still effective at reducing mortality, but their work confirms that roughly three times more early stage, potentially overdiagnosed slow- or non-growing cancers were being found than life-threatening invasive cancers.

The Bleyer and Welch estimate that roughly one-third of breast cancer detected by mammography is overdiagnosed was challenged in a

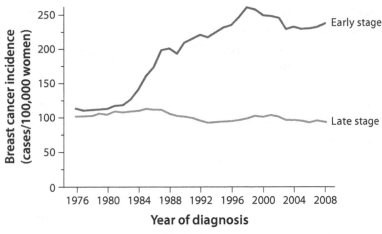

FIGURE 4.1

Early and late stage breast cancer incidence, 1976–2008.
*Adapted from A. Bleyer and H. G. Welch, "Effect of Three Decades of Screening
Mammography on Breast-Cancer Incidence,"* New England Journal of Medicine
*367 (2012): 1998–2005. Copyright © 2012 Massachusetts Medical Society.
Reprinted with permission from Massachusetts Medical Society*

study published in 2022, in which several leading experts estimated that
the actual rate is only 15%.

But Kathy didn't get these details. She was told, simply, that most
DCIS like hers is highly unlikely to ever cause any harm. "My doctor told
me that one of my options was not doing any surgery and just regular ongoing surveillance, 'watchful waiting,' she called it," But Kathy chose
surgery anyway, a lumpectomy with follow-up radiation. She was cautioned about the risks of such treatment; infection, long-term pain, body
image issues, and in rare cases, death. But "it was an easy choice," she
said. "I wanted to do everything I could to be around for my kids."

Overtreatment

False Positives

Few women are more fully informed about mammography's modest
benefits and significant risks than Elayne (she asked that her name
be changed and full name not be used). She is a journalist who
writes a lot about science and health issues and has written extensively about overscreening. Yet, fully aware of the USPSTF recommendation that screening not start until age 50, Elayne scheduled

her first mammogram at age 43. Some women under 50 have additional clinical risk factors for breast cancer that warrant such screening, like family history. Elayne didn't. But she did have a 3-year-old daughter.

"I understood all the numbers about the downsides of screening," she said. "I had talked to a lot of the experts for my stories. But now I had a kid, and now it was an existential thing. It wasn't just a numbers thing. I needed to do everything I could to make sure my daughter had a mother as she was growing up."

Two days after her exam, Elayne got a call with the results. Because of dense breasts and a suspicious shadow, she was asked to come back for a follow-up exam. She had to wait four days before going back in. It was a long four days.

"I knew this would almost certainly be nothing. But I'm a worrying sort of person. Give me something to worry about, and I will. As I went to sleep at night, my mind was filled with thoughts of worst-case scenarios and my daughter not knowing her mother when she grew up.

"I went in, and yeah, I was a little nervous. They do the ultrasound, and you look at the eyes and faces of the people doing the exam, trying to get some sort of a clue as they watch the screen. But they can't say anything. After they were done, the radiologist came in pretty quickly and said, "It's fine. You're fine. There's nothing of concern, nothing to worry about." And I just burst into tears. I just sat there, and it was like this tension burst, and I just wept.

"When I got back outside, the sun was shining, and the sky was blue, and I felt great, and everything felt great. It's not the best analogy, but you know how when you go in to get your teeth cleaned, and then you're done and you leave, and you feel great because it's over with and you don't have to face that again for a while? It felt like that, just a relief."

Elayne is hardly alone. It's sometimes hard for a radiologist to tell whether the tiny spots and vague shadows in a mammogram might be cancer, so frightening false positives, in which women are told they might have cancer only to learn after additional mammograms or a biopsy that they don't, are common. And because modern advanced screening technology is designed to increase the likelihood that nothing is missed ("sensitivity," in academic jargon), advances like digital mammography and MRI as adjunct to mammography are finding more and more of these dubious spots and shadows. Seek better, and ye shall find more. A 2021 meta-analysis of studies from around the world found that the shift from film to digital mammography, for example, increased the rate at which women like Elayne were called back for another screen or a biopsy by 7%.[40] Another study on that shift found that digital mammography increased the overall cancer detection rate from 25 to 35 per 1,000, but it didn't decrease the breast cancer *mortality* rate, since most of those extra cancers detected were DCIS.[41] New 3D technology is even better at spotting things, but as yet there is no evidence it's any better at saving lives.[42]

The same thing is happening with MRI screening as an adjunct to mammography. It is increasing the rate of false positives, follow-up screenings, biopsies, and hospitalizations from testing procedures with no evidence it reduces mortality rates.[43] But as evidence of how hungry we are for the latest and supposedly most perceptive screening technology, women are ignoring the risk criteria intended to guide who gets these tests. MRI in addition to mammography is recommended by the ACS only for women with at least a 20% lifetime risk of breast cancer because of family history or dense breasts. The Society of Surgical Oncology, the American College of Physicians, and other groups specifically recommend against adjunct MRI screening in women with low to average risk. But fear of cancer, belief in screening, and the desire for the best new technology are driving much broader use. A 2017 study found that in community hospitals (as opposed to national cancer centers, where guidelines are followed more closely), 83% of the women getting these screens did not meet the risk-based recommendations.[44]

All this screening produces an enormous number of women experiencing false positives. According to the US Breast Cancer Surveillance Consortium (BCSC), one woman in eight who had a mammogram between 2003 and 2011 had a false positive.[45] And the likelihood of a false positive rises the more scans a woman has over the years. A woman who starts screening at age 40 (recommended by the American College of Radiology) and screens every year (which the American College of Radiology recommends) has a 6 in 10 chance of a false positive over 10 years, and a woman who screens every other year starting at age 50 (which the USPSTF recommends) has a 4 in 10 chance per decade.[46]

To translate these percentages into actual people, according to the Centers for Disease Control and Prevention, 39.3 million mammograms were done in the United States in 2018.[47] That means 4.9 million women went through what Elayne did *in just one year.*

False positives do psychological damage. A literature review of the various effects of false positives found four studies focused on "distress" reported that women showed significantly more general symptoms of distress after a false alarm; four of eleven studies looking at "anxiety" found that women with false-positive results had significantly higher levels than women with normal results; four of six studies focused on "worry / intrusive thoughts / perceived risk" reported that false-positive results led to significantly higher levels of worry; and two of four studies found that women with false positives had significantly greater ongoing fear of breast cancer than women who never got a false positive.[48]

In one study of Swedish women who got false-positive mammogram results, the authors report that at one month, six months, and one year after the participants' final all clear, "The odds for experiencing short- and long-term psychosocial consequences regarding sense of dejection, anxiety, impact on behavior, sleep, and existential values were at least twice as high for the recalled women compared with controls at all study assessments."[49] Another that followed women for three years found the same thing.[50] Researchers asked Danish women who had mammograms to fill out a "Consequences of Screening in Breast Cancer" questionnaire. The authors reported: "Three years after being declared free of cancer, women with false-positive results consistently reported greater negative psychosocial consequences compared with women who had normal findings in all 12 psychosocial outcomes."

Most dramatically, that study reported that women's false-positive experiences—their brushes with cancer—seemed to exacerbate their general worries about life. "Six months after final diagnosis, women with false-positive findings reported changes in existential values and inner calmness *as great as those reported by women with a diagnosis of breast cancer*" (my emphasis). For most women these effects were modest and more acute in the six months after the experience and lower after that. For a sizable minority, however, the effects were persistent three years later.

Harm from Treatment

> For every woman who avoids a death from breast cancer
> through screening, 2 to 3 women will be treated unnecessarily.
> —USPSTF

The psychological harms of false positives are just the beginning. The physical harm from overtreatment of low-grade, low-risk DCIS is also enormous. Again, some cautions are important. Treatment for DCIS is not always *over*treatment. BCT (lumpectomy) and full mastectomies do catch some cases, particularly high-grade DCIS, which might have eventually become life-threatening. Further, whether something feels like *over*treatment is in the eye of the beholder. Facing uncertainty about their individual cases, and their fear of cancer, most of the roughly 60,000 women a year in the United States who choose surgery for their DCIS don't *feel over*treated. Even though survival rates from lumpectomy and from mastectomy are the same (98%–99% of women treated by either method are alive 10 years after surgery), a more extensive full mastectomy, with the potential for more serious side effects than BCT, is still not *over*treatment for women worried their DCIS will recur. (Mastectomy slightly reduces the rate of recurrence compared to lumpectomy.) When DCIS is found in one breast, the chance of cancer showing up in the other breast is under 5%, but a prophylactic double mastectomy—a far riskier treatment than clinical conditions require and beyond the standard of care that doctors recommend—is still not *over*treatment to the woman who fears cancer so much that she wants everything done to reduce the risk as much as possible.

But those choices have costs. Treatment for DCIS has short- and long-term side effects. The likelihood of these harms is low for any individual, but at the population level, the numbers are sobering. Far more people treated for low-grade DCIS are harmed than are saved.

First, there are risks from the surgery itself. (Another caveat is in order. This discussion generalizes, but there are all sorts of different mastectomies and lumpectomies, and side effects vary with each, in most cases being higher with mastectomy than lumpectomy.) Let's start with the worst of these risks and, thankfully, the rarest. One-quarter of one percent of mastectomy patients die within 30 days from postsurgical complications, according to a study by El-Tamer et al., which reported that the mortality rate after lumpectomy is near zero.[51] That's a tiny risk for an individual. But let's do the math for the entire population.

1. An estimated 60,000 women in the United States were diagnosed with DCIS in 2017.[52]
2. Of these women, 97%, or 58,200, had some kind of surgery.[53]
3. Based on several studies, it is estimated that roughly half of those surgeries, 29,100, removed the high-grade DCIS that had a greater likelihood of progressing, and half removed the low- and intermediate-grade disease most likely to be overdiagnosed.[54]
4. Roughly 30% of all surgeries were mastectomies.
5. So this mortality analysis conservatively considers only the 8,730 women who had mastectomies for the intermediate and lower grades of the disease, the less-threatening cases that are almost all overdiagnosed.
6. *One-quarter of one percent of those women **died** as a result of postsurgical complications from single or double mastectomy. That's 22 women, dead from surgery to remove a cancer that would never have harmed them. Just in 2017.*

The number of women choosing mastectomies rather than lumpectomies for DCIS is rising, even though full removal of the breast does not reduce mortality compared to BCT. The percentage of women in the United States eligible for BCT who instead chose full mastectomy rose 34% from 2003 to 2011.[55]

To be accurate as we now calculate this harm over the lifetime of mammography, we have to modify our formula, since it's based on 2017 figures. Between 1977, when popular mammography began, and 2017, the average annual number of women between 40 and 84 having mammograms was roughly 28 million, about 35% fewer than in 2017.[56] So we'll reduce the 2017 annual death toll estimate by that same percentage, to an average of 14 deaths per year from postoperative complications following surgery for DCIS.

That means that, quite roughly, over the 41-year lifetime of popular mammography (as of the end of 2017), an estimated 574 women have died as a result of overtreatment by mastectomy for an overdiagnosed case of DCIS.

And that estimate is conservative, because though we have eliminated all the high-grade cases, a significant number of them in fact never progress either. Further, the estimate doesn't factor in the greater risks from double mastectomies, from which surgical complications—including death—are between 5% and 35% more likely than from removal of just one breast.[57] More women are choosing that option. The rate of *bi*lateral mastectomy for *uni*lateral disease increased from 2% in 1998 to 11% in 2011, another 2,000 more women per year choosing this aggressive treatment.[58] (The choice of double mastectomy is more common among younger, more educated white women of higher socioeconomic status, with private insurance.) In a study of those who had chosen bilateral mastectomy for DCIS, women said the physical and emotional costs of the surgery were higher than they expected, but 41 of the 45 women interviewed said they'd make the same choice again.[59]

Fortunately, death from surgery is rare. A far more common side effect—from either mastectomy or BCT—is lasting pain, which can be mild or severe, can come on immediately after surgery or weeks or months later, and can last a short time or a lifetime. This pain is so common, affecting two to three breast cancer surgery patients out of ten, that it has a name: post-mastectomy pain syndrome (PMPS), which is actually a misnomer, since it affects women who undergo BCT as well.[60] (It's more common in women whose surgery involves one or more lymph nodes, which many surgeries for DCIS do not.)

1. Based on the estimated average of 28 million mammograms per year from 1977 to 2017, and the rate at which DCIS was diagnosed from those exams (0.15%, the rate in 2017), roughly 42,000 women in the United States per year have been diagnosed with DCIS over that period. (Not all breast cancer is found via mammography, but most DCIS is.)

2. Assuming that 97% of these women had surgery of some kind (BCT, mastectomy, double mastectomy), then 40,740 per year had surgery—a total over the lifetime of mammography of 1.7 million surgeries for DCIS.

3. Again eliminating the cases of high-grade disease more likely to progress (though many don't and are also overdiagnosed), then 50% of those women, 20,370 per year, for a total of

835,000, had surgery to remove a low- or intermediate-grade DCIS, the kind of breast cancer that almost certainly never would have harmed them.

4. *Conservatively assuming the lowest rate of PMPS, 20%, general population screening with mammography condemns roughly 4,100 women per year to some degree of long-term pain as the result of a surgery that relieved them of their fear but provided no mortality benefit. That's a total of roughly 168,000 over the lifetime of mammography (as of 2017).*

In addition to death and lasting pain, breast cancer surgery has other potential side effects. One is infection, immediately after the operation or from what is known as breast cellulitis, which can occur months or even years later. Infection affects 4%–13% of breast surgery patients (we'll assume the middle, 8%). It can cause swelling and pain, in rare cases so severe that it requires surgical treatment, though most patients are successfully treated with antibiotics. Breast cellulitis recurs *repeatedly* in one patient out of five. Of the 835,000 women who, over the lifetime of mammography, had surgery to remove a kind of breast cancer that never would have harmed them, *roughly 67,000 suffered some type of serious postsurgical infection, 1,600 women per year.*

The radiation or drug treatment many women have after surgery to reduce the likelihood of recurrence also has side effects. (Two-thirds of BCT patients, like Kathy, have follow-up radiation.[61]) Radiation treatment increases the likelihood of breast cellulitis.[62] In the short term, radiation often causes heavy fatigue, swelling in the breast or chest wall, and skin burns where the external beams are focused. Longer term side effects include the breast becoming smaller and harder, problems breastfeeding, and nerve damage, causing permanent numbness, pain, and weakness in the shoulder, arm, and hand. Radiation treatments, which have to be done in a hospital, also require a lot of time, a significant cost for many women who have trouble scheduling such treatments without missing work or who have to be home parenting their children.

Yet DCIS patients who endure all this achieve no lifesaving benefit. While radiation cuts the rate of DCIS recurrence from roughly 16% of cases to 8%, radiation follow-up after BCT *does not reduce long-term mortality from DCIS.*[63] (Radiation and hormone therapy following DCIS surgery cause other side effects: fatigue, vaginal dryness, hot flashes, increased risk of uterine cancer, stroke, cataracts, and heart disease. But while these effects are worth noting, they are rare, so they aren't quantified here.)

And then there are the long-term effects of BCT or mastectomy on body image, sexuality, and psychological health. Once again, a caveat: It's hard to accurately generalize about how many women may have endured such effects, because there is wide variation by age, culture, relationship status, and other factors that determine how an individual woman feels about breasts, and how their partners and society do. But it is safe to say that thousands of women have endured these harms following surgical treatment for a disease that was unlikely to ever cause them any physical harm.

A 2017 meta-analysis of the research on the psychosocial aspects of surgical DCIS treatment summarized 17 studies from various countries. The surgery caused a range of negative psychosocial consequences that lasted for several months, but fortunately, for most women these effects were minor and faded with time. Nonetheless, the study reported, "A minority of women experienced considerable impact, including depression and sexual issues associated with body image problems."[64]

The meta-analysis also had one profoundly disturbing finding. A substantial number of women who had what were essentially fear-ectomies, trading the risks of surgery for peace of mind, didn't get it.

- Five studies reported persistent exaggerated fear of death from cancer in women who had been treated for DCIS.
- Approximately 40% of these women suffered clinically significant anxiety at 4 to 6 weeks after initial surgery, dropping to 12% at 6 and 9 months.
- Two studies reported long-term anxiety and depression at 6, 9, and 18 months, as well as at 15 years postsurgery.[65]

This nagging fear of death was the same for women who opted for BCT, unilateral mastectomy, or even double mastectomies. No matter how cautious they had chosen to be, their worries about cancer persisted even after the cancer was gone. Cruelly, for these women, their fear-ectomies cut out their cancer but not their fear.

After that long list of its harms, it would be easy to lose sight of the benefits of mammography. So it bears repeating: research finds that mammography saves lives. It is recommended by several national government health organizations for women of certain ages, at either annual or biennial rates depending on other risk factors, because for those subpopulations, the lifesaving benefits, though modest, still outweigh the harms. But by finding more and more cancers that are unlikely to ever cause any harm, mammography does serious damage as well, both physical and psychological, from moderate to severe, ranging from loss of peace of mind up to and including death. Without carefully considering those costs along with the modest benefits of breast cancer screening, millions of women who fear what is sometimes—but not always—a deadly disease and who blindly believe in mammography face the very real risk that the procedure will do them more harm than good.

Men face that same risk too, so fearful of prostate cancer that they overlook the potential risks involved in screening for that disease, another common type of cancer that in many cases will never cause any harm. That issue is next.

prostate cancer

When Worry Causes Us to Do Too Much

Don't look too hard
Might hurt ya' self.
—Bruno Mars, "24K Magic"

Michael is soft spoken, warm, and sincere. He smiles readily. But he grimaces and his voice tightens as he thinks back to what he calls the most frightening day of his life, when he got the results of his prostate biopsy. He remembers walking into the urologist's office, his mind spinning, imagining his death. "As we suspected from the physical exam and your PSA score," the doctor told him, "the biopsy indicates you do have cancer of the prostate. But it's a slow-growing type, and we've detected it at an early stage. The prognosis for a case like yours is very good."

Michael remembers how it hit him, shocked him, hearing it confirmed that he had cancer—how he suddenly felt far away, how the doctor's voice seemed muffled, instinctive fight or flight responses to learning what he believed he was being told, that he might die.

The doctor gave Michael the details. "Your Gleason score was a 6. That's the lowest possible score. Basically this means that your tumor is not aggressive. It's slow growing. And there is no sign it has spread. And your PSA level was only a little elevated. Based on all of that, your prognosis is good. The 10-year survival rate for a case like yours is nearly 100%. There is no need to rush," he said. "You have plenty of time to figure out what you want to do." Michael recalls leaving in a fog, unable to remember much of what the doctor had said.

There were tears when he told his wife, from both of them. There was talk of hope, against the unspoken specter of death. There were days of research, learning about different kinds of treatment and the frighteningly high rate of serious side effects they all involved. He kept seeing the same phrase: "More men die with prostate cancer than of it." There was confusion about what to do. In the end, he recalls, it just felt wrong to think of waiting and watching, one of the options the doctor suggested. That felt like not doing anything at all. So he opted for brachytherapy, the insertion of radioactive pellets in the prostate gland to burn it away from the inside out. The treatment worked. Five years later a biopsy found no signs of any remaining cancer.

But at age 58, Michael no longer has sex. His treatment destroyed his erectile function. And his bladder constantly leaks. He has to sleep in diapers. During the day he can't be far from a bathroom. Michael says he accepts all this as the cost of treatment for the two conditions he knows he was suffering from: cancer and cancerphobia. And he knows he chose aggressive treatment, and risked all its harms, more to treat the fear than the disease.

Overscreening

The entire problem analyzed in this section of the book, regardless of the type of cancer, is typified in just three letters: PSA. In that simple little acronym, which stands for prostate-specific antigen, lies a sobering example of how our deep fear of this family of diseases contributes in some cases to vastly more harm than the disease itself. But the PSA story also offers cautious encouragement, because it illustrates how the medical community can, after a lot of resistance, recognize the problem and rein in at least some of the damage it does.

The History

Michael's case began with his annual physical. He had no symptoms, and no history of prostate cancer in his family. But without asking Michael, and as a matter of standard practice, his doctor ordered an analysis of the PSA level in Michael's blood. The results came in slightly above 4, the numerical threshold of concern, and brought the first mention of cancer, the frightening tripwire for all that followed.

PSA is almost synonymous with prostate cancer now, but when this protein was first identified in the sixties, its initial application had nothing to do with that disease. The prostate gland wraps around the urethra and produces liquid to carry and nourish sperm. Japanese investigators realized that PSA levels are elevated after sex and used it in forensic analysis of semen samples in rape investigations. Other researchers later investigated PSA as a possible tool to screen for and help treat prostate cancer *once it had already been diagnosed*, but they discovered a critical fact: prostate-specific antigen is not *cancer*-specific. It's produced by healthy prostate cells as well as cancerous ones, and stimulation or irritation of the prostate, whether from sex, benign prostatic hyperplasia (an enlarged prostate gland common in aging men), cancer, or just a bumpy bike ride, can raise PSA levels in the blood. So while an elevated PSA level can tell an asymptomatic man if he has an irritated prostate, it can't by itself tell him if he has prostate cancer.

But bear in mind the historical context in which these discoveries were being made. This was the late sixties and early seventies, when cancer death rates were rising (largely from lung cancer in men), and the general topic of cancer was getting ever more alarming coverage in the news media. The war on cancer was declared in the United States, and billions of government dollars were becoming available for research. The nascent environmental movement was raising alarms about the ubiquity of environmental carcinogens. Then in the late seventies and early eighties, mammography became widely available. Women had a way to screen for one the most common cancers they faced. The public pressure was immense to provide the same thing for men: an easy, affordable test to detect the second most common cancer in males (after skin cancer) as early as possible, when it would be more treatable.

A test like that would be worth a fortune to its inventor. In 1984 T. Ming Chu of Roswell Park Comprehensive Cancer Center in Buffalo, New York, won a patent for a type of PSA analysis that could be used to monitor men *already diagnosed* and being treated. This was *not* intended to screen asymptomatic men to detect cancer in the first place. But after the FDA approved it for use in 1986 as a tool to monitor men undergoing treatment, off-label application of PSA as a screen for prostate cancer in asymptomatic men soared.

The pharmaceutical company Schering-Plough, which was making one version of the test, hired a public relations firm to create Prostate

Cancer Awareness Week in 1989 (now Prostate Awareness Month). The number of centers providing (and profiting from) off-label PSA screening jumped from 100 in 1989 to 1,800 just three years later.[1] In 1987 fewer than 1 American man per 100 had had a PSA test. By 2000 45% of white men and 43% of Black men between the ages of 40 and 84 years had at least one PSA test.[2]

Prostate cancer incidence soared. The age-adjusted rate of prostate cancer in men 65 and older rose a frightening 82% in just the five years from 1986 to 1991. From 1990 to 1991 alone, prostate cancer incidence in the United States jumped a remarkable 25%.[3] In just that one year, the odds that an American man would be diagnosed with prostate cancer in his lifetime more than doubled, from 8% to 17%.

Famous men came forward with their stories of prostate cancer, all of them praising screening: US senators Bob Dole and Jesse Helms, financier Michael Milken, rock star Frank Zappa. Demand for formal approval of PSA as a screening test exploded. Men wanted what women had. An early prostate cancer advocacy group even called itself Us Too.[4] And as breast cancer advocates had their emblem, a pink ribbon, Us Too had a ribbon as well. Theirs was blue.

The pressure on the FDA to approve the PSA test for screening was intense. The 1993 hearing at which a panel of experts heard public testimony was heavily attended by patient advocates, pharmaceutical company lobbyists, and the news media. The hearing was long, contentious, and frequently emotional. But the experts had little scientific information to go on. They knew that most prostate cancers grow slowly, or not at all, and that they rarely spread out into the body and kill. They knew then what remains true, that more than 90% of diagnosed prostate cancers are "localized," meaning they haven't metastasized. The 15-year survival rate for these types of disease is an astonishing 96%–98%.

The experts at that meeting were also aware of the rising controversy about what would come to be known as overdiagnosis, how mammography was finding more slow-growing and nonthreatening kinds of breast cancer and scaring women into medically unnecessary but often harmful treatments without lowering the mortality rate for that disease. They didn't want to cause the same thing for this cancer.

But just as with mammography, which fear of cancer rushed into common use before careful trials had determined whether it provided a net benefit and whether it caused harm, no randomized clinical trial had been done to measure whether the PSA screen was actually beneficial, or safe. The only research the FDA experts heard had been done by Hybritech, the company making the test. That research showed that the company's Tandem PSA assay was better than other potential screening methods, but it didn't compare men who were screened against those who weren't, the only real way to determine whether PSA screening saves lives.

Several panel experts and witnesses warned of danger. Representing the US Preventive Services Task Force (USPSTF), Dr. Steven Woolf testified: "There is little evidence that early detection of prostate cancer improves patient outcomes, and there is mounting evidence of the adverse effects of testing and treatment, which range from patient anxiety and discomfort to the substantial physical complications of surgery, such as incontinence, impotence, and even death."[5] He warned that if the test was approved as a screen for cancer, "the lives of millions of American men will be negatively affected." Woolf was prophetic. And remarkably perceptive about how fear, and the need to take control when we're afraid, drives overscreening in general: "There is a tendency to want to do something to prevent this disease even if there is no proven benefit and even if it means ignoring potential harms. There is also a tendency to dismiss the physical and psychological harms that screening imposes on millions of healthy men, and the billions of dollars in potential costs for the sake of those with actual disease. Although this is an understandable viewpoint for advocates of screening, it is not a sound basis for making public policy."

A panel member, Dr. Alexander Baumgarten, was blunt about what approval of the PSA test for screening would mean: "We cannot, like Pontius Pilate, wash our hands of guilt. We must accept the consequences for what we are doing, and that is creating a large number of people subjected to radical prostatectomy who will be adversely affected in large numbers."[6] But wash their hands of potential guilt is essentially what the panel did. The majority recommended approval of the test, and in the years since 1994, when the FDA commissioner formally approved it (as long as the patient also received a digital rectal exam), the predictions of Woolf and Baumgartner have tragically come to pass.

The Controversy

Concerns erupted almost immediately. Articles began to show up in the medical literature, and then in the news media, questioning the test's accuracy and raising concern about whether finding more cases was saving more lives or unnecessarily harming men from the side effects of treatment they didn't really need. Within a decade books came out with titles like *Invasion of the Prostate Snatchers*, by Mark Scholz; *The Great Prostate Hoax: How Big Medicine Hijacked the PSA Test and Caused a Public Health Disaster*, by Richard Ablin (who first identified PSA); and *How We Do Harm*, by Otis Brawley, then the chief medical officer of the American Cancer Society.

Against this growing body of criticism of the PSA test, urologists—the medical specialists who perform the biopsies and treatments often prompted by that first PSA finding—adamantly defended it, noting that it was only one of several tools they used to diagnose prostate cancer, along with the digital rectal exam and the Gleason score rating system used to assess biopsy samples. Developed in 1960 by Donald Gleason, that system tries to answer perhaps the most critical question about cancer: not what it is, but what it is going to do. By inspecting prostate tissue looking not just for cells with the internal hallmarks of cancer, but more broadly at how the cells are arranged and how the tissue around those cells looks, the Gleason score helps predict which cancers are more or less likely to grow, spread, and kill. It combines two separate grades (for different aspects of the cells being inspected) to come up with the total score. A Gleason 6, for example, the lowest score on the scale, is actually a 3 + 3. Decades of research has established that a Gleason score of 6 or 7 reliably means the cancer is slow growing and highly unlikely to cause any symptoms in the lifetime of the patient.

Urologists defended widespread use of PSA screening. But research found that while mortality from prostate cancer was indeed dropping—in part because screening was saving a small number of men with more threatening metastatic disease, and in part because treatment of unscreened but symptomatic men had improved—it was also catching vastly more men with prostate cancer that was unlikely to ever cause the patient any harm.[7] As with all cancer-screening programs, PSA screening had both benefits and risks, and research established that the risks from overdiagnosis were far greater. Which is why in 2012 the USPSTF gave the PSA test a D rating, essentially a "D as in Don't," recommending that the test not be used because it caused more harm than benefit.

Patient advocacy organizations, and several prominent politicians who had experienced prostate cancer, were furious. It was the same reaction the USPSTF got for its tepid recommendation about mammography: outrage, in the press, in Congress, and among advocacy groups. But despite support for the test from urologists and patient advocates, the evidence against the use of PSA continued to pile up and point ever more clearly in one direction: the general practice of relying on the test to screen asymptomatic men for prostate cancer was doing far more harm than good.

The Evidence

As use of the PSA test exploded, it was finally possible to do the thorough research on its efficacy that had not been done prior to its approval. One key study published in 2017, nicknamed CAP (for Cluster Randomized Trial of PSA Testing for Prostate Cancer), included more than 400,000 British men aged 50–69.[8] Some were invited to an appointment with a registered nurse, who offered them information on a PSA test and, if they chose, the test itself. They were compared with a control group of men who weren't offered the test. After 10 years more prostate cancers were detected among the one-time testing group, but the prostate cancer mortality rate was the same in both.

Also published that year, a follow-up to an earlier trial in the United States named PLCO (for Prostate, Lung, Colorectal, and Ovarian Cancer Screening Trial) reported: "Extended follow-up of the PLCO trial over a median of 15 years continues to indicate no reduction in prostate cancer mortality for the intervention arm (screened) versus the control arm (not screened)."[9] (In the controversy over PSA testing within the medical community, supporters of the test questioned the accuracy of the PLCO trial.)

In late 2018 a meta-analysis of five respected clinical trials (CAP, PLCO, ERSPC, or European Randomized Study of Screening for Prostate Cancer, and two others), reported in the British Medical Journal: "When considering the whole body of evidence, screening . . . may have no effect on prostate-specific mortality . . . one less death from prostate cancer per 1,000 men screened over 10 years."[10] That was essentially what another highly regarded meta-analysis, a Cochrane Review (by some of the same authors of the 2018 BMJ study) had reported in 2013: "Pooled data currently demonstrates no significant reduction in prostate cancer-specific or overall mortality. Harms associated with PSA-based screening and subsequent diagnostic evaluations are frequent and moderate in severity."[11]

A PSA test is astonishingly inaccurate at identifying cancer. The 2018 *BMJ* study reported, "Two thirds of men with an elevated PSA level (above the threshold of 4 nanograms per milliliter of blood—4ng/mL) can expect a false positive test result," meaning two men in three will face the frightening initial news that Michael got, that they may have prostate cancer and should have a biopsy—a painful needles-through-the-rectum procedure that carries significant risk of infection—but learn from that procedure that they don't have prostate cancer at all. Another 15% of men tested with PSA will get a false negative, a PSA result *below* the threshold of concern that says they don't have cancer when in fact they do. In total, PSA tests correctly identify cancer only about 25% of the time, just one test in four.[12]

Nonetheless, in 2018 the USPSTF, under intense pressure, changed its 2012 D rating of the PSA test to a C, recommending neither for nor against its use but leaving it up to the man and his doctor to decide. That seemed almost like a C as in Cop out to Cancel Controversy, given how the USPSTF summarized the evidence: "For every 1,000 men ages 55 to 69 years who are screened every 1 to 4 years for 10 to 15 years . . . screening offers a small potential benefit of reducing the chance of death from prostate cancer in some men (about one death per 1,000 men screened). However, many men will experience potential harms of screening, including false-positive results that require additional testing and possible prostate biopsy; overdiagnosis and overtreatment; and treatment complications, such as incontinence and erectile dysfunction."[13] The *New York Times* reported:

> The new USPSTF results suggest that of every 1,000 men offered PSA screening, 240 will receive a positive result that may indicate prostate cancer and be referred for a biopsy. Only 100 will get a positive biopsy result showing cancer; others who have false positives may still suffer side effects or harm from the biopsy.
>
> Of the 100 found to have cancer, 80 will have treatment like surgery and radiation, and 60 will experience complications, even though up to half of those men will have a cancer that never grows, spreads, or becomes life-threatening. But over the course of 10 to 15 years, three cancers will be prevented from spreading, and one to two deaths of prostate cancer will be prevented.[14]

The USPSTF reported that across all the studies it reviewed, between 16% and 50% of the prostate cancers identified by PSA testing were overdiagnosed.

Fortunately, all this evidence has made a difference. All but the most adamant advocates of the PSA test eventually backed off. After decades of actively recommending it, in 2013 the American Urologists Association dropped their recommendation of annual screening for men aged 40 and up and, like the USPSTF and most other medical groups, recommended only that men between 55 and 70 consult their doctors. The professional guidelines for general practitioners and family doctors, who actually do most of the PSA screening, said the same thing.

As a result, the use of the test as a screen for cancer in asymptomatic men has declined. An analysis of PSA screening rates before and after the USPSTF D recommendations reported that the percentage of men 50 years and older who'd had PSA screening in the previous 12 months was as high as 41% in 2008, but dropped to 31% in 2013. A 2017 survey of family medicine and internal medicine practitioners found that six in ten no longer routinely recommend PSA, and now do so only based on their patient's individual risk factors.[15] A survey of 400,000 men with no history of prostate cancer found that the number who said they had had a PSA test dropped from 30% in 2012 to 20% in 2018.[16]

Not surprisingly, prostate cancer incidence also dropped. In 1992, at the peak of the PSA boom, 163 men per 100,000 were diagnosed with prostate cancer. In 2016 incidence was down to 103 per 100,000.[17] The drop has been particularly dramatic for men 50 and older, the group at higher risk because of their age. In just 2011–2012, the number of men 50 years and older in the United States diagnosed with prostate cancer declined from 214,000 to 180,000.[18]

Yet the frightening warnings from patient advocates and urologists that prostate cancer deaths would rise if PSA testing decline have not materialized. Even as screening and incidence dropped, so did the mortality rate, from 39 men per 100,000 in 1992 to 19 per 100,000 men in 2016.[19] (There has been a slight increase since then.) Screening *was* finding prostate cancer earlier, but as with mammography and DCIS, it was mostly finding slow-growing localized cancers that didn't need anything more than ongoing surveillance.

Despite that progress, however, PSA screening for asymptomatic men remains remarkably common. As of 2018, among men 55–69 years, four in ten—11.5 million—were being tested annually.[20] According to the CDC, 11% of men *below* the recommended testing range—3.9 million— were getting tested. And a staggering 65% of men over age 74–6.24 million—were still getting tested.[21] That flies squarely in the face of rec- ommendations from every major medical group that men of this more advanced age *not* get PSA tests, because they are far more likely to die of something else before prostate cancer would kill them.

(Famously, 81-year-old billionaire investor Warren Buffett followed the advice of his doctors and had a PSA test in 2012, even though the USPSTF recommendation against testing men older than 75 had been out for four years. Buffett then had a biopsy and was found to have a low-grade cancer, yet he underwent radiation therapy. He was widely criticized, as were his doctors. A cancer specialist from the University of Pittsburgh School of Medicine said, "If one of my residents biopsied an 81 yo (with no mets [metastases]) I would fire them on the spot."[22]

After the USPSTF change in 2018 from a D as in Don't rating to a C as in Consider it, screening increased: 10% among men 40–54 years old, for whom the recommendation remained a D; 12% for men aged 55–69, to whom that change applied; and 16% for men 70 and older, for whom the recommendation also continued to be a D.[23]

Why? Why does a screening test for cancer that is clearly likely to do more harm than good remain so popular? Certainly, fear plays a part. In a survey one month after the USPSTF rated the PSA test a D in 2008, 54% of men said they'd ignore that recommendation and have the test, and 33% were undecided. Only 13% of men said they would avoid PSA screen- ing.[24] In 2012 three doctors in four said the biggest reason they contin- ued to prescribe a PSA test was because patients still wanted it.[25] In 2015 general practitioners in the United States who still recommended the test said, "I would say that [PSA screening], that's mostly to satisfy the pa- tients," and "Most of the studies show that PSA is not a reliable trigger for intervention. And so we get it but then we don't know what to do with it, and it just ends up scaring patients."[26]

Why do patients still want it, despite the statistics and all the warn- ings? As we've seen, screening provides a sense of control against the deep fear of cancer. Listen to the comments of African American men, who are at twice the risk of dying from prostate cancer as non-Black men. Interviewed in 2015 in focus groups in North Carolina community health centers and churches, most said they knew of, and worried about, all the harm the PSA test might lead to. But no matter. Most had one anyway. Researchers reported, "Most of them cited staying alive as a critical benefit to screening . . . When confronted with the possibility of losing sexual function, commonly believed to be a consequence of a biopsy, someone noted, 'What's more important: your sex life, or your real life?' " Not only does PSA screening offer a sense of empowerment and control, but it also reduces the "fear factor" of uncertainty. Despite its imprecision, the test provides at least some knowledge. "Many participants indicated that they would prefer the risks of screening to not knowing that they have a potentially dangerous and aggressive cancer."[27]

(As I was writing this book, at age 68, I had a PSA test, not so much to know my level but to see how I would feel about and react to the results—a sort of self-test about the way fear of cancer would affect me. I knew all about the imprecision of the test and how unreliable it is. Yet I confess that when my results came in—0.04—I was slightly relieved. I also confess that had the number come in at 10 or 12 or dramatically above the threshold of concern—4—I'm not sure what I would have done. As I've said several times, this book looks at things from the population level, where statistics are abstract and more readily seen objectively, rationally, but at the personal level, where we make choices as individuals, things are much more subjective. For all of us.)

There is another reason the test is still so frequently used. While doctors say they still prescribe it mostly in response to patient demand, remember that doctors are people too, and many male doctors have a long-standing *personal* belief in the PSA test. A survey done in 2006, before the USPSTF D recommendations but well after serious questions had arisen about the efficacy of the test, found that among doctors 50 years old or older, 78% of general practitioners and 95% of urologists had had a PSA screen themselves.[28]

And the profit motive remains real too. Many of the doctors and hospitals that make money from doing the PSA test and performing the biopsies and treatments it often leads to are still actively promoting its use. Many cancer centers and other hospitals and clinics offer free prostate cancer screening, promoting the test (a cheap simple blood test) with the mantra of "Find cancer early" but with little or no mention of its imprecision or harms, because men diagnosed with prostate cancer usually turn to the same facility for their treatment. Free PSA testing turns many men into paying customers.

Overdiagnosis

Like tens of thousands of men, Michael's PSA test sent him into a fear-driven medical cascade without having had the chance to decide for himself whether to take that first step. He was screened as a matter of standard practice, without his knowledge or any sort of prior conversation about the pros and cons of a PSA test. Word that his PSA level was slightly elevated caught him completely by surprise. That experience is common.

At that point Michael was given a choice. He could simply wait and have another test in six months or a year, or he could undergo a biopsy to harvest cells from his prostate gland. This is no casual procedure. It involves the insertion of a device up the anus that shoots hollow needles through the wall of the rectum into the prostate to collect samples of tissue from various areas. It's a frequently painful procedure that has a roughly 5% chance of a serious infection, lasting weeks or months, and a roughly 2% chance of causing sepsis, a life-threatening infection that requires hospitalization.[29] But it provides more certainty.

So Michael did what most men do who face that choice. He had a biopsy. It confirmed he had cancer, but it also confirmed that his cancer was unlikely to ever harm him, because his Gleason score was a 6.

But now imagine you are Michael, sitting there in the urologist's office having just heard that you have CANCER! Your mind is swimming. The fight or flight response triggered by this threatening news is flooding your brain with stress hormones and literally making it hard to think clearly. Your doctor says that you can just wait and monitor things, or have your prostate gland removed with either surgery or radiation. The doctor cautions that those treatments often cause serious side effects, like loss of erectile function, urinary and bowel incontinence, and in rare cases serious infections or death from the surgery itself—for a cancer almost certain to never harm you. But it's CANCER! What would you do?

Like most people, Michael sought more information. He learned that between 20% and 50% of men diagnosed with prostate cancer—as many as one man in two—are overdiagnosed, told they have a frightening disease that in fact would never harm them and that requires no immediate clinical treatment.[30] He learned that while 11 men in 100 (in the United States) will develop prostate cancer in their lifetimes, only 2–3 in 100 will die from it, because the majority of prostate cancers are slow growing. He learned that the 15-year survival rate from diagnosis of his kind of cancer was close to 100% *whether he had treatment* or didn't. In other words, given that he had a disease that was highly unlikely to develop symptoms or to harm him even if left alone, surgery or radiation might well harm him but probably wouldn't improve his chances of living longer.

Probably. But not for sure. And as we've said, that's the whole problem with overdiagnosis of cancer in general. Despite the reassuring numbers, Michael couldn't be absolutely certain whether he would be one of the majority of men who are overdiagnosed and overtreated, or one of the very few men in his circumstances whose life would be saved by treatment. The odds were low, but not zero, that he might die a long, slow, painful death.

Michael did his best to rationally weigh the pros and cons of each option and make an objective evidence-based choice. He talked to friends who had experienced something similar, to learn how they dealt with their situation. He called me to ask how the psychology of risk perception influences people's judgments in cases like this. "I've done all the homework," he said. "I know most of the facts I need to know. It's just, I need help trying to figure out how to decide what to do. I mean, I know I probably don't need to do anything. But it's cancer. *Cancer*!"

I asked him a bunch of "How would you feel if" questions about his various options, the way good medical decision aids do. (More on them in part four.) I cautioned him about how psychological factors like control, uncertainty, and pain and suffering shape our fears. But in the end, I could only offer my friend the suggestion that he should do what felt right to him. Ultimately his fear of cancer was more powerful than his fear of the side effects of treatment, and it overpowered the evidence that watchful waiting would be enough as a start. So he had brachytherapy—to kill his entire prostate gland. The cancer was eliminated, but he could no longer achieve an erection, and erectile dysfunction medication had little benefit. He suffered urinary leakage that requires him to have to be near a bathroom at all times and he has to sleep in diapers.

Profound costs. But Michael says he accepts them as the price he was willing to pay to rid himself not just of his cancer but of his fear of that disease as well.

Overtreatment

As Michael researched his options, the statistics about survival were mostly good, but the data about side effects were decidedly worrisome.

He learned that roughly two men in every three who undergo prostate surgery end up with long-term, often permanent, erectile dysfunction.[31] Roughly two in ten suffer some degree of urinary incontinence that can last for several years.[32] And 15% suffer some degree of bowel incontinence that also can last for several years.[33] Furthermore, as with all surgery, he learned there is a tiny but real risk of death.

In the end, Michael's decision to risk these harms in exchange for peace of mind was the right one for him. But now let's step back from the individual level and consider things from the broader overall public health perspective. From that view the harm done by overtreatment of prostate cancer is staggering.

To quantify that harm, we'll use the period between 1992, when PSA testing began to peak, through 2017. (Remember, though the FDA approved the PSA test for already-diagnosed patients in 1986, off-label use for screening of asymptomatic individuals began immediately and spread quickly, causing that frightening 82% leap in the age-adjusted rate of prostate cancer in men 65 and older from 1986 to 1991. So using 1992 as our starting point means the figures that follow are conservative.) No records detail how many men have PSA tests each year, but to be conservative, let's estimate that one man out of four aged 45–84 had an annual PSA test over the period we're looking at, a yearly uptake rate of just 25%. (Most studies suggest that the screening rate was higher, especially before the 2008 USPSTF D recommendations.) The average annual population of men in that age group for that period was 49 million. So if only one in four of those men had an annual PSA test, that means that 12.3 million men had a test each year, or a total—very roughly—of 306 million men tested over those 25 years. Some of these were the same men, testing repeatedly as part of their annual physicals, but for our purposes, the total is the same: 306 million tests were done on men over that time, each one exposing the man to the potential harms the test could lead to. (A caveat about estimating how many people screened over 25 years: Over a long period screening will identify some men with cancer who will then leave the ongoing population being screened, bringing the total number screened down. But over those years, other men will enter the population, undergoing screening for the first time, so this analysis assumes, crudely, that these rates are roughly similar and cancel each other out.)

The harms of overtreatment begin with false positives. For that calculation, this analysis relies on the CAP trial. The most common threshold of concern from a PSA finding is 4 (nanograms per milliliter of blood, or 4 ng/mL), but the CAP trial used a lower standard, 3, and reported that 11% of the men who had PSA tests had levels of 3 or above. Since 4 is the more common figure in the United States, however, we'll adjust the CAP number downward and estimate that 10% of men in the United States who had a PSA test produced a result of 4 ng/mL or higher. That brings the total number of men tested over the 25 years who had a level of 4 or higher to roughly 30.6 million.

But false positives aren't confirmed until after a biopsy. The CAP trial reported that 85% of the men who got PSA levels above the threshold of concern (usually confirmed by a second PSA test) went on to have biopsies. That means 26 million men in the United States had biopsies as a result of PSA tests over the period of 1992–2017.

Two-thirds of them—17.4 million—got the worrying news that they might have prostate cancer but in the end did not.

As with mammograms, false positives cause both physical and psychological harm. One study comparing men who had false-positive PSA findings with a control group of men who had normal findings found that "men who received false-positive PSA test results reported having thought more about prostate cancer (49% compared to the control group at 18%) and worried more (40% compared to 8%) despite receiving a negative biopsy result on follow-up. The false-positive result also led many to believe they were more likely to develop prostate cancer (36% to 18% among controls)."[34] As the authors of that study said, "Screening can be detrimental to the mental health of our patients."[35]

Another study on the psychological impact of false-positive PSA tests found that 26% of the men whose biopsy results told them they were cancer-free worried "a lot" or "some of the time" that they may develop prostate cancer in the future, compared with 6% of men who got normal PSAs and didn't need a biopsy at all. Among the biopsy group, 46% reported worrying that their wife or significant other was concerned about prostate cancer developing in the future, versus 14% in the normal PSA group.[36] And yet another study reported that men who receive a false-positive PSA test report more problems with sexual function compared with men with normal screening results.[37]

These concerns take a psychosocial toll, but they also raise the risk of physical harm from chronically elevated stress, which changes the body's hormone levels, raises blood pressure, weakens the immune system, and increases the likelihood of developing diabetes and clinical depression. A study of men 67 and older who got a prostate cancer diagnosis found that 38% were more likely to be hospitalized for *noncancerous* health conditions in the year after they were diagnosed compared with the year before.[38] These hospitalizations were more likely in the four months after diagnosis. The authors wrote, "It has been documented that the diagnosis of prostate cancer can trigger psychological distress, anxiety, and suicidal ideations. This increase in psychological stress may increase blood levels of epinephrine and norepinephrine, resulting in increased heart rate, blood pressure, and blood sugar levels."[39]

Let's move on to Michael's next step, biopsy. Using needles to puncture a part of the body rich in blood vessels and adjacent to the organs carrying solid and liquid waste out of the body runs a risk of serious infection. One study reported that prostate biopsies cause infection requiring treatment in 0.5%–7% of patients.[40] Assuming that most of the 17.4 million false positives from 1992–2017 led to biopsies, *between 87,000 and 1.2 million men suffered side effects of biopsies serious enough to warrant ongoing medical treatment.* The USPSTF estimates that 1% of biopsies lead to hospitalization. Based on that conservative figure, of the 17.4 million men who got a false positive over the lifetime of the PSA test, *174,000 were hospitalized after false-positive PSA results led them to undergo a painful and risky procedure because they feared they might have a disease that it turns out they did not have.*[41]

False negatives—when the initial PSA level is below the threshold of concern—also cause harm.[42] The imprecise PSA screen produces them 15% of the time. In the 25-year sample period used here, when roughly 306 million men had a PSA test, roughly 46 million got a false "all clear" but were eventually found in other ways to have prostate cancer. That surely delayed the diagnosis of their disease, contributing to worse outcomes, including potentially avoidable death. It would be difficult, however, to quantify with any accuracy the specific harms those cases caused.

———

PSA testing finds a huge number of overdiagnosed cancers, frightening many men into fear-ectomies, surgery or other treatments to "just get it out" that they don't clinically require. The side effects of surgery or radiation treatment are serious, and common. Using National Cancer Institute data on the annual incidence rate of prostate cancer per

100,000 men for each of the years from 1992 through 2017 and multiplying that by the total population of men of screening ages, 45-74, for those years, roughly 1.9 million American men were diagnosed with prostate cancer, of all grades.[43] Using the range cited above, that between 20% and 50% of men diagnosed with prostate cancer are *overdiagnosed*, and conservatively taking the middle of that range—35%—from 1992 to 2017, 665,000 men were diagnosed with a type of prostate cancer that was unlikely to ever cause them harm.

According to a national disease registry of men with prostate cancer, known as CaPSURE, as of 2008, roughly 90% of men diagnosed with prostate cancer chose some sort of aggressive treatment to remove their prostate gland.[44] Another study reported that between 2010 and 2015, roughly 70% of men diagnosed with prostate cancer—of any type—chose radical prostatectomy (33%) or radiotherapy (34%) treatment.[45] So let's assume for our crude calculations that over the period being considered, 80% of the 665,000 men with overdiagnosed prostate cancer—565,000—chose some type of aggressive treatment.

Note that there are several ways to treat lower risk prostate cancer, either surgically removing it or "burning" it out with radiation. With external radiation, beams from outside the body are pointed at the one spot in the prostate where the biopsy has found cancerous cells to be burned away. With brachytherapy, ultrasound-directed needles are inserted through the rectum to place radioactive pellets in the prostate gland itself.

There is much debate about the mortality risks from various form of treatment, and only scant data on the postsurgical death rate from prostatectomy surgery alone. This analysis relies on a study of outcomes in Sweden between 1998 and 2012, which estimated the mortality rate from this type of treatment at roughly 0.17%.[46] How many men in the United States with overdiagnosed prostate cancer had this surgery? Again, the data are thin. One study reported that from 2004 to 2013, about the same number of men had prostatectomy by surgical excision as had external beam radiation therapy to kill the gland.[47] So from 1992 to 2017, it's estimated that roughly 280,000 men had radical prostatectomies for low-grade overdiagnosed prostate cancer. Based on the many assumptions that go into this rough calculation, *from 1992 through 2017 roughly 500 men in the United States were **killed** by prostatectomy surgery to remove a disease that scared them but would never have harmed them.*

But death from surgery is the rarest of the harms from aggressive treatment of prostate cancer. Far more frequent are the other serious side effects, which are common regardless of the type of procedure. Based on the estimate that 565,000 men had some kind of surgery to remove low-grade, low-risk prostate cancer from 1992 to 2017, *overtreatment caused an estimated 375,000 cases of long-term erectile dysfunction (two-thirds of surgical patients), 113,000 cases of long-term urinary incontinence (20% of patients), and 85,000 cases of men left with trouble controlling their bowels (15% of patients).*

To put this in perspective, remember that PSA testing is estimated to save roughly one life per 1,000 men *over 10 years.* (Some research suggests that this estimate may be low.)[48] That means *for the entire population of 306 million men who got PSA tests over 25 years, screening saved an estimated 31,000 lives, killed 500, and left more than half a million men seriously harmed.*

There is one last harm from overtreatment to consider: regret. Michael is like the majority of men who undergo surgery or radiation for low-grade cancer who, despite the side effects, are content with their choice. But a significant minority are not. One study found that among 400 men who'd had surgery, 19% regretted their choice.[49] Regret was lowest right after the treatment but rose over time, as men had to face the long-term consequences of the side effects they were suffering, and as the acute fear of death that made a fear-ectomy so appealing at first faded. Regret was also higher for men who had robotic surgery on the assumption—and often on the promise of the doctors and hospitals providing such surgery—that this supposedly more advanced technique causes fewer side effects. It doesn't.[50]

If 19% of the 565,000 men who had surgery for low-grade prostate cancer from 1992 to 2017 have experienced regret, that means *roughly 107,000 men look back on the choice they made, a choice largely driven by fear, and have to live with the psychologically corrosive feeling that, in retrospect, they chose wrong.*

Progress

As noted at the outset, the story of prostate cancer also offers hope, because important changes are being made to reduce the harm of overdiagnosis and overtreatment. The full details are explored in part four, but one key point is worth noting here: the number of men choosing active surveillance rather than risky surgery or radiation is rising rapidly.

Between 2010 and 2015, the number of men over 55 choosing either active surveillance or watchful waiting nearly tripled, from 22% to about 60%. Among men 55 and younger, the rate rose more sharply, from 9% in 2010 to 35% in 2015.[51] Many of these men still had biopsies, part of the active surveillance protocol, and biopsies carry their own risks. But even after those biopsies confirmed that they had prostate cancer, an increasing number of men still chose to just watch and wait. And among those 55 and under whose biopsies produced only 1 or 2 positive tissue samples out of the 10 to 12 normally taken—a strong indicator that the cancer is low-grade—13% were willing to accept active surveillance in 2010, but by 2015 nearly half were. As of 2019 between one-third and one-half of all men in the United States with low-grade prostate cancer have been on an active surveillance or watchful waiting protocol.[52] That is remarkable progress.

In large measure this is the result of acceptance by the medical community, including urologists, that more aggressive treatment for low-grade prostate cancer does more harm than good. This acceptance has been possible because, unlike the case of DCIS breast cancer, studies have been done comparing surgery and radiation versus active surveillance, confirming that for low-grade prostate cancer, both approaches produce similar reductions in prostate-specific mortality.[53] A study named ProtecT found, "At a median of 10 years, prostate cancer–specific mortality was low irrespective of the treatment assigned, with no significant difference among treatments."[54] Another, named PIVOT, came up with similar results: "After nearly 20 years of follow-up among men with localized prostate cancer, surgery was not associated with significantly lower all-cause or prostate-cancer mortality than observation."[55]

In light of that evidence, in 2018 the National Comprehensive Cancer Network, a consortium of leading cancer hospitals in the United States, officially made either active surveillance (more follow-up testing with biopsies) or watchful waiting the guideline-approved standards of care. That offers legal protection to physicians who recommend less aggressive treatment should a patient later decide that this approach wasn't enough. Many general practitioners and urologists now recommend some version of "wait and monitor" more often. Many even actively discourage men with low-risk prostate cancer from choosing surgery or radiation.

But despite all the progress, roughly half the men diagnosed with low-grade prostate cancer are still making Michael's choice, opting for surgery or radiation. Further, not everyone who initially chooses surveillance stays with it, even men whose follow-up tests confirm that they still have only low-grade disease. Some just can't live with the fear, and they switch to more aggressive treatment.[56]

Another hurdle remains. Despite the professional guidelines certifying surveillance as an option for certain low-grade cases, many doctors still recommend the more aggressive path, for various reasons.[57] One is medical training. In 2015 urologists in the United States told interviewers: "We train people to do something. We are by nature doers and active surveillance is not really part of what a surgeon is wired to do." Then there is concern about being sued for not doing everything possible. "There's obviously some degree of liability because you're at some point fundamentally telling the patient not to seek treatment because of our experience and understanding." And then there is the profit motive. "Guys in practice make their money doing things. They don't make nearly as much money doing surveillance and I think that that plays a lot into it. I think there is this attitude that I have heard expressed many times which is, you know, I believe in surveillance, you watch the tumour all the way to the time you wheel the patient in the operating room." Another said, "We as an industry, as a large corporation, we have to meet certain benchmarks. And certainly on our side if we don't do radiation we're not really doing things, you know, that's what they pay me to do, to put it mildly. There is always an incentive."[58] (To be fair, remember that these comments were made in 2015, when the expanded treatment options had just begun.)

The evidence that profit motivates some doctors is everywhere. Major cancer centers still actively promote free prostate cancer–screening programs, which generate no revenue by themselves but produce enormous earnings later because many people who are screened seek treatment at the same facility. The prominent Roswell Park Comprehensive Cancer Center, which patented the PSA screening test and encouraged the FDA to approve it, is among many leading cancer centers that still tout the test as far more effective than most research has found: "The PSA serum test," it says on its website, "is an invaluable tool for prostate cancer diagnosis that, when used intelligently, can significantly reduce the mortality rate of this disease," which flies squarely in the face of the evidence, 1 life per 1,000 screened over 10 years. They add, "Roswell Park physicians are well aware of the risks of over-treating this disease," a curious caveat given that the risks they say they're concerned about stem directly from the PSA test they promote.

But things are changing, faster for PSA and prostate cancer than for mammography and breast cancer. Doctors are more aware of the harms being done by overscreening and overdiagnosis and are trying to reduce those harms. Even more importantly, the public has begun to accept that prostate cancer is not always a death sentence. There are hopeful signs that with time, continuing attention, and persistent pushback against those promoting screening for profit, the problem of overscreening, overdiagnosis, and overtreatment of prostate cancer might eventually be brought under control.

Despite that hope, however, these remain early days in our shifting emotional relationship with the Emperor of All Maladies. Cancerphobia runs deep, and fear is often impervious to reason, as we'll see in the coming chapters.

Chapter 6

thyroid cancer

When Worry Causes Us to Do Too Much

A poem begins as a lump in the throat.
—Robert Frost

The Korean word for cancer is 암—it's pronounced "ahm." The Korean word for phobia is 공포증 (cohn-PUT-zin). There is probably no more clarion example of 암공포증 (ahm cohn-PUT-zin)—cancerphobia—than the recent epidemic of thyroid cancer in South Korea. It left thousands injured unnecessarily, billions of dollars spent on health care that did not have to be spent, and clear lessons for all of us about the harm caused by excessive fear of nonthreatening cancers, lessons that are being heeded by some, but sadly, ignored by most. What happened in South Korea is also happening in the United States and elsewhere.

In 1999, the South Korean government began an aggressive campaign against cancer—the most common cause of death in that country since 1983. The National Health Insurance (NHI) program provided free screening for the top cancer killers—stomach, breast, and cervical. Screening became a major new line of business for the health care industry in South Korea. New cancer-screening centers sprang up across the country. Major hospitals, health care clinics, and private medical practices invested in new equipment. To maximize revenues from that equipment, many of these facilities promoted an inexpensive $30–$50 examination for thyroid cancer to go along with the free screening. That affordable, fast, noninvasive screening was performed by ultrasound.

The incidence of thyroid cancer in South Korea shot up, especially in women, who are more prone to this disease. So did the rate of surgeries to treat it, partial or total thyroidectomies—removal of either one or both lobes, "wings," of the thyroid gland, which has the basic shape of a butterfly. Nothing obvious explained this precipitous rise. There had been no increase in the risk factors for thyroid cancer. There had been, though, an early warning flag about a possible cause.

A curious epidemiologist had noticed a sharp rise in thyroid cancer in the city of Yeonggwang, where a few years earlier a doctor had started doing thyroid exams with ultrasound. The public health researcher investigated whether the local nuclear plant might be the cause, but he found nothing implicating the reactors. No accidents, no leaks—nothing unusual. He proposed that the rising number of thyroid cancers in that area might simply be an artifact of the increased use of ultrasound screening, which can find much smaller lumps and growths than manual examination. Sensitive screening technology, he suggested, was only finding what had been there all along.

But his research got little attention. And his implication, that there might be too much cancer screening, offended common wisdom, that the most effective way to fight cancer is to catch it as early as possible, so doing as much screening as possible with the most sensitive technology available just makes sense. It made sense to Kim Jung-mi.[1] She is in her 50s now, having raised young kids and taken care of her home and family. That work was tiring, but Jung-mi felt especially fatigued after her thyroidectomy in 2011, a surgery she regrets having.

She was one of the 40,000 South Koreans diagnosed with thyroid cancer that year, part of a frightening epidemic of the disease.[2] Fifteen times more people were diagnosed in 2011 than just 20 years earlier. Curiously, it was an epidemic of only one type of thyroid cancer, papillary carcinoma, by far the most common type and, critically, the kind least likely to do any harm. Eighty-five percent of thyroid cancers are papillary, 11% are follicular, 3% are medullary, and 1% are anaplastic.[3] Those latter three types are more dangerous. Papillary thyroid cancer is so slow growing that it almost never causes any symptoms in the patient's lifetime.

Jung-mi had no symptoms to warrant screening in the first place: no neck pain or problems with breathing or swallowing that might have suggested some sort of nodule or growth in her thyroid; no problems with her metabolism, which is regulated by hormones produced in the thyroid; no lump accidentally noticed while buttoning a collar or washing her neck.

But Jung-mi had heard that thyroid cancer was becoming more and more common. (Remember from chapter 2 how the psychological factor of "awareness" can create fear that exceeds the risk.) Some of her friends had been diagnosed. (Remember too the psychological factor of "personification.") And she had heard advertisements from the rapidly expanding cancer-screening industry in South Korea, offering screening they said was fast, easy, and cheap. So though she had no symptoms, Jung-mi chose to have her thyroid examined.

A few years later she told the *Korea Times* that she wished she hadn't. "After getting an ultrasound, I was diagnosed with thyroid cancer. It was about one centimeter in diameter. A doctor recommended surgery. Scared by the word, cancer, I just had it," she said. "Now it feels like my body recovers from fatigue much slower than before the surgery. I wish I did more research before making the decision."

The sensitive ultrasound had found in Jung-mi what hundreds of millions of people all around the world have, what you may well have in your neck as you read this: a tiny asymptomatic nodule in the thyroid gland highly unlikely to ever cause any harm. Nine out of every ten of these nodules are benign, meaning they don't even meet the cellular criteria for cancer. The vast majority of those that are cancerous (based on microscopic examination of cells acquired through biopsy) rarely cause any problems. Most people who have papillary thyroid cancer never know they do. Nearly everyone with these growths who does not have them removed dies of something else.[4]

The great majority of these nodules, especially the ones detected by ultrasound, are tiny, like Jung-mi's, less than 1 centimeter wide (about the width of a pencil)—what the medical community calls micropapillary thyroid cancer, or mPTC. The 10-year survival rate for mPTC is 100% *both for those who have treatment and for those who choose to do nothing at all.*[5] Standard medical recommendation for such cases is active surveillance, nothing more than periodic monitoring. From 1999 to 2008, 94% of the increase in thyroid cancer incidence in South Korea was tiny papillary growths of 2 centimeters or smaller.[6]

These statistics explain why, even though the incidence of this type of cancer was becoming more common in South Korea and around the world, death from thyroid cancer remains rare. In 2014, 77,000 people in South Korea died of cancer of all types. Only 346 died of thyroid cancer. That same year in the United States, cancer of all kinds killed 592,000 people. Thyroid cancer killed just 1,832.

So ultrasound screening was finding way more disease, almost none of which posed any health threat—except that the name of the disease included the word "cancer."

Ultrasound was first used to look for cancer by neurologist George Dussik in 1942, when he scanned patient's skulls looking for brain tumors. But it came into wider use in medicine in the eighties, especially for monitoring fetal development, after technological advances made the images much sharper. Ultrasound for detecting thyroid cancer came into common use in the midnineties, and just as mammography had done for DCIS microtumors that weren't big enough to feel by hand, ultrasound detected many papillary micronodules too small to be detected by palpation. Ultrasound can also reveal other characteristics of the nodules, such as whether the tissue is more solid or liquid, important additional clues about whether it may contain cancerous cells. But like mammography, it can't *confirm* that a suspicious growth is cancer. Only microscopic examination of cells from a biopsy can do that. So if a growth is found that has any suspicious characteristics, even if it's tiny, doctors recommend to patients like Jung-mi that they have a biopsy. Facing the frightening possibility that they may have cancer, the vast majority of people who get a recommendation to have a biopsy do. The cascade has begun.

The fine-needle biopsy of a thyroid is a low-risk affair. Medically. But there is plenty of risk created by the findings. About 5 in 100 find papillary carcinoma, which puts people like Jung-mi in a fearful spot, where they have to choose between active surveillance—coming back in for periodic checkups—or surgery, even though that carries its own risks and in most cases will only eliminate a small clump of abnormal cells that pose essentially no threat. A thyroidectomy for small papillary cancer is in almost every case truly a fear-ectomy. The statistics clearly favor the less risky option of watching and waiting, but the choice that people like Jung-mi face isn't just about the numbers.

Had Jung-mi been fully informed by her health care providers, she would have learned that all patients who have their thyroid removed suffer hypothyroidism—the absence of hormones the thyroid produces that are critical for maintaining normal metabolism. Hypothyroidism is treatable with synthetic replacement hormone, but many patients complain of short- and long-term symptoms as they struggle to determine the right dose to match the fine-tuned levels the body produced naturally. That struggle is complicated by the fact that the effectiveness of the synthetic hormone is diminished by variables like eating anything containing soy, drinking coffee, or just taking it on a full stomach.

These symptoms are not uncommon. In the North American Thyroid Cancer Survivorship Survey (NATCSS), of 1,174 post-thyroidectomy patients asked about their quality of life in the months and years after surgery, 45% reported one or more of the following symptoms: fatigue, hair loss, bone pain, memory problems / brain fog, constipation, dry eyes, and sensitivity to cold. Jung-mi suffers from several of these symptoms.[7]

The NATCSS found that surgery also had psychosocial consequences. On a 10 point scale of various quality of life issues, with 0 indicating that surgery had no effect and 10 being maximum effect, respondents rated worry about a second cancer at 6.4, fear of recurrence of thyroid cancer at 5.8, their "total psychological well-being" at only 5.5, and their "spiritual well-being" at 5.2. Seventy percent of these respondents were suffering these costs after surgery to remove nonthreatening small papillary thyroid cancer tumors. The authors of that study summarized their findings this way: "Survival for patients with thyroid cancer has been perceived in the past as a relatively benign experience, particularly when compared with survivors of other cancers. This perception is likely because thyroid cancer has a good five-year survival rate. The current findings illustrate that this perception is unfounded, and that thyroid cancer survivors experience several adverse physical, psychological, social, and spiritual challenges that linger for many years following treatment."[8]

Jung-mi would have also been warned that thyroidectomy surgery poses other risks. There is sometimes damage to the parathyroid glands, which are adjacent to the thyroid. These glands control levels of calcium in the body critical for bone growth and nerve activity. Calcium supplements solve this condition, hypoparathyroidism, for most patients, but 8% of surgery patients are left with calcium levels so low that they have to be rehospitalized, and 2% of thyroidectomy patients end up with permanently depressed levels of calcium. Many of the respondents to the NATCSS reported several common symptoms of hypoparathyroidism: seizures and mood change; painful muscle spasms in the face, hands, and feet; cramping, tingling, and burning sensations in the hands, feet, lips, and tongue; rough, dry skin; brittle nails; and coarse, easily breakable hair.[9]

Another side effect Jung-mi would have learned about is that between 1 and 2 surgery patients out of every 100 suffer partial or total vocal cord paralysis, since the nerves and muscles controlling the voice lie just above the thyroid gland in the neck. In the NATCSS, 55% of respondents reported some degree of voice change, 10% required treatment to repair damage to their vocal cords, and 62% reported dysphagia—dry mouth or problems swallowing, sometimes persisting for several months, a surgical side effect of damaged salivary glands.

Jung-mi also had postsurgery treatment with radioactive iodine to kill off any cancerous cells the surgeon missed. (Thyroid cells attract radioactive iodine like a magnet, causing cancer in a healthy gland but burning off any cancerous cells the surgeon missed in a thyroidectomy.) That has its own risks. The short-term side effects include impaired taste and inflammation of salivary glands in roughly 30% of patients, as well as temporarily reduced fertility (mostly in males, lasting up to nine months) in half.[10] Occasionally some of these side effects are permanent. A close friend of mine has lost a lot of her sense of smell and taste as a result of postsurgical radioactive iodine treatment following a thyroidectomy, an outcome her endocrinologist never warned her about. Longer term, radioactive iodine is associated with secondary malignancies. In 14,589 patients who received radioactive iodine from 1973 to 2007 in the United States, there was a 13% increase in salivary gland malignancies and a roughly sixfold increase in leukemia, compared with a reference group without thyroid cancer.[11]

In addition, as with any surgery, there are low but real risks of infection, heart attacks, strokes, and blood clots, which in this case can be fatal, blocking the ability to breathe. One small study of 517 thyroidectomy patients reported that 0.2% of them, a rate of 2 people per 1,000, died as a result of the surgery.[12]

Any fully informed patient would have all those numbers, so they could objectively weigh the risk of their disease against the risks associated with surgery. But like Jung-mi, many thyroid cancer patients are not fully warned about all the side effects, especially those that are less medically distinct like fatigue, weight gain, bone and muscle pain, voice changes, dry mouth, problems swallowing, and sensitivity to heat or cold. In part this lack of warning is because some physicians don't take those side effects as seriously as their patients do. A study of doctors that followed up on what patients said in the NATCSS reported: "Physicians consistently underestimated the prevalence of physical symptoms in thyroid cancer survivors compared with what was actually found in NATCSS."[13] Another found that the test doctors use to measure voice changes (the Voice Handicap Index) underestimates the real world experience of patients.[14]

Yet, even had Jung-mi had all the information about side effects, the choice she faced—a choice that felt literally like a matter of life or death—was based on more than just an objective statistical analysis. You can hear this in how she described her experience. She remembers hearing only that her doctor recommended surgery and the frightening word "cancer." At that point fear took over and essentially made the decision for her. Looking back with the clarity of hindsight, Jung-mi realizes regretfully that she essentially opted for a fear-ectomy as much as for a thyroidectomy, and she is paying a price for that choice.

She is hardly alone.

Let's step back from the individual level and consider the effects of this excessive fear of cancer on the overall population of South Korea. (It's happening in countries around the world. More on that in a moment.) First, and most important, all the extra screening is not saving lives. The age-adjusted 10-year survival rate for thyroid cancer in South Korea is right where it was before the ultrasound screening began, 99.2%.[15] But the surgeries themselves have taken a sobering toll.

The International Agency for Research on Cancer (IARC), part of the World Health Organization, estimates that 90% of the thyroid surgeries in South Korea since 2000 were the result of overdiagnosis.[16] Based on that 90% estimate, in just 2013, the peak year of this epidemic, roughly 45,000 thyroidectomies in South Korea were not clinically necessary.[17] Given the general rate of side effects listed above, those surgeries left approximately 10,000 people like Jung-mi with some degree of hypothyroidism symptoms, 900 people with some degree of vocal cord paralysis, and 9 people dead, from operations to remove a tiny nodule that posed little or no clinical threat. And that was just one year.

From 2000 through 2014, approximately 300,000 medically unnecessary thyroid surgeries were performed in South Korea. That means 60,000 people ended up suffering from some degree of hypothyroidism symptoms, 6,000 people ended up with partially or totally paralyzed vocal cords, and 600 people died—as a result of surgeries for overdiagnosed disease.

Then there is the financial cost. A review by South Korean doctors found, "The economic burden of thyroid cancer in South Korea increased about sevenfold, from $257 million in 2000 to $1.724 billion in 2010."[18] Another study estimated that by 2015, the epidemic had cost the South Korea health care system roughly $2 billion, an enormous investment in treating an essentially nonthreatening disease.[19]

The lesson from these costs—that excessive fear of a nonthreatening type of cancer can do more harm than the disease itself—is clear. But the South Korea example teaches another important point in the larger context of this book. Even after the overscreening, overdiagnosis, and overtreatment problem with thyroid cancer was widely reported in the national press, and its harms were recognized not only by the medical community but by the public and the government as well, change came slowly, for three reasons: the deep fear of cancer, the public's absolute faith in screening, and the resistance of those with vested interests.

In March 2014, a group of eight South Korean doctors calling themselves the Physician Coalition for Prevention of Overdiagnosis of Thyroid Cancer published an open letter warning their medical colleagues that ultrasound testing of thyroid cancer was doing vastly more harm than good. That warning got a lot of public attention. Broadcasters ran in-depth reports on television, public TV carried a series of debates, and both the South Korean National Assembly and the nation's health ministry held a series of hearings to investigate. That rising public awareness helped. Surgeries fell from roughly 11,000 in the first three months of 2014 to 8,000 in the second three months, then down to roughly 7,000 per quarter for the rest of the year. A panel of the nation's top experts issued new recommendations in 2015, stating that "thyroid ultrasonography is not routinely recommended for healthy subjects."[20]

But the Korean Thyroid Association, the endocrinologists and thyroid surgeons making the most money from the screening and surgery, fought back. In an article that ran in a widely read national newspaper, "Early Detection/Treatment of Cancer Is the Right of Patients, Thyroid Society Rejects Overdiagnosis," they argued, "The surge in thyroid cancer patients is not an over diagnosis, but a medical explanation (for the fact that) in East Asia, Korea is much more likely to develop thyroid cancer than other regions."[21] The doctors offered no explanation for why, if that was the case, thyroid incidence only skyrocketed in South Korea *after* the ultrasound screening began. The doctors also criticized new national health service recommendations for who should or shouldn't consider screening, arguing that people had a right to screening: "No one can restrict the rights of patients to detect and treat thyroid cancer early." This is the same false criticism of recommendations from the US Preventive Services Task Force (USPSTF) and similar advisory panels in other countries. They are not rules, just suggestions—based on thorough research—for whom screening is likely to benefit more than harm. The South Korea guidelines were entirely voluntary.

But even flexible guidelines against screening challenge the fundamental belief that early detection of all cancer is always beneficial. So while thyroid cancer incidence in South Korean women dropped a remarkable 50% between 2012 and 2015, from roughly 120 per 100,000 to just 60, massive screening continued, and thyroid remained the most commonly detected cancer among South Korean women as of 2015. In 2016 South Korea still had the highest rate of thyroid cancer incidence in the world, almost tenfold higher than the global average, six times higher than the United States, fifteen times higher than England.[22] It was still twice as high as it had been back in 1999. Why?

A study that tried to find out is revealing. In "A Qualitative Study of Women's Views on Overdiagnosis and Screening for Thyroid Cancer in Korea," 29 women were interviewed in depth.[23] Half had not been screened; half had. Of those who had been screened, all but one were asymptomatic at the time. Seven of the women had had surgery.

Even though most of the 29 knew that thyroid cancer is slow growing and "not serious," researchers reported that "hearing about the risks of overdiagnosis had limited impact on the participants' attitudes and intentions to undergo thyroid cancer screening, as many women expressed willingness to undergoing continued screening in the future." And their reasons were clear:

> "Thyroid cancer is still a cancer, and screening is required for prevention, no matter how big or small the cancer is."
> "Because all diseases have a possibility to become a threat to my life, I myself will go on with thyroid cancer screening, regardless of the debate surrounding it."

"Every single disease must be identified. Whether or not one should be treated is up to the individual, but just finding disease is not unreasonable."[24]

Researchers asked the women about the issue of overdiagnosis and overtreatment, and the damage it causes. Fear of the disease trumped fear of those far more likely harms.

"The word 'overdiagnosis' is inappropriate. I think finding disease early and seeking timely treatment is very important."

"For preventive purposes, early discovery of disease is necessary, though it may cause overdiagnosis."

"People have stated that thyroid cancer is unnecessarily overdiagnosed; however, I do not agree."

Another aspect of the South Korea thyroid story reinforces what we found with mammography and PSA testing. Though active surveillance was an approved treatment option, most of the women said their doctors had recommended surgery. The women said they trusted their doctors and followed their recommendations, but several questioned whether they had been fully informed.

"Doctors should give and share well-documented information with patients, so that laypeople might be able to make an informed decision."

"After my surgery, I gained more than 30 kg, and my nails and hair are not the same as before. The huge scar left by the surgery is also stressful. I often have to go on business trips, and whenever I go abroad, I need to get up and take pills at the specified time, which is annoying. Had I known about overdiagnosis and the side effects of the surgery, I would have thought about other options. Sufficient and accurate information about thyroid cancer and the side effects of surgery should be provided."[25]

A Global Problem

What happened in South Korea is chilling, but it's happening elsewhere. The incidence of thyroid cancer is now five times greater around the

world than in 1953.[26] In many countries thyroid cancer incidence is rising faster than any other type of the disease. Since ultrasound screening
came into more common use, the incidence of thyroid cancer in women
has doubled in Canada and China; tripled in the United States, France,
and Italy; and quadrupled in Israel and Costa Rica.[27] And that increase is
expected to continue. At present rates, thyroid cancer will be the fourth
most common type of cancer in the United States by 2030.

In none of these countries has mortality from thyroid cancer
changed much. It remains one of the least likely types of cancer to kill. But
the number of people harmed not by thyroid cancer but by fear of the disease has jumped dramatically. According to the IARC, at least three
people in four who get the diagnosis Jung-mi got make the same choice
she did: surgery. "The majority of the overdiagnosed thyroid cancer cases
undergo total thyroidectomy and frequently other harmful treatments,
like neck lymph node dissection and radiotherapy, without proven benefits in terms of improved survival," according to the IARC. The number
of people who suffer is enormous.

In just the 12 countries included in the IARC 2016 report, *Cancer Incidence in Five Continents* (Australia, Denmark, England, Finland, France,
Italy, Japan, Norway, Republic of Korea, Scotland, Sweden, and the United
States), 550,000 people (460,000 women and 90,000 men) were overdiagnosed with low-risk papillary thyroid cancer in the past 20 years.[28] If
three in four of these people had surgery, 412,500 people were exposed
to greater risk from an operation to remove a disease than from the disease they were removing. Based on the average rate of side effects, that
means that across those 12 countries, 41,250 people are now suffering
some of the general symptoms of hypothyroidism (despite being on synthetic hormone), 8,250 are living with partially or fully paralyzed vocal
cords, several hundred who took radioactive iodine postsurgically are living with an increased risk of salivary gland cancer and leukemia, and
825 are dead, because of choices shaped by an excessive fear of a nonthreatening disease.

An evidence review in 2017 for the USPSTF reported that incidence
of thyroid cancer nearly tripled in the United States between 1975 and
2014, from 5 cases per 100,000 to 14.3/100,000.[29] Yet the mortality rate
of 0.5 per 100,000 did not change. (A separate study reported that mortality *rose* 1%.)[30] Incidence began to jump in 1995 and persisted long after
the USPSTF recommended against ultrasound thyroid screening with a

D rating in 1999. The USPSTF evidence review reported, "Although ultrasonography of the neck using high-risk sonographic characteristics plus follow-up cytology from fine-needle aspiration can identify thyroid cancers, it is unclear if population-based or targeted screening can decrease mortality rates or improve important patient health outcomes. Screening that results in the identification of indolent thyroid cancers, and treatment of these overdiagnosed cancers, may increase the risk of patient harms."[31]

The United States has no formal ultrasound thyroid screening program, but even without it, thyroid cancer is still being found and overdiagnosed, in part because ultrasound is still used by some doctors and in part because CT or other scans of the head, neck, and chest for other conditions incidentally detect tiny thyroid growths too. And the use of that sort of scanning is increasing. From 1985 to 2010, the annual use of CT scans increased 8%, MRI use went up 10%, and PET scan use went up 57%.[32] (The incidence of these "incidentalomas" is rising for several abdominal organs as well, like the kidneys and liver, and a portion of these cancers also turn out to be overdiagnosed.)

As a result, until 2017 thyroid cancer was the most rapidly increasing cancer in the United States, growing faster in the 65 and older age group than in any other.[33] There were an estimated 44,280 cases in 2020, roughly twice as many as in 2000.[34]

Overdiagnosis, Overtreatment

Federal statistics report that in 2018, 89% of thyroid cancers were papillary, and 90% of *those*, 35,470, were small.[35] These are the overdiagnosed cases with a close to 100% 20-year survival rate with or without surgery. As of 2014, an average of 85% of papillary thyroid cancer patients had total thyroidectomies.[36] Assuming that rate has stayed roughly the same, it means that in 2020, 30,150 people diagnosed with a cancer that was almost certain to never harm them had surgery to remove it anyway. A review of 67 studies found that between 2 and 6 partial or total thyroidectomies out of 100 (with no involvement of the lymph nodes, the least invasive type of surgery) led to permanent hypoparathyroidism, the condition that depletes the body's calcium levels and requires people to take calcium supplements several times a day to avoid what can be severe muscle spasms and cramping. Assuming the middle of that range—4%—that comes to 1,200 people per year. Between 1 and 2 surgeries per 100

caused permanent damage to the laryngeal nerve that controls the ability to speak. That comes to about 450 people per year. The use of radioactive iodine as a follow-up to surgery caused damage to salivary glands
in between 2% and 35% of all cases. Assuming the middle of that range
(18%), and assuming that only 70% of surgical patients had follow-up radiation, that comes to 3,800 people annually.

And recall the rate of other side effects discussed earlier: 62% of thyroidectomy survivors reported short- or long-term dry mouth or problems swallowing (18,700 people), 55% reported a change to their voice
(16,600 people), 10% needed treatment to repair damaged vocal cords
(3,000), and 45% (13,600 people) reported one or more of the following:
fatigue, hair loss, bone pain, memory problems/brain fog, constipation,
dry eyes, or sensitivity to cold.

That's in just one year. From 1995, when the use of ultrasound to
screen for thyroid cancer in the United States began to climb, through
2016, 10.7 cases of thyroid cancer were diagnosed per 100,000 people, a
total of 520,000 cases. Of those, 85% were papillary, 90% of *those* were
small, and 85% of *those* were surgically removed.[37] That means there were
roughly 338,000 surgeries on overdiagnosed disease over that 22-year
period, about 15,400 surgeries per year. So based on the rates for various
side effects described earlier, treatment for a nonthreatening type of thyroid cancer left 27,000 rehospitalized with severe hypoparathyroidism
and 13,520 people with that condition permanently; 186,000 with some
degree of voice change, 34,000 who required treatment to repair damage to their vocal cords, 5,100 with some degree of permanent damage
to their ability to speak, and roughly 209,000 with damaged salivary
glands. (That last number is probably higher, however, since some
patients who receive follow-up iodine treatment—a population not included here—also experience this side effect.)

Now let's add the number of people living on synthetic thyroid
hormone who are suffering from low-grade hypothyroidism-like symptoms. Based on the rough estimate of how many patients reported such
symptoms on the NATCSS, from 1995 to 2016 152,000 people suffered
one or more of the following—fatigue, hair loss, bone pain, memory prob-
lems/brain fog, constipation, dry eyes, or sensitivity to cold—months or
years after their surgery.

Finally, we have to add the death toll from surgery, a rare—2 per
1,000—but real outcome. From 1995 through 2016, the 338,000 clinically

unnecessary thyroid surgeries for overdiagnosed thyroid cancer in the United States caused 676 deaths and saved very few lives, if any.

Progress

The dramatic lessons of South Korea have prompted change. Screening for thyroid cancer has declined. Thyroid cancer incidence in the United States had risen at a rate of 7% per year from 2000 to 2010 (as of 2014, it was up an incredible 500% since 1975), but it only went up 1.5% between 2011 and 2015.[38] In 2017 the USPSTF strongly recommended *against* screening asymptomatic adults for thyroid cancer, with ultrasound or any other method. Seek less and ye shall find less—and do less harm. Professionals in this field have also made noteworthy changes, more progressive in some ways than those in the fields of breast, prostate, lung, or colon cancer care—other areas in which overdiagnosis of cancer is a problem.

In 2015 the professional guidelines of the American Thyroid Association issued new standards of care formally recognizing the harm of overdiagnosis of thyroid cancer. "A major goal of these guidelines," they wrote, "is to minimize potential harm from overtreatment in a majority of patients at low risk for disease-specific mortality and morbidity."[39] The new guidelines said that there was no evidence to support screening at all and recommended that if a tumor was somehow detected but was small (<1 centimeter), no biopsy be done. Not long afterward, the Thyroid Association took an even more dramatic step.

───────

In 1986 the Chernobyl nuclear accident spread radioactive iodine over a wide, mostly agricultural region around the plant. Cows ate grass coated in the fallout. For a time, as the Soviet government tried to play down the fear, kids in the region drank milk from those cows. The number of kids with thyroid cancer, normally a rare disease among the young, shot up. One of the doctors treating those children was a resident in Belarus, Yuri Nikiforov.

Years later, after emigrating to the United States, Dr. Nikiforov got a call from a colleague about a 19-year-old girl who had been diagnosed with a common type of noninvasive papillary thyroid cancer called EFVPTC (encapsulated follicular variant of papillary thyroid carcinoma; between 10% and 20% of cases are this type). At that time the standard of care for this diagnosis was removal of the thyroid gland, followed by radioactive iodine treatment, and then a lifetime on hormone replacement medication. But the surgeon wanted Dr. Nikiforov's opinion as a now world-renowned pathologist: Did the young woman need such radical treatment for a noninvasive tumor whose cells had only *some* hallmarks of cancer under a microscope, and which had a less than 1% chance of growing, spreading, or causing any harm at all?

Dr. Nikiforov had seen too many such cases. "Something had to be done," he said. "We are doing more harm than good by treating these tumors in the same way that we treat aggressive cancers."[40] He assembled a team of experts, including Ronald Ghossein, who had been writing about this problem for years, and three years later, doctors Nikiforov and Ghossein published a paper proposing a new name for EFVPTC, to remove the reference to cancer.[41] Since 2016 EFVPTC has been called noninvasive follicular thyroid neoplasm with papillary-like nuclear features (NIFTP). The frightening C-word (carcinoma) is gone. Buried in the paper suggesting the name change was one sentence that speaks volumes about the significance of this seemingly small step: "The outcome data obtained in this study support renaming this tumor in a manner that *more accurately reflects its behaviour*" (my emphasis).

Making this seemingly simple change was no easy feat. From the time it was first proposed, it took 15 years for endocrinologists to adopt it. A study reported that among 22 clinicians who treat thyroid cancer, interviewed *before* the change in the diagnostic language, "The majority of clinicians did not believe that changing the terminology of this diagnosis was a viable strategy to reduce patients' anxiety and their perceived preference for more aggressive treatments."[42] Those doctors resisted the whole idea that overdiagnosis of low-risk thyroid cancers may do more harm than good. "There was little acceptance of active surveillance to manage . . . patients. Clinicians did not feel comfortable recommending this management approach, as they were worried about the risk of metastases, did not feel that evidence to support this approach was strong enough, and also believed that patients currently have a high preference for surgery."[43] (Remember Dr. George Crile, whom we met earlier? In his 1955 book *Cancer and Common Sense*, he writes, "it takes courage to refuse to operate. More of this courage is needed in the profession. Not every surgeon dares to follow his best judgment in the face of popular opinion. The physicians are as afraid of cancer as are their patients.")[44]

While the semantic change was being discussed, however, some physicians *had* begun to find the courage to recognize the problem of overdiagnosis and realize that they were violating their oath to "first, do no harm." More of them started offering less aggressive treatment for low-risk cases, partial "lobectomies" to remove the wing of the thyroid containing the cancerous growth rather than the whole gland. These operations produce fewer side effects. A study of patient choice from 2000 to 2014 reported that most patients were declining this option and still wanted the more thorough but riskier full thyroidectomy.[45] Since the name change, however, early research has found that 5%–10% of papillary thyroid cancers are now being diagnosed as NIFTP, and that more patients with that diagnosis are willing to forgo complete removal of the thyroid gland and accept less aggressive excision of just one lobe.[46]

The change in diagnostic language is progress against overdiagnosis all by itself. But far more important is the modern approach of diagnosing a cancer based not just on what its cells look like under a microscope, but also on its behavior—what it's likely to do. As Bryan Haugen, a prominent endocrinologist who also worked on the name change, said, "If it's not behaving like cancer, why call it cancer?" That is the conceptual leap that some experts say must happen to rein in the problem of overdiagnosis of DCIS breast cancer and low-grade prostate cancer—even slow-growing, nonthreatening types of lung cancer, the subject of the next chapter. While professionals in those other fields debate the very idea of overdiagnosis, the medical specialists who deal with thyroid cancer have already started to lead the way.

Chapter 7

lung cancer

When Worry Causes Us to Do Too Much

All last breaths happen for the first time.
—Aniekee Tochukwu Ezekiel

Mark was 78, still carrying those extra 25 pounds, still struggling to control his high blood pressure, when his doctor asked the same question he always asked at Mark's annual physical:

"Still smoking?"

"Same as always," Mark replied in his droll Maine accent. "Just a pack a week. Not too bad."

"Bad enough," the doctor replied as he moved his stethoscope across Mark's chest. "Deep breath."

Finished, Dr. Owens added something new. "Sounds clear. But we should get you screened. Just to be safe."

"Screened?!" Mark asked, annoyed. He was never one for doctors, much less hospitals. "Yup," Dr. Owens answered. "The government just recommended it for people like you, long-time heavy smokers."

Five weeks later, after a CT scan of Mark's chest found a small suspicious spot in his lung, and a follow-up biopsy confirmed that he had small stage 0 (in situ) lung cancer, Mark was back in the hospital, lying on a gurney and looking up at the bright overhead lights of the operating theater, counting down from 100 as the anesthesia took effect and the surgical team prepared for Mark's lobectomy, the surgical removal of the middle lobe of his right lung. He had been told his cancer was small and slow growing, and he had been given the option of just periodically coming back to monitor the

158

tumor's growth. "No, let's just get it out and get it over with," he had told his physician. "I don't wanna have to keep coming back to the hospital," he said.

But the hospital is where Mark spent the next five weeks, the last weeks of his life. He had expected to go home after three or four days, but breathing problems and heart arrhythmia after surgery prolonged his recovery. Then a serious antibiotic-resistant infection developed. He weakened, needed mechanical assistance breathing, and then suffered a devastating stroke he barely survived, only because he was already in the hospital. But he never regained consciousness, and 26 days after his lung surgery, Mary, his wife of 52 years, told doctors to turn off the machinery that was keeping Mark alive. His cause of death was listed as irreversible loss of brain function, with underlying causes of hypertension, postsurgical pneumonia, and transient ischemic stroke. Not lung cancer.

Lung cancer kills more people than any other type of the disease: globally, 1.8 million people a year, nearly one-fifth of all cancer deaths. It kills roughly 50% more women than breast cancer, more than twice as many men as prostate cancer. More people in the United States die of lung cancer every year than colon, breast, and prostate cancers combined. Lung cancer killed 139,603 Americans in 2019, 74,860 men and 64,743 women. That made lung cancer alone the fifth leading cause of death in the United States that year.

It's not just how deadly lung cancer is that makes it so frightening. It's also one of the hardest cancers to catch early because it doesn't cause symptoms—unexplained shortness of breath, weight loss, persistent chest pain, coughing up blood—until it's more advanced and harder to treat. By the time most lung cancer is found, it has spread, and the odds that the patient will live more than five years are low. In general lung cancer is found at stage 3, and only one person in five lives more than five years after diagnosis. For small cell lung cancer, the most aggressive type of disease, the five-year survival rate is 6%, just 1 person in 16.[1]

So if one kind of cancer needs screening to catch it early, it's lung cancer. Fortunately, one form of screening has provided hope: low-dose computed tomography (LDCT), a CT scan that can use less radiation than normal CT by looking at the patient from various angles and using a computer to develop a detailed image of the lungs. But that hope has not come without controversy.

Several studies find that LDCT lung cancer screening saves lives. But several others find that it doesn't. Those studies agree on one thing, though: LDCT has a high rate of false positives—growths that look suspicious but don't turn out to be cancer—and it causes overdiagnosis, by finding cases of lung cancer that are so slow growing, or in some cases non-growing, that they would never cause any symptoms in the person's lifetime. Incredible as it sounds, there are indeed types of lung cancer unlikely to ever cause the patient any harm.

That overdiagnosis leads to overtreatment. So along with the lives LDCT screening apparently saves come significant harms, including many deaths, like Mark's.

Overscreening

The Evidence

Three studies have found that LDCT for lung cancer screening saves lives. The most significant is called the National Lung Screening Trial (NLST). It assigned roughly 53,000 subjects to either LDCT or chest x-ray, which hadn't been found to be very effective. Criteria for screening included asymptomatic people between 55 and 74 who had smoked at least 30 "pack years" (a pack a day for 30 years) and were current smokers or had quit within the past 15 years. After being followed for 10 years, those screened with LDCT had a 15%–20% lower chance of dying from lung cancer compared to those screened with chest x-rays.[2]

But in terms of the actual number of people saved, the benefit was small. Lung cancer mortality was reduced by just half of one percent, or 133 actual people out of the 26,000 people screened in the study.[3] That would come to about 5 fewer deaths from lung cancer per 1,000 people.

Another study, NELSON (the Dutch acronym for Dutch-Belgian Randomized Lung Cancer Screening Trial), had broader standards for who it accepted, and it compared LDCT to no screening at all, not just against x-rays. It found that of roughly 15,000 people in the study, after 10 years, 157 men died of lung cancer among the approximately 7,500 who had been screened, compared to 214 out of the roughly 7,500 who hadn't, a solid *relative* mortality reduction of 27%. But the actual number of lives saved was still modest, 57 out of 15,000 people in the trial, slightly fewer than 4 per 1,000. Good, certainly, and important progress in the fight against lung cancer, but modest.[4]

A third study, the LUSI Trial, conducted in Germany, reported in 2019 that after five annual rounds of LDCT and roughly nine years of follow-up, screening reduced the risk of lung cancer mortality by 60% among women compared to an unscreened control group, though puzzlingly, hardly at all among men.[5]

The Danish Lung Cancer Screening Trial (DLCST), which split 4,104 heavy smokers into groups that got screening or didn't, reported that at the end of screening, 15 people in the screening group died of lung cancer, and *fewer* died of lung cancer in the *unscreened* control group, only 11. The authors concluded, "CT screening for lung cancer detects more cancers and early disease, but *does not significantly reduce mortality due to lung cancer*" (my emphasis).[6] Similarly, the Multicentric Italian Lung Detection (MILD) study, another one with a smaller sample size than the NLST, assigned 4,099 people who had been or still were heavy smokers to either annual screening, biennial screening, or no screening at all. The researchers reported, "There was no evidence of a protective effect of annual or biennial LDCT screening. Furthermore, a meta-analysis of the four published randomized trials showed similar overall mortality in the LDCT arms compared with the control arm."[7]

A still smaller Italian study (DANTE, for Detection and Screening of Early Lung Cancer with Novel Imaging Technology) of 2,450 Italian men who had been or still were heavy smokers found no difference in lung cancer mortality between those who were screened and those who weren't. The authors acknowledged that their study was too small to make a definitive statement one way or another about whether LDCT saved lives.[8] So did the authors of a study of 2,027 people in England, the UK Lung Screening Trial (UKLST), which also found no lung cancer mortality reduction from LDCT screening.

Finally, a study of 2,106 patients of the US Veterans Health Administration who underwent lung cancer screening did not report directly on how many lives screening might save but did find that screening led to harm: "For every 1000 people screened . . . 20 will undergo unnecessary invasive procedures (bronchoscopy and thoracotomy) directly related to the screening; and 550 will experience unnecessary alarm and repeated CT scanning." Of the 2,106 patients screened, 1,257 (60%) had suspicious nodules, but only 31 of them turned out to be lung cancer. The rest, the vast majority of people with initially suspicious nodules, turned out after follow-up testing to have had false positives—97% of the people told they might have lung cancer didn't.[9] All the other LDCT studies reported similar results. LDCT is yet another modern screening technology designed to be so sensitive that it can find anything that might be cancer, and as a result it finds a lot that looks frightening but isn't cancer at all.

Based on all the available studies in 2013, the USPSTF gave LDCT lung cancer screening a B grade, a recommendation that people at high risk—aged 55–80 who had smoked at least 30 pack years and were current smokers or had quit within the past 15 years—should be screened. (In 2020 the task force expanded the criteria to ages 50 to 80 years who had a 20 *pack-year* smoking history.) Expert panels in some countries made similar recommendations: South Korea in 2015, Canada in 2016, China in 2018. But the recommendations in Canada were so weak that the Canadian government still didn't have an organized screening program in place as of early 2021. Neither did the UK initially, because even though the disease strikes more than 44,000 people there per year and kills roughly 36,000, as Cancer Research UK put it, "It isn't clear that screening saves lives from lung cancer, the tests have risks, and they can be expensive."[10] (The National Health Service in the UK did recommend the implementation of lung cancer screening in late 2022.) The Japanese government says that the evidence about lung cancer screening is insufficient to recommend it, and the European Union suggests only that member states *consider* screening programs, which most of those 23 countries—where lung cancer incidence and mortality is the highest in the world—had not yet begun as of 2022.[11]

Let's quantify what this muddle of evidence means in terms of overscreening in the United States and what that overscreening leads to. A study by researchers at the Centers for Disease Control and Prevention (CDC) reported that in 2015, 2,166,000 Americans were screened for lung cancer by CT scan. (Illustrating the popularity of screening in general, many more chose x-ray exams, though that's been proved ineffective at saving lives when used as a prophylactic scan for asymptomatic individuals.) Of those, 360,000 met the USPSTF at-risk criteria for such screening, but five times more, 1,806,000, did not but screened anyway.[12] Based on the NLST findings, that means screening saved a remarkable 10,830 lives (at the rate of 5 per 1,000 screened). But since 25% of those screens

(541,500) produced suspicious findings of which 95% were false positives, it also subjected more than 514,000 people to a frightening initial result and, in many cases, invasive and sometimes harmful follow-up procedures.

The more serious harms from overtreatment of overdiagnosed cases include invasive procedures to investigate suspicious findings and chest surgery on patients that average 65 years old and often have comorbidities, to remove disease that would almost certainly never have gone on to harm the patient in their remaining lifetime. More on those harms shortly.

As was true for PSA testing and remains the case for mammography, some supporters of LDCT lung cancer screening resist claims that it causes any serious harm and fail to fully inform their patients about the damage LDCT screening can lead to. Many doctors and lung cancer advocates, for example, dismiss the damage from false positives as inconsequential and downplay or dismiss the serious harm from overtreatment. The American Lung Association (ALA) "Saved by the Scan" campaign, for example, lauds the benefits of scanning and barely mentions any potential harms.[13] The website offers people's stories about how screening saved their lives, but no stories about false positives or overdiagnosis and overtreatment. A study comparing pulmonologists and primary care physicians found that 60% of general physicians worry about the medical complications from LDCT scans, while only 47% of pulmonologists do.[14] One leading lung cancer specialist, Nasser Altorki, highly respected chief of thoracic surgery at Weill Cornell Medicine, suggested that the medical community play up the benefits and minimize the harms: "The uptake of CT screening nationwide has been slow. This may be largely due to the overemphasis on the potential harms resulting from false-positive findings while minimizing the potential benefits of preventing lung cancer–related deaths. We need to increase awareness among primary care physicians of the benefits of screening and the various approaches that mitigate against potential harms."[15]

A lot of doctors are taking up Dr. Altorki's suggestion. The USPSTF recommendations supporting screening stress the need for a full discussion of risks and benefits between doctors and patients (Medicare requires it as one condition for payment), but a study in 2018 found that, in

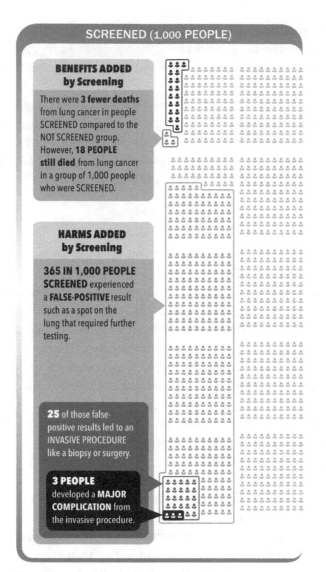

FIGURE 7.1
A graphic decision aid about lung cancer screening,
adapted from a guide produced with data available in 2016.
*Adapted with permission of the American Thoracic Society. Copyright © 2021
American Thoracic Society. All rights reserved. From Slatore et al.,*
Decision Aid for Lung Cancer Screening with Computerized Tomography (CT),
*American Thoracic Society, 2015, p. 10, https://www.thoracic.org
/patients/patient-resources/resources/decision-guide-lcs.pdf*

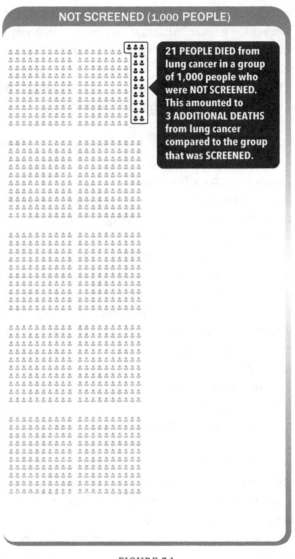

FIGURE 7.1
(Continued)

at least one small sample, doctors were not having those conversations.[16] On a scale of 0 to 100, with 100 meaning they covered all the key benefits and risks, this small sample of doctors rated a dismal 6. And they were mostly leaving out the risks. The study found that "even in the highest-rated discussions there was no mention of possible harms from the screening."[17] In an accompanying editorial in the journal that published that study, the editor wrote: "Although Brenner et al. analyzed a small sample of conversations, there is no reason to believe that these conversations were atypical . . . Evidence from other areas suggests that there are many instances where SDM [shared decision making] is not happening as widely as necessary, including mammography, prostate cancer screening," and other areas of medicine.[18]

Clinicians are not without tools to help them fully inform their patients about both the benefits and the risks of LDCT lung cancer screening. The American Thoracic Society, for example, published a decision aid that doctors can use with their patients, including a chart that helps bring the statistics of lung cancer screening into focus.[19]

Doctors could just show this chart to their patients. It appears that most don't. In the study that rated doctors a 6 on a 0–100 scale, none of them showed patients any kind of decision aid. Research suggests that if patients *were* fully informed, they might choose less screening than their doctors advocate. In a study of 4,246 Veterans Health Administration patients who met the criteria for lung cancer screening, after they were given patient education materials, electronic tools, and the assistance of full-time LCS coordinators, 2,452 agreed to screening. Just 58%.[20]

As with breast and prostate cancer, it's understandable that health care providers and advocates working to reduce the terrible death toll from lung cancer want more people to be screened. They are trying to save lives. They are also, of course, protecting themselves against legal action for not providing enough care. And providing care is how they earn their living. Screening produces patients who need treatment. Customers. All those motivations contribute to screening advocacy that fails to provide patients with balanced information.

But doctors are sworn to do no harm, and biased promotion of lung cancer screening without commensurate cautions indisputably contributes to the harms of overscreening. After the USPSTF B recommendation in 2013, the total number of people screening rose by 50% (comparing 2010 to 2015), albeit to still dismally low actual numbers, rising from 1.8% to just 2.3%. Yet while some of the additional people being screened were in the high-risk eligible category as defined by the NLST criteria, most were not.[21] In the CDC study mentioned earlier, which reported that in 2015, 2,166,000 people were screened by LDCT for lung cancer, 1,806,000 who did not meet the risk criteria screened anyway, five times more than those who were high risk. Another part of that study, an analysis of lung cancer screening in 10 states in 2017, found that lung cancer screening was reported "by 12.5% of smokers who met USPSTF criteria and 7.9% of smokers aged 55–80 years who did not meet USPSTF criteria." The CDC report concludes that "avoidance of screening inconsistent with USPSTF criteria could reduce the potential for harms such as overdiagnosis and overtreatment."[22]

This overscreening of those who don't meet the established risk-based criteria is remarkable given that Medicare requires, as a condition of insurance payment, that doctors referring patients for a lung cancer scan certify that the patient meets the risk criteria for screening. Those cautions were built into the Medicare qualifications for insurance coverage because when the experts reviewed all the evidence to determine whether coverage was warranted, they had "low confidence" (2.22 on a 1–5 scale) that the benefits of lung cancer screening would exceed the harms for the Medicare population, so they tried to build in ways to limit those harms. Nonetheless, the statistic suggests that the Medicare requirement for doctors to certify that a patient recommended for LDCT screening meets the risk criteria is clearly being commonly circumvented.

But that's just overscreening, the first step that triggers the cascade of harm that sometimes follows. In addition to a huge number of worrying false positives, roughly one lung cancer case in five initially identified by LDCT screening is being overdiagnosed. Those cases usually lead to harmful diagnostic procedures and clinically unnecessary surgeries, which in some cases cause serious health damage, including death.

Overdiagnosis

From the moment he heard that his initial LDCT scan had found "something suspicious," Mark worried about the frightening prospect of lung cancer. By the time he got the results of his biopsy, he was more than ready to undergo surgery to get the frightening disease out of his body, even though the doctor said it was slow growing and hadn't spread, warned him that given his comorbidities surgery was risky, and suggested the possibility of ongoing monitoring, with surgery down the road only if necessary. Mark's choice was right for him in the context of his life, but essentially his fear, triggered by his overdiagnosis, killed him.

An analysis of the NLST results by Edward Patz and colleagues found that the rate of overdiagnosis—in the major study on which most lung cancer–screening recommendations are based—was 18.5%.[23] A 2020 update of the NELSON study reported an overdiagnosis rate of 19.7%.[24] An analysis of the Danish DLCST study reported a staggering rate of overdiagnosis, 67%.[25] In the major studies that support lung cancer screening, at a minimum roughly one in five cancers detected by LDCT turned out to be cancer that would not have produced any symptoms in the patient's lifetime. That is the very definition of overdiagnosis.

How can this be? Lung cancer is such a lethal form of the disease. How can there be a type that is essentially nonthreatening? This is one of the central messages of this book. Not all cancers are alike, and not all cancers, even if left untreated, go on to kill. Lung cancer *is* often lethal *if* it gets to later stages and spreads, or if a slow-growing type strikes someone young. But like breast, prostate, and thyroid cancer, some lung cancers have the cellular features of cancer when inspected under a microscope but don't grow or spread, or they grow so slowly that they would never cause any symptoms in the remaining lifetime of the patient. (It's important to remember here that the average patient who undergoes an LDCT lung cancer scan is 65, with an average remaining life span of less than 15 years.) By looking ever more closely for the tiniest hints of cancer, LDCT screening finds a greater number of these early, slower growing, less dangerous types of disease.

The Patz analysis describes the research that explains how we know this:

- Earlier screening trials using chest x-rays found more cancers among those screened than among those not screened *but did not reduce lung cancer deaths.* In other words, x-ray screening found many lung cancers that weren't fatal.
- Autopsy studies have shown that some people who die of other causes have undiagnosed lung cancer that never produced any symptoms. Like prostate or thyroid cancers, some people die *with* lung cancer, but not *from* it.
- And finally, Patz and coauthors note a small Italian study (of only 175 patients) in which researchers reviewed the records of people diagnosed with lung cancer. Based on the metric of "volume doubling time," by which doctors monitor the

growth rate of small tumors over time to try to predict which ones will become life-threatening, the Italian researchers reported that one cancer in four detected by screening was slow growing or indolent, "many of which may have been overdiagnosed."[26]

All this evidence makes clear that, while most people still believe that all cancers—especially lung cancer—kill, this is just not the case. And as contrary as it is to the universal assumption that finding all cancers as early as possible is always best, that is not the case either. But try telling that to Mark. You could reassure him after his initial scan that 95% of suspicious lung scans like his turn out to be false positives, so he might not even want to risk a biopsy. Or after his biopsy, you could reassure him that 99% of tumors like his—small with smooth edges and mostly solid bright appearance—are indolent, slow or nongrowing, and not immediately threatening, so he might want to wait and have follow-up scans to monitor volume-doubling time.[27] But those statistics are population averages. Mark wasn't thinking about everybody else, just himself, and 99% is not 100%. Doctors cannot say with absolute certainty what any given case will do.

So if you are Mark, worried you might *die*, you're probably not going to take even a tiny chance that your cancer will be the slow-growing overdiagnosed kind. Your understandable fear, fueled by all the unique psychological factors that make cancer so particularly frightening, will likely push you to choose surgery. That's what most people choose. And that is where the most serious damage caused by overscreening for lung cancer occurs.

Overtreatment

The NLST is the benchmark study on which recommendations for lung cancer screening, for appropriate individuals, are based. Its finding of a 20% mortality improvement with LDCT compared to x-ray screening is the highlight of nearly every campaign to encourage more LDCT lung exams. But the NLST might also be held as the benchmark for the overtreatment cancer screening can cause. The study's authors were asked how many *major* side effects, such as lung collapse, heart attack, stroke, and death, were caused as a result of treatment triggered by screening of their roughly 26,500 subjects. (That treatment included both invasive diagnostic tests to confirm the results of the scan—like tube-down-the-throat bronchoscopies or needle-through-the-chest-into-the-lung biopsies—and surgeries to remove cancers that were confirmed.) They told then assistant professor Vinay Prasad that there were "27,034 major complications that follow(ed) a positive screening test."[28] (These complications affected only 9 people out of every 100 screened, however, because in many cases, the same people suffered several of these complications.)

But these harms may be occurring at an even higher rate. NLST subjects were screened and treated in the most advanced health care facilities, by the most experienced experts. The care there is often better than in community hospitals, where more people go. A study by Jinhai Huo and colleagues, looking only at invasive postscan procedures and biopsies but not surgeries, analyzed medical insurance claims of more than 300,000 individuals treated in regular community medical practices or hospitals and found that "the complication rates of such procedures were roughly *double* those reported among participants in the more controlled clinical trial setting of the NCI-sponsored National Lung Screening Trial" (my emphasis).[29] Compared to the rate of 9 people per 100 in the NLST, they estimated that nearly 25 people per 100–1 in 4—suffered these complications when the procedure was done at a less advanced hospital. So while the evidence suggests that LDCT lung cancer screening for some people does save lives and has what the USPSTF describes as "a modest benefit," it also causes significant harm, in several ways.

Again, let's crudely quantify the effects of overtreatment, beginning with the damage caused by a false positive—being told you may have lung cancer only to find out later that you don't. Most people, like Mark, are not warned before their scan about the possibility of false positives. Using our baseline figure from the CDC of 2,166,000 Americans a year being screened by CT, as of 2015, and the NLST finding that one in four of those tests produces a suspicious result, and that 95% of *those* turn out to be false positives, at least 514,000 people a year in the United States endure that worrying experience. And that worry takes a toll. In a study of 244 patients from three hospitals who experienced a false positive about a nodule found in their lungs by a CT scan, one person in four reported mild emotional distress, and another quarter described distress that was clinically significant.[30] (Distress was measured using the Impact of Event Scale, a psychological tool initially designed to help diagnose PTSD.)[31]

Eighteen percent of respondents said, "I feel sad more often"; 24% said, "I generally feel more anxious"; 12% cut back on time at work; 31% began spending more time with loved ones; and 32% said they felt closer to God. In perhaps the clearest evidence of the emotional impact of a false positive about lung cancer—as hard as it is to quit smoking, the scare motivated 35% of those patients to stop.[32]

Even though these people ultimately got an all clear, the frightening experience exacerbated their cancerphobia. As a whole, the group estimated their future risk of cancer to be three times higher than it actually was. Most were told that they would need to be scanned for only two or three more years as a follow-up, but 32% said they would be worried if they weren't scanned for the rest of their lives.

Another study found similar results, reporting that people who had false positives rated their risk of cancer as higher than it actually was for more than a year after that frightening experience, and they had a higher general sense of anxiety a year after the screen than they'd had before the test.[33] A related study found that 25% of people who experienced a false-positive lung cancer finding reported elevated distress two years later.[34] This means that in just one year, roughly 129,000 Americans experience serious emotional distress as a result of false positives from lung cancer screening. And that is based on screening levels in 2015.

Now let's quantify the total number harmed in this way over the lifetime of LDCT lung cancer screening since it began to rise in 2010 through 2020. Based on the CDC estimate that 2.2 million people were screened per year between 2010 and 2015, and the fact that participation rates were probably lower at the beginning and have risen since then, to be conservative, we'll take that 2.2 million figure as the average screened per year for the decade of 2010–2020, a total of 22 million people. In 10 years of LDCT lung cancer screening, based on the finding that 25% of those tests found suspicious results but 95% of those were false positives, 5.2 million people suffered clinical levels of anxiety and psychological distress as a result of screening that frightened them into believing, even if only temporarily, that they had lung cancer, a disease almost universally assumed to be fatal.

Let's move to the next harm from overscreening, radiation exposure. LDCT exposes people to slightly more ionizing radiation than x-ray exams, and some medical experts believe even those tiny doses of radiation may slightly raise a person's risk of cancer in general. But many radiation biologists question whether this risk exists at all. Since medical experts assume the risk is real, however, it bears a bit of discussion (see box).

Another set of harms comes from diagnostic procedures and biopsies to check out the initial results of a suspicious scan. According to one study, by Zhao et al., roughly 4% of those who undergo CT lung cancer screening end up needing some sort of invasive follow-up diagnostic test: a needle biopsy through the chest wall, a bronchoscope down the trachea into the lung, or open lung surgery.[35] That's 880,000 people over 10 years of LDCT screening. These procedures occasionally cause harm, ranging from infection and collapsed lung to cardiac arrest and stroke. In the

"Radiation" is a scary word—a fear closely linked, in fact, to cancerphobia—but the radiation dose from each screening scan is tiny. (Remember that the LD in LDCT stands for low dose.) Radiation biologists disagree about whether tiny doses of ionizing radiation raise the risk of developing cancer. Some think they do, while many think low doses of ionizing radiation pose no cancer risk at all. But they all agree that even if the risk is real, at the doses a patient is exposed to in a scan like an x-ray or LDCT, the risk is infinitesimal. This is based on the ongoing Life Span Study of 86,000 survivors of the atomic bombs dropped on Japan, which found that even at high doses, this sort of radiation is a surprisingly weak mutagen.[1] That study found that even at doses massively higher than a normal CT scan, ionizing radiation does not increase the rates of any disease, cancer or otherwise, beyond normal rates for those diseases among the general population. Even at the frighteningly highest dose exposures, to people who were within one kilometer of where the atomic bombs detonated, ionizing radiation raised the overall lifetime cancer death rate among survivors by only about two-thirds of one percent. And it caused no inheritable genetic damage.

Note that this is just true for scans. The risk from the higher doses of radiation used as treatment, like follow-up radiation after mastectomy or thyroidectomy, or the radiation used to remove a prostate gland, is greater.

1. "Life Span Study (LSS)," Radiation Effects Research Institute, accessed Jan. 25, 2023, https://www.rerf.or.jp/en/programs/research_activities_e/outline_e/proglss-en/.

NLST the rate of harmful side effects from lung biopsies was 9%, 9 people in 100. But remember, participants in the NLST research were treated at the very best and most experienced hospitals. According to the paper by Zhao et al., the overall rate of complications from invasive diagnostic procedures triggered by LDCT lung cancer screening in community hospitals was 17%.[36] Conservatively combining those two rates, let's assume that 10% of people who have these procedures suffer medical problems as a result. That means that over the 10-year lifetime of LDCT screening, 88,000 people have suffered minor to life-threatening medical complications from the diagnostic tests prompted by a suspicious scan, and in 95% of those cases—83,600—patients suffered those outcomes only to find that the warning prompting their test was a false alarm.

The most serious harms caused by overdiagnosed lung cancer, however, are from surgery. Remember, the average person who undergoes lung cancer screening is 65, in many cases a current or past heavy smoker, and like Mark often has comorbidities (other serious health problems), all of which make the risk of surgery greater than for the average person. The standard of care for stage 1 or 2 lung cancer is resection, an operation to cut the tumor out, and almost everyone who gets such a diagnosis has surgery. Very few opt for ongoing surveillance, which is rarely even offered. (Encouragingly, this is changing, as the problem of overdiagnosis from lung cancer screening is becoming clear, and as doctors are getting better at predicting which lung cancers are likely to progress and which ones aren't. The standard of care for the least threatening types of lung cancer now includes the option of watchful waiting, an option being offered more frequently, at least at the most advanced cancer care centers.)

Lung cancer surgery is done in various ways, but it usually involves opening the chest wall, spreading the ribs, and removing some part of the lungs, often one whole lobe. One of the most common side effects of such surgery is pain that can last for years. It is so common it has a name, post-thoracotomy pain syndrome.[37] Nearly half of all lung cancer surgery patients suffer some degree of long-lasting chest pain, shoulder pain, or shortness of breath.

Based on the estimates that 22 million people a year were screened between 2010 and 2020, that 25% of them have suspicious findings, that 5% of *those* (275,000) are diagnosed as having cancer and have surgery, and 18.5% (51,000) of those surgically removed cancers were *over*diagnosed, that means that from 2010 to 2020, 25,500 people have suffered long-term pain as a result of surgery for a disease that would probably never have harmed them.

And then there are the more serious side effects of surgery, the major complications discussed at the beginning of this section, complications including death.

- A study of 374 patients who underwent pulmonary resection from 1995 to 1999 found that eight patients (2%) died, and of the 366 discharged, 73 (20%) had to be readmitted to a hospital because of serious complications, 27 of them more than once.[38]
- A study of 1,023 patients who underwent surgical removal of stage 1 or 2 lung cancer between 1999 and 2004 found that the operation killed 14 people (1.4%), and that 38% had one or more serious complication (heart attacks, pneumonia, hemorrhage requiring another operation).[39]
- A review of 83,700 lung cancer surgeries for stage 1 or 2 cancer found a mortality rate of 3.5%, and 9% of the patients had to stay in the hospital more than 14 days due to serious complications.[40]
- Another study of 287 patients who underwent lung cancer surgery for stage 1 or 2 cancer found that 12 died (4%) and 135 (47%) suffered serious complications.[41]
- A meta-analysis of the entire literature on the outcomes of all types of lung cancer surgery found a mortality rate of 2% and a rate of serious complications between 10% and 50%.[42]

These studies provide the basis for estimates of the most serious harms of overtreatment for overdiagnosed lung cancer discovered by LDCT scanning. From 2010 to 2020, roughly 51,000 people had surgeries for a disease that would probably never have harmed them. Approximately 1,000 of those people (2%) died, and roughly 19,000 (37%) suffered serious complications.

(We need to briefly revisit all-cause mortality here, discussed in chapter 6. Deaths from surgery don't count as deaths from cancer. They fall into the all-cause category. This is worth noting because the NELSON study, which found that screening saved 3 lives per 1,000 screened if you measure just deaths from cancer, reported that, factoring in these other all-cause deaths, after 10 years there was no difference in the number of people who had died between those who were screened and those who weren't.[43] A study published in 2019 looking at eight randomized controlled trials of LDCT lung cancer screening asserted the same thing: considering not just cancer mortality averted but all-cause mortality on a population-wide basis, LDCT screening does not save lives.)[44]

─────

As in previous chapters, this one closes by putting things in perspective. The USPSTF review of the evidence finds moderate support for the belief that LDCT lung cancer screening for the highest risk population does save lives. Over 10 years of such screening, it has prevented an estimated 66,000 deaths from lung cancer (22 million people screened per year, 3 lives saved per 1,000, multiplied by 10 years). That is incredible progress against the cancer that kills more than any other. And the number of people being screened who meet the eligibility criteria is still low. More lives could be saved if more people screened, even if those criteria don't change.

But those gains have not come without cost. The issue is not whether screening for lung cancer should be done. The issue is that its benefits come with significant harm, harm that is being overlooked, harm that patients are rarely even warned about, harm that is to a significant degree the result of our fear of cancer.

colorectal cancer

When Worry Causes Us to Do Too Much

The road to health is paved with good intestines.
—Dr. Sherry A. Rogers

Call it the Case of the Stolen Colon, or the largest colectomy ever. An inflatable pink plastic tunnel designed to represent a human colon, big enough to walk through, was removed by thieves from an outdoor plaza at the University of Kansas Medical Center in October 2018. The "Super Colon" was touring the country as part of a campaign to raise awareness about colon cancer. A thorough probe (sorry) by local police recovered it in an abandoned building several days later.

Kidding aside, this effective teaching device helps us get past our disgust with the lower parts of the digestive system to teach people about the second leading cause of cancer death in the United States. According to the American Cancer Society, colorectal cancer was expected to kill 53,200 people in 2020, a huge number given that incidence was expected to be only roughly twice that, 104,610.[1] That ratio of mortality to incidence is so high in part because colon cancer is often found very late, when it's harder to treat, so early detection by screening is vital for saving lives.

Colorectal cancer screening has been doing just that since it was first approved in the late 1990s. The US Preventive Services Task Force (USPSTF) reports that it saves 22 lives per 1,000 people screened, a far better rate than any other form of cancer screening. The USPSTF gives it the top rating, an A (the only other cancer screening with that rating is cervical), recommending it for people between ages 50 and 75 with no risk factors, and they give it a B rating for people 45–49. It is also recommended for a wider age range among those at higher risk, like African Americans (starting at age 45), those with a family history, and people up to age 85 who have not yet screened at least once.

There are several kinds of screening tests. There are the well-known endoscopic exams (by a flexible tube with a video camera and other equipment on the tip) of the whole colon, a colonoscopy, or just the lower third of the colon, a sigmoidoscopy. There are also do-it-yourself-at-home kits to collect stool samples for a lab to analyze, looking for signs indicating the need for a follow-up endoscopic examination. Suggested frequencies for each method vary: every year to every five or ten years, depending on the various kinds of tests, the results of your previous exam, and your risk characteristics.

The endoscopic exams are more than just screening, though. They sometimes involve treatment at the same time. Most colorectal cancer starts as polyps, small slow-growing nodules on the inner wall of the organ. The tube that's inserted into the colon to find them carries a device that can remove worrisome polyps. There are three kinds of polyps: adenomas (nonadvanced or advanced), sessile serrated, and hyperplastic. Hyperplastic polyps don't go on to cause cancer. Adenomas and sessile serrated polyps sometimes do, especially those larger than 1 centimeter, about the size of a pea. Those are the ones that are removed. Two-thirds of the polyps found during colonoscopies are adenomas. But even most of these don't go on to cause cancer.

The problem is, doctors can't tell for sure which ones will and which ones won't. So to be safe, they remove any that might—and that turns out to be many more than would ever have caused disease. (Removing *potentially* dangerous tissue before it's cancerous reduces the incidence of colorectal cancer, one big reason that the incidence and mortality rates for colorectal cancer are so close.)

In most cases the patient wakes up after the exam and finds out if any polyps were removed during the procedure, then waits to clear the cobwebs from the anesthesia while someone comes to pick them up. In most cases, but not all. In rare cases the exam causes serious harms. Both the visual inspection itself and the removal of any suspicious polyps can cause perforations of the colon wall, major bleeding, and infections. Infrequently, patients develop cardiovascular problems from the anesthesia. Some patients have to stay in the hospital for treatment. Some have to return after symptoms develop. That's why this brief chapter is included.

Millions more screen for colorectal cancer than have the risk factors that
warrant such screening, and many of them experience overdiagnosis and
harm. Fear of cancer plays a big role in all of this, particularly for one age
group: the elderly.

Overscreening

Doctors have been looking down patient's throats and up their digestive
systems for nearly three hundred years. Phillip Bozzini's 1805 invention
of the first endoscope for examining the inside of a patient—the Licht-
leiter, or "light conductor"—was a rigid tube that couldn't be maneuvered
more than ten inches up the twists and turns of the five-foot-long colon.
Endoscopy only advanced in the 1960s and '70s when more flexible and
narrower tubes improved how far into the colon the device could pene-
trate, and fiber optics improved how clearly the examiner could see. The
critical development that made colonoscopy a procedure that could both
screen *and* treat came in 1966, at a time when chemotherapy was just
starting to save lives, public pressure for "the cure" was rising, and colon
cancer was the fourth most common cause of cancer mortality in the
United States. William Woolf and Hiromi Shinya figured out how to equip
the tip of an endoscope with a snare that could lop off polyps and cauter-
ize the wound.

Over the eighties and nineties, what was initially seen as a disgusting and uncomfortable procedure gained growing acceptance as another
weapon in the "war on cancer," another tool to provide some sense of
control over a disease that was then, and still is, widely believed to be a
death sentence. Colonoscopies among the famous helped. President
Ronald Reagan's colonoscopy in 1985 was highly publicized. *Today Show*
host Katie Couric had one on live TV in 2000 to promote colorectal cancer screening after the disease killed her husband, prompting a spike in
participation that researchers called "the Couric Effect."[2] In 2018 Harry
Connick Jr. and his wife had a "colonoscopy date" on video. Stars like
Jimmy Kimmel and Will Smith have posted videos of their procedures,
and Tom Hanks, Steve Martin, and Martin Short have well-publicized
"colonoscopy parties"—a social get-together on the night before their si-
multaneously scheduled procedures—to promote participation, which is
now an estimated 65% among those in the age groups for which such
screening is recommended by the USPSTF.[3]

But vastly more people choose to undergo colonoscopy than those in that age group. According to the CDC (in research done for this book), based on people's replies to the National Health Interview Survey, 2.3 million people aged 40–44 and 10.4 million over age 75 reported that they had had colonoscopies at some point during the ten years between 2008 and 2017. Because more precise data are not available, this analysis simply divides those decadal totals by 10 to come up with a crude annual rate: 230,000 people aged 40–44 and 1,040,000 over age 75 had colonoscopies per year in the United States over that period.[4] The health care research firm iData estimates that a total of 15.8 million colonoscopies were done in 2017.[5] So roughly 1.5% of those procedures are done per year on people younger than the recommended age, and roughly 6.5% are done on people above the recommended age. Research suggests that for those cohorts, screening does more harm than good.

Overdiagnosis

Following medical recommendations, I've had three colonoscopies. After the first two, the doctor told me a couple polyps had been removed, without any complications. I was told they were nothing to worry about and were removed as a precaution. I felt reassured that something that may have caused cancer one day was removed from my body.

Yet I might have been overdiagnosed and overtreated. There was only a small chance that those polyps would eventually cause cancer. Most don't, but as a precaution, they are removed anyway, according to Mette Kalager and colleagues, who described the theoretical problem discussed here in a 2018 paper, "Overdiagnosis in Colorectal Cancer Screening: Time to Acknowledge a Blind Spot":

> The prevalence of precancerous polyps in the average screening population is high, namely, 32% in a recent international, population-based screening study including individuals 60 years of age, and higher than 50% in older individuals. In comparison, the lifetime risk of colorectal cancer for an average risk individual is relatively low; approximately 5%.
>
> Thus, although most cancers arise from polyps, the proportion of polyps that would progress to clinically symptomatic cancer if not removed is low. Consequently, most precancerous

polyps diagnosed during colorectal cancer-screening interventions are removed with no clinical gain. All such nonprogressing polyps are, by definition, overdiagnosed because they would not progress to give clinical symptoms or cancer.[6]

There are, however, important qualifications to the conceptual argument that Kalager et al. make, which is basically that if 32% of the people in the screening population have precancerous polyps but only 5% die, the gap between those numbers reflects some measure of overdiagnosis. First, their data come from just a few northern and central European countries, and the incidence and mortality rates for colorectal cancer vary widely internationally and by demographics. In the United States, for example, the rates are higher for Blacks than whites, and higher for men than women.[7] More importantly, Kalager et al. note that the lifetime risk of colorectal cancer is 5% (again, in a few select European countries). But remember, colonoscopies save lives. *Some* of the precancerous polyps excised during colonoscopies likely *would* have developed into life-threatening disease. According to the National Cancer Institute, the mortality rate for this type of cancer (in the United States) has dropped 50% since 1975, roughly when this procedure started to be used. (It has also dropped elsewhere, at different rates.) Without colonoscopies, the lifetime risk of colorectal cancer mortality might be higher than 5%.

So the statistical comparison on which Kalager et al. base their case for overdiagnosis is a persuasive but merely theoretical argument. The Kalager paper suggests only that some polyps are overdiagnosed, probably many, but it can't say how many. Nonetheless, they are not the first to raise concern about the gap between the higher prevalence of polyps and the lower rate of colorectal cancer mortality. Back in 2002, years before the general problem of overdiagnosis was recognized, the *New York Times* ran a story about the rising popularity of colonoscopies in which it quoted Michael Pignone, then an assistant professor of medicine at the University of North Carolina, who noted just what Kalager et al. did, worrying that as colonoscopies were being widely promoted, their side effects were ignored. "Ninety-five percent of the population will never get colorectal cancer . . . so why subject everyone to a risky procedure?"[8]

While overdiagnosis in colonoscopy may be real when considered from the statistical general population perspective, it's challenging for doctors to recognize on a patient-by-patient basis, because the only thing they have to go on when deciding whether to remove a polyp, bump, or irregularity is what it looks like. There are guidelines for which growths are more dangerous and warrant removal, based on the type of polyp, its size, its shape, and whether it is partially embedded in the colon wall (an indication cancer may have begun). But these are only guidelines, not hard biological evidence of which growths will go on to cause cancer and which ones won't. So the doctor has to make an on-the-spot decision. There is no waiting around while tissue samples are harvested and taken to a lab for microscopic examination. Colonoscopy skips that crucial step. By the time the tissue is finally inspected in a lab, days later, determining whether the polyp was cancerous, precancerous, or unlikely to ever cause any harm (overdiagnosed), the patient is either up and gone, or in some cases being treated for the damage that occurred when the polyp was removed, a removal of tissue that in some cases was never going to cause any damage.

Colonoscopy and sigmoidoscopy are by their very nature precautionary. That seemingly reassuring approach almost guarantees overdiagnosis and overtreatment, but it is also precisely why these procedures save so many lives, as Kalager and colleagues recognize: "Because it is unknown which polyps would progress to symptomatic cancer, the success of screening depends on a high detection and removal rate of all precancerous polyps."

That detection rate is rising. When screening programs get their professional ratings, one of the measures on which they're judged is the adenoma detection rate (ADR), and the more the better, because in general, the more polyps found and removed, the less likely the patient will develop colon cancer. But a higher ADR also means a greater chance that polyps will be removed that don't need to be. Evidence suggests that "a worldwide race for higher ADR values" is well underway.[9]

To be sure, that race is driven in part by doctors' dedication to saving lives. But the race has an economic as well as a medical incentive. As of 2021, when a colonoscopy started as a screening exam of an asymptomatic patient, an investigation merely to determine whether there were any polyps at all, Medicare paid doctors $190 and hospitals $790. (Ambulatory surgical care centers not affiliated with hospitals get a lower rate.)

But if any polyps were found *and* removed, the procedure was then called a "therapeutic" exam, and the doctor was paid either $204 or $258, depending on how the removal was done, and the hospital was paid $1,000. Those payments are even larger if the patient is covered by commercial insurance. In short, doctors and hospitals are paid much more to remove polyps than to just find them.

In addition, Medicare provides general economic incentives to health care providers that meet or exceed certain standards and penalizes those that don't with reductions in how much they can bill. The goal of these rules is to encourage quality care, and finding more polyps is considered a key indicator of better quality. In 2020 when the ADR standard was removed as a basis for those potential incentives (for reasons having nothing to do with overdiagnosis), the professional societies representing doctors who perform colonoscopies erupted in protest.[10] Meeting or exceeding the ADR makes them money.

So in a tangible way, there are potential dollar signs on every suspicious polyp spotted during a colonoscopy, an incentive that reduces cancer mortality but also increases the possibility of overdiagnosis and overtreatment.

Overtreatment

There is a greater likelihood that overdiagnosis and overtreatment are occurring among the elderly because colon cancer is slow growing. It can take 10 years or more for a precancerous polyp to develop into symptomatic cancer, and most people at age 75 or above are statistically in the final several years of their lives. From that age on, a person with this type of cancer is likely to die of something else first. So at or beyond that age, the potential harms of the screening outweigh the benefits, which is why the USPSTF does not recommend colonoscopy for people 75 and older (for those who have already had such an exam with negative results).

And if overdiagnosis and overtreatment are occurring, as seems to be the case, the elderly are at greater risk of harm. Older people are more likely to have other health problems and weaker immune systems, so they are more vulnerable to the various things that can go wrong during a colonoscopy. As the author of "Performing Colonoscopy in Elderly and Very Elderly Patients: Risks, Costs and Benefits" wrote: "Colonoscopy in very elderly patients carries a greater risk of complications and morbidity than in younger patients. Thus, colonoscopy in elderly patients should be performed only after careful consideration of potential benefits, risks and patient preferences."[11]

Infrequently, colonoscopies have side effects, sometimes from the anesthesia but mostly related to the excision of polyps. A literature review reported: "Clinically significant adverse events during (flexible colonoscopy) were seen in 2.9 per 1,000 asymptomatic individuals in 12 combined studies. This included perforation, hemorrhage, diverticulitis, cardiovascular events, severe abdominal pain, and death."[12] These effects are rare, but they do happen, and given the huge number of people who undergo colonoscopy, there are a lot of victims.

For people over 65, for every 10,000 colonoscopies, 14 lead to infections serious enough to require a visit to the emergency room or rehospitalization, 10 result in perforations of the colon wall (requiring follow-up surgery if the hole is big enough), 63 result in gastrointestinal bleeding, 191 produce cardiovascular or pulmonary complications from anesthesia, and 10 lead to death (officially from other causes—part of all-cause mortality—but triggered by the procedure).[13] These events are more common for those over 75.[14]

Again, those rates are very low for any individual, but now let's apply them to the estimated 1,040,000 people over the cutoff age of 75 who, according to the CDC, had colonoscopies in 2017. To be conservative, let's reduce the total number of people who screened by 10%, to account for those who had exams because they had symptoms or specific risk factors like family history. That means that very roughly, 940,000 asymptomatic people 75 and older with no risk factors had a screening colonoscopy in 2017. (To be even more conservative while calculating side effects, this analysis uses only the rate of those side effects noted above, for people over 65, though the rate for those over 75 is higher.)

These assumptions mean that 13,200 people 75 and older suffered an infection that required an emergency room visit or rehospitalization, 9,400 suffered perforations of the colon wall (sometimes requiring follow-up surgery), 59,200 suffered gastrointestinal bleeding, 180,000 had cardiovascular or pulmonary complications from anesthesia, and *9,400 people died* as a result of cancer screening that experts say is more likely to harm than help for that age group. In one year. (These numbers are not cumulative. Some who died may have been in the groups initially suffering other side effects.)

Now let's consider what that means for the 21 years from 1997, when colonoscopy was first formally recommended by professional medical organizations, through 2017. Once again, specific data are not available, but the following numbers provide a rough idea of the total number of screening colonoscopies of asymptomatic average-risk individuals, of all ages, performed in that period:

- The *New York Times* in 2002 cited figures from the journal *Gastrointestinal Endoscopy* reporting that in 1999, before Medicare added routine screening colonoscopy as a benefit, 4.4 million Americans had colonoscopies.[15]
- A study estimated that in 2012, 15 million colonoscopies were done in the United States.[16]
- Another analysis estimated that 14 million colonoscopies were done in the United States in 2013; 10.7 million were screening exams on asymptomatic patients.[17]
- The medical research firm iData reported that the total had risen to 16.6 million by 2021.[18]

Based on those figures, it is estimated that an average of roughly 10 million people a year, of all ages, have had a colonoscopy in the United States since 1997. Again, let's reduce the total number of exams by 10% to account for those who had symptoms or specific risk factors like family history. That comes to 9 million asymptomatic people per year, 189 million exams from 1997 through 2017 on people of all ages.

At the rate of 22 lives saved per 1,000 (of all ages) according to the USPSTF, colorectal cancer screening has saved a remarkable 4.2 million lives. But now let's consider the lives it has taken, just among the overscreened population 75 and over, the age beyond which the USPSTF finds that the harm from colonoscopy outweighs the benefit, and therefore the age group in which all treatment—from a statistical population-level perspective—can be considered overtreatment.

As noted earlier, the annual rate of overscreening in this age group (as of 2017) was roughly 6.5%. So very roughly, of the 189 million procedures done on asymptomatic individuals in those 21 years, 11.3 million were done on people older than the recommended age for such tests, people for whom the procedure was more likely to harm them than provide benefit.

The mortality rate from this procedure is low for any given individual, just 10 in every 10,000 screened for those above age 65. But on a population basis, that means that from 1997 through 2017, overscreening and overtreatment of colon cancer by colonoscopy led to the death of roughly 11,300 people 75 and older, people so worried about colon cancer that they tried to lengthen their lives by undergoing a procedure that shortened their lives instead.

And that's just on the overscreened population 75 and over. The statistical gap that Kalager et al. have observed between the rate of polyps removed (32%) and lifetime colorectal cancer mortality rates (5%) suggests that overdiagnosis and overtreatment affects those *within* the recommended ages for screening too. The CDC figures for 2017 that found that 8% of those screening were below or above the recommended age suggests that of the 16.6 million total such exams being done each year (as of 2021, according to iData Research), roughly 15.3 million are done on age-appropriate individuals. Again reducing that by 10% to eliminate those done on people who are symptomatic or have elevated risk factors, then very roughly, 13.7 million asymptomatic average risk individuals who *are* within the recommended ages of 50-75 currently have screening colonoscopies in the United States per year. Some of them are overdiagnosed and overtreated and endure side effects too, though at a lower rate than among the elderly, for whom any kind of surgery is higher risk.

In "Complications of Colonoscopy," the American Society for Gastrointestinal Endoscopy reports the overall rate of side effects at 0.9% for cardiovascular complications, 0.3% for perforations, 0.4% for serious bleeding, and death at 0.03%.[19]

That means that as a result of screening colonoscopies on *age-appropriate asymptomatic individuals*, an estimated 108,000 people experience cardiovascular complications, 36,000 suffer perforations, 48,000 suffer serious bleeding, and 3,600 die in the United States *per year* at the current rate of colonoscopy screening. And over the 21 years from 1997 through 2017, when an average of 8.3 million such tests were done per year on this population, a total of 174.3 million, roughly 756,000 experienced cardiovascular complications, 252,000 suffered perforations, 33,600 suffered serious bleeding, and 25,200 died.

Now to maintain focus on the main topic of this book—the harm caused not by cancer but by fear of cancer—we have to estimate how many of these side effects are caused by the overdiagnosis among age-appropriate patients that Kalagher et al. suggest. The problem is, we can't. As explained earlier, there is no way to quantify how many polyps are removed during colonoscopies that don't need to be. The rate of overdiagnosis that Kalagher et al. theorize is unknown. But in an effort to provide some numerical perspective, based on the figures from Kalager et al.—32% removal versus only a 5% lifetime colorectal cancer mortality rate—this analysis very conservatively theorizes that just 1 polyp removed for every 20 colonoscopies, just 5%, involves overdiagnosis and over-treatment. Five percent of 8.3 million procedures per year comes to 415,000 overdiagnosed cases annually. On that crude, conservative, and theoretical assumption, 3,700 age-appropriate asymptomatic individuals suffer cardiovascular problems, 1,200 suffer perforations, 1,700 suffer serious bleeding, and 125 die per year from overdiagnosis and overtreatment of colorectal cancer caused by colonoscopy.

It bears repeating that these numbers are theoretical, crude, and based on numerous assumptions. Even more, it must be emphasized that colonoscopy saves far more people than it harms. As with the data in previous chapters, the numbers presented here are only offered to add to the general point—that even the most effective cancer screening, which under the dark cloud of our fears we've come to believe in so blindly, has costs as well as benefits.

Chapter 9

underscreening

When Fear Scares Us Out of Doing Enough

What you don't know can't hurt you. A dubious maxim: sometimes what you don't know can hurt you very much.
—Margaret Atwood

Lara had plenty of reason to fear cancer. When she was 20 she
watched as, over 13 emotionally torturous months, breast cancer cruelly killed her 58-year-old mother. Now Lara was 35. She was in good
health and knew that mammography was not recommended until
age 40 for women like her. But she had a newborn daughter and
understood that, given her family history, her doctor's recommendation for an initial baseline mammogram made sense—made
sense intellectually, anyway.

But fear of what that test might find was so strong that it was two
years before Lara had the courage to go in for a scan. When she did,
in the dressing room at the hospital, as she changed into the gown
preparing for the exam, she melted into tears of apprehension.

Two hours later she learned that the scan had found nothing
suspicious.

Given all the evidence of screening's potential harms, it must be
repeated that some types of screening, for some people, do save lives.
Breast, cervical, prostate, colorectal, and lung cancer screening are recommended by some medical authorities for people with certain characteristics because, at the population level, those examinations have net benefit
for those people. The statistics about participation seem encouraging.

Many asymptomatic people *are* being checked (table 9.1). But a huge number are *not* being screened (table 9.2). More than 70 million people who should screen for various kinds of cancer don't.

There are many reasons that people who should be screening for cancer don't. Fear of cancer is only one of them.

TABLE 9.1.

Participation in Recommended Cancer Screening (USPSTF A and B Ratings), United States, 2015

TYPE OF CANCER	TOTAL NUMBER SCREENED	TOTAL POPULATION IN THE RECOMMENDED GROUP (%)
CERVICAL (Pap smear within the last 3 years)	78.5 million women aged 21–65	82
BREAST (mammography within the past 2 years)	33.7 million women aged 50–74	72
COLON—WOMEN (colonoscopy within the past 10 years, sigmoidoscopy within the past 5 years, FOBT within the past year)	29.5 million women aged 50–75	63
COLON—MEN (colonoscopy within the past 10 years, sigmoidoscopy within the past 5 years, FOBT within the past year)	29 million men aged 50–75	62
LUNG (figures predate USPSTF recommendations broadened in late 2020)	320,000	4

Source: *I. J. Hall, F. K. L. Tangka, S. A. Sabatino, T. D. Thompson, B. I. Graubard, and N. Breen, "Patterns and Trends in Cancer Screening in the United States,"* CME Activity 15 (2018), *https://www.cdc.gov/pcd/issues/2018/17_0465.htm.*

TABLE 9.2.

Lack of Participation in Recommended Cancer Screening by People for Whom Screening Was Recommended (USPSTF A and B Ratings), United States, 2015

TYPE OF CANCER	TOTAL NUMBER *NOT* SCREENED	TOTAL POPULATION IN THE RECOMMENDED GROUP (%)
CERVICAL (Pap smear within the last 3 years)	17.2 million	18
BREAST (mammography within the past 2 years)	13.1 million women aged 50–74	28
COLON—WOMEN (colonoscopy within the past 10 years, sigmoidoscopy within the past 5 years, FOBT within the past year)	17.3 million women aged 50–75	37
COLON—MEN (colonoscopy within the past 10 years, sigmoidoscopy within the past 5 years, FOBT within the past year)	17.8 million men aged 50–75	38
LUNG	7.7 million	96

- Some people think that their healthy lifestyle or lack of cancer in their immediate family makes screening unnecessary.
- Millions of people, particularly in lower socioeconomic groups, don't know many of the cancer risk factors, such as age, genetics, obesity, alcohol consumption, and others.
- Some are put off by the uncomfortable or unpleasant nature of the screening process.
- Many are not insured and can't afford it.
- Many have no easy access to screening facilities.

- Some don't trust the health care system.
- Some cancers are still so socially stigmatized (lung cancer, breast cancer for some cultures) that people don't screen because they fear being shunned if they have it.
- And finally, there is fear of cancer itself. Some people are so afraid of cancer that they simply don't want to face finding out they have it. People like Lara.

These factors don't just keep many people away from initial screening. The same factors also help explain why many women who are notified of abnormal mammography results never come back for the recommended follow-up screen. A literature review of 17 studies reported in 2021, "Failure to follow-up abnormal screening mammograms within 3 and at 6 months ranged from 7.2%–33% and 27.3%–71.6%, respectively."[1]

In general, fear of cancer motivates most people *toward* screening. But it also scares a huge number of people away, and that form of cancerphobia also causes real harm. Lara was lucky. No cancer was found. But thousands—probably more—whose fear leads them to forgo screening do indeed have threatening types of cancer that screening might have caught. Those people are ultimately diagnosed later and suffer worse outcomes—sometimes death—than they would have had their disease been detected earlier, when it could have been treated more effectively. These are people whom screening might have saved but who end up as victims not only of cancer, but of their fear of the disease.

What the Research Says

An initial caveat: there are dozens of studies on this issue, but generalizing about their findings has to be done carefully. Different studies use different semantics—fear, worry, anxiety, concern, distress—and they measure these similar but distinct emotions differently. Further, most studies focus only on mammography and breast cancer and only interrogate specific subpopulations, targeting groups based on gender, age, location, race, ethnicity, or socioeconomic class.

Making generalization even harder, this research has been done in various countries, where health care systems and cultural norms differ widely. The studies have also been done at different times, and attitudes about PSA testing, mammography, and other types of cancer screening have shifted over the years. So what follows is a cautious effort to cite a few key studies whose findings identify the overall patterns this research has found.

One of the most revealing studies features a chart showing the correspondence between worry about cancer and screening rate among women with average risk and high risk for breast cancer.[2] The study focuses only on mammography, and captures only the attitudes of women between 50 and 80 years old living in mostly rural areas of the state of Washington in 2003. But the shape of the curves in the chart reflect what other research has found. Low or moderate worry, going left to right along the horizontal axis, encourages screening participation, which initially rises on the vertical axis. But after worry gets high enough, participation declines. Fear starts to keep people away.

Reinforcing this finding, the darker line, representing women at greater risk because of family history—people like Lara who have real reason to worry and more reason to screen—drops more dramatically than the lighter line, representing women of average risk. The greater fear of women at higher risk prompts a more dramatic drop in participation. The authors reported, "Severe worry may be a barrier to mammography use for all women, not only those with a family history."[3]

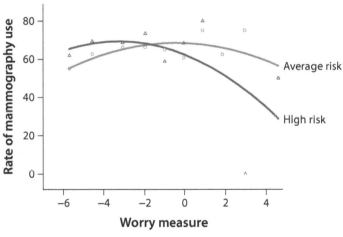

FIGURE 9.1
The "curved line" effect.
Adapted from M. R. Andersen, R. Smith, H. Meischke, D. Bowen, and N. Urban,
"Breast Cancer Worry and Mammography Use by Women with and without a
Family History in a Population-Based Sample," Cancer Epidemiology,
Biomarkers, and Prevention *12, no. 4 (2003): 314-20*

The finding that at some point fear of breast cancer gets so strong that it discourages mammography participation is not just true for women aged 50–80 in rural Washington state. A 1992 study of 247 women with one or more first-degree relatives with the disease, meaning they are at higher risk, found that 94% of the women came in for a recommended annual mammogram starting at age 40, but only 69% came in for a clinical breast examination every six months, and only 50% did regular breast self-examination, both of which are also recommended for women in this elevated risk category. Greater worry helps explain these choices. That study reported, "Higher anxiety was directly related to poor attendance at a clinical breast examination and poor adherence to monthly breast self-examination." That study also found evidence of the "curved line" effect. As worry reached progressively higher levels, screening decreased more dramatically. "Women who perceived their risk as high, had high anxiety, and felt they could do little about developing breast cancer were less compliant with surveillance by breast self-examination, regular clinical breast examinations, and other preventive behaviours."[4]

A 2004 literature review of 29 studies about fear of mammography offers more insight into why this fear deters some people from screening. It's fear of a diagnosis—the idea of hearing those terrifying words "You have cancer"—that scares people away. The authors wrote that studies "have tended to return a positive relation between non-specified cancer worry and screening behavior. Conversely, however, fear of a *breast cancer diagnosis* seems likely to deter screening" (my emphasis).[5] The literature review cited studies like "Underutilizers of Mammography Screening Today: Characteristics of Women Planning, Undecided about, and Not Planning a Mammogram," which reported that one reason some women chose to avoid mammography was "being too fearful to know results": and "Knowledge, Perceptions, and Mammography Stage of Adoption among Older Urban Women," which found that "worry about finding a lump in the breast is related to reduced mammography utilization."[6]

An even more comprehensive review of 155 studies done over 30 years, "The Role of Cancer Worry in Cancer Screening: A Theoretical and Empirical Review of the Literature," reported, "Among women who have refused mammography screening, from 4 to 39% state that fear about finding cancer was an important reason for their refusal of screening."[7] Again, this review found that it wasn't fear of cancer in general, nor fear of the uncomfortable experience of the mammogram, that kept some women away. It was fear of a positive finding, of being told, "You have cancer." (The review cited several studies that found the curved line effect.) Most of the research on how fear shapes people's choices about cancer screening has looked at mammography. But this review included research on colorectal, prostate, and cervical cancer, and it found the same general pattern.

Additional evidence does too.

Colorectal

- One meta-analysis reported that 14% of women and 4% of men said fear kept them from participating in colorectal screening: "In three studies cancer worry inhibited intentions to undergo colorectal cancer screening."[8]
- A survey for the Colon Cancer Alliance found that fear of both the test and the test results were why some older people didn't screen for colorectal cancer. A *New York Times* article about that study reported, "Some respondents were afraid because they had witnessed the ravages of colon cancer." The article quoted one person over 50 who hadn't had a colonoscopy, despite a worrisome family history, saying the reason was "pure fear": "My grandfather, aunt and sister died from colon cancer." Referring to the sister, the person said: "I saw everything that she went through. I saw her fear, her pain, her humiliation, her sadness."[9]
- The US National Cancer Institute's Health Information National Trends Survey (HINTS), a huge annual survey of American attitudes about cancer, asked people in 2017 to respond to the statement "I'd rather not know my chance of getting cancer," 10% strongly agreed, and 20% agreed "somewhat."[10] When asked specifically about colon cancer screening in 2003—"You are afraid of finding colon cancer if you were checked"—15% strongly agreed, and 20% agreed "somewhat."[11]

Lung

- In the HINTS survey, 14% of respondents agreed with the statement "You are reluctant to get checked for lung cancer because you fear you may have it."[12]

- A study of UK attitudes toward a lung cancer–screening program being considered by the government reported that "frequent worriers actually had lower intentions to be screened, and that infrequent worriers had the highest intentions in the NHS invitation scenario. Although preliminary, these results are consistent with evidence for a curvilinear association (the 'curved line' effect)."[13]

Prostate

- A survey by the Prostate Cancer Foundation in 2018 reported that the three top reasons that men don't screen for prostate cancer were (1) discomfort with the procedure (42%), (2) fear of the results (37%), and denial ("it won't happen to me," a psychological coping mechanism reflecting worry that it *will*; 32%).[14]
- Another study found that the more stressed men felt in general, the less they participated in prostate cancer screening, another instance of the curved line effect.[15]
- A study of Swedish men with a family history of prostate cancer reported that while most men wanted to be screened with genetic testing, "subjects with high levels of cancer-specific stress were less likely to opt for screening."[16]

Cervical

- Swedish women reported in 2008 that fear was one of several reasons they chose to avoid Pap testing. "Some women explicitly expressed fear of knowing the results of the cervical cancer screen (CCS). They argued they were aware of the necessity to go and knew their behaviour was considered irrational. Other women more implicitly mentioned that by avoiding CCS, one source of distress was diminished in situations when they had private trouble. Swedish women above 50 described some kind of fatalism, i.e., 'what is to be will be.' CCS was not worthwhile as it could cause anxiety, and some women added that anxiety was unhealthy."[17]

From all these studies, a pattern is clear: while general cancer concern, worry, fear, or anxiety motivates most people toward screening, the fear that screening might confirm that you have cancer scares some people away, especially people like Lara, who are more worried to begin with. The evidence also reveals other patterns. Fear of cancer discourages screening even more among certain groups of people: those at lower socioeconomic levels; in certain ethnic, cultural, or racial groups; and some people of deep religious faith. Distinct as these communities are, one psychosocial element seems to magnify fear of cancer in all of them. People in these groups are more fatalistic, more likely to feel powerless against the big threats, like cancer, that life throws our way. That powerlessness makes any threat more frightening, and some people deal with that fear by choosing not to face the threat at all.

Socioeconomic Status

People with lower incomes and less education participate less in cancer screening. A literature review of 19 studies done between 1998 and 2007 reported, "Low-income, less educated, and working-class populations are less likely to have obtained and maintained cancer screening than their counterparts."[18] A study by C. von Wagner, A. Good, K. L. Whitaker, and Jane Wardle of Cancer Research UK, a leading researcher about fear of cancer who died of chronic lymphocytic leukemia in 2015, confirmed: "Cancer screening participation shows a strong, graded association with socioeconomic status (SES) not only in countries such as the United States, where insurance status can be a barrier for lower-income groups, but also in the United Kingdom, where the National Health Service provides all health care to residents, including screening, for free."[19]

People with lower income and less education screen less for many reasons, including general mistrust of the health care system, less access to the system, and fewer resources that would let them spend time away from work. But it appears that a greater sense of powerlessness also plays a role. Recall from chapter 2, about the psychology of why we fear cancer so much, that a threat evokes more worry if we feel powerless to do anything about it. The von Wagner et al. study found, "There is evidence for an association between lower SES (socioeconomic status) and a subjective sense of powerlessness, as well as a greater tendency to believe in the influence of chance."[20] Another study, of the findings in HINTS, described something similar: "Low educational attainment and low income were associated with higher fatalistic cancer beliefs."[21] Fatalism is another way of describing powerlessness, a lack of personal control.

Another psychological component of cancer fear also appears to carry extra weight in this population. Recall that cancer is particularly frightening because it is perceived to always cause great pain and suffering. Wardle and colleagues found, "Lower SES is also associated with perceiving the physical, social, and emotional consequences of a diagnosis of cancer to be worse."[22] This makes sense given that health outcomes in general are worse for people in lower socioeconomic groups, for many reasons. So it's likely that the suffering of the cancer patients they know is greater than the suffering of those in higher socioeconomic groups, who have more access to better care. That would also exacerbate the psychological fear factor from chapter 2 called "personification"—what we have witnessed personally has greater emotional power—among those with lower SES.

While we know that those of lower SES screen less, there is little quantitative evidence specifically measuring how much of a role the fear of cancer plays in these choices. A 2015 study by Smith and colleagues offers a glimpse. They found that though most people said they would participate in FOBT (the kit that lets you send in a fecal sample for analysis) colorectal cancer screening, people with lower education were more worried about what they might find. Of those with college degrees, 14% said that the test "would make me worry more about bowel cancer," while among those with less income and education, almost twice as many, 26%, said they'd worry more. Only 4% of those with college degrees said, "doing the FOBT would be tempting fate" versus 16% of those with no formal education.[23] "Tempting fate," of course, is a way of describing a sense of "I can't do anything about it" fatalism.

Another glimpse comes from a study of 140 American women done in 1993. More educated women—beyond high school—were five times more likely to screen than women with a high school education or less. Worry was one reason. The study found that those with lower education levels worried more: "Breast cancer worries may pose a barrier to mammography adherence among high-risk women, *particularly those with less formal education*" (my emphasis).[24]

Ethnicity, Race, Religion

In addition to those of lower SES, or some like Lara at high risk, people in certain ethnic and cultural groups, and those of deep religious faith, are also less likely to screen for cancer. Here too fatalism seems to play a significant role.

As of 2010, Latino men were less likely to participate in prostate cancer screening, either by PSA or by digital rectal exam (41%), than white men (57%) or African American men (59%), even though prostate cancer was the most commonly diagnosed cancer among Latino men in the United States (131 per 100,000). One reason, researchers report, is the powerful cultural norm among Latino men of manliness—machismo. As several subjects in the study told Z. A. Rivera-Ramos and L. P. Buki, they feared finding out that they had prostate cancer because "if I have prostate cancer I will no longer be a man." One Mexican American man described his fatalism this way: "Machismo is always machismo, right? But if one has a [serious] illness like this one [prostate cancer], holding machista views doesn't help . . . [In that case] one may as well die because, due to machismo, one will not want to get [medical] care."[25] Finding out that they had prostate cancer would mean facing a frightening choice, between the cultural importance of manliness versus treatment that might save their lives but that would threaten that manliness. So to avoid the sense of powerlessness that such a no-win choice would create, they choose not to screen, not to know—avoiding that difficult decision altogether. The research is clear about the effect this form of cancer fear has on health. As Rivera-Ramos and Buki reported, "Due, in part, to lower rates of screening . . . Latinos are almost four times as likely to be diagnosed at an advanced stage than non-Latino Whites."[26]

Fatalism also seems to discourage some Latina women from mammography. One study reported: "In Hispanic women, great fear of cancer is associated with extreme fatalism about the disease. Most believe that cancer cannot be cured, and a diagnosis is considered a death sentence. This fear leads to the avoidance of the subject (and mammography)."[27] A literature review found, "Many Hispanic women strongly believe that the fear of finding cancer would deter them from screening," and noted, "Several studies report that many Hispanic women would prefer not to know the diagnosis of breast or cervical cancer."[28] In interviews with American women who had moved from Mexico or from Central or South America, researchers found, "Because informants believed that breast cancer is fatal, they anticipated that knowledge of a breast cancer diagnosis would render them terribly hopeless."[29] This fear scared some women away from mammography.

> Participant 1: "I'd rather not go, that way the doctor can't tell me that I have cancer, because just by knowing, that I will, that I will die, just from knowing . . . if I go to the doctor tomorrow and he tells me 'You have breast cancer,' I would die."
> Interviewer: "You would die from knowing or . . ."
> Participant 1: "From knowing. From the fear."[30]

Again, this fear takes a physical toll. One study reported, "Hispanic women have lower incidence rates of breast cancer than white women; however, they are more likely to have larger tumors or metastatic disease when diagnosed."[31]

Fatalism also plays a role in low mammography rates for lower-income African American women. Until recently mammography participation by black women in the United States was lower than by other groups, but that gap has closed.[32] It remains, however, for those at lower income and education levels, in whom health outcomes are generally worse, and fear and fatalism are part of the explanation. That fatalism is understandable—though breast cancer incidence for black women in the United States is lower than for white women, a higher percentage of black women who get breast cancer die from it. So based on their personal experiences, breast cancer seems more like a death sentence, something they can't do anything about. Focus group interviewees in one study of black women told researchers why that they had not gotten mammograms:

> "I just thought you just died; if you had breast cancer you was gonna die anyway."
> "I didn't know that it was a possibility to live after you had breast cancer or had been found having breast cancer."
> "Everybody I know who had breast cancer [has] died. I [wasn't aware] of anything different."[33]

Research about how religiousness and fear combine to influence people's cancer-screening choices finds that in most cases, religious belief encourages screening, in part because it helps people cope with their fears. As one woman told researchers, "Even before I have an exam that I go to, I pray . . . because I have somewhat of a fear that they are going to say stuff that I don't want to hear. And it helps me to be able to go and be calm."[34] But for those whose spiritual beliefs are more deeply fatalistic, who believe that "Everything is in God's hands," their beliefs combine with fear of cancer—specifically fear of being told that "You have cancer"—to discourage screening. A 2012 study of 481 African American men reported, "Men who held more fatalistic attitudes about prostate cancer were more likely to be afraid that a prostate cancer screening test would reveal a diagnosis of prostate cancer." While most of these men said their religious beliefs allowed them to cope with fear of cancer and encouraged screening, the study found a small but direct correlation between religion, fatalism, and reduced prostate cancer screening. "Fatalistic beliefs about cancer cause individuals to feel that they have no personal control over cancer, as if death is inevitable, and . . . fear arousal is then expected to affect actions taken against the threat."[35]

A study of 682 black, white, and Hispanic women 40 and older in North Carolina found the same thing: a majority "believe that God works through doctors to cure breast cancer" and said that their beliefs helped them face mammography and the fear of a potential diagnosis. But a minority, more commonly African American women who were less educated and older, said that the fear of going in for screening—and even going in for treatment of symptoms ("delayed presentation" is the focus of the next chapter)—was something they didn't need to face, because "only God could cure breast cancer." The study reported that "the odds of not having been screened were 1.42 times higher for women with greater levels of religious and spiritual values."[36]

Another study, of African American women in the St. Louis, Missouri, area, reported similar findings: some women said faith helped them with the fear of mammography and a possible cancer diagnosis, but some avoided screening because of religious fatalism. One woman said she wouldn't screen because "a lot of times . . . if we name it, we're claiming it. My mama always says, 'Don't claim it.'" Another woman in the focus group said, "If it was in some way I was to get breast cancer . . . I'm not claiming it . . . If you're a strong individual and you believe in God, and you keep your faith, you can get through anything." Another added, "I think a lot of times if you really have faith, I do believe you can be healed. But other times, you just need to go get checked out. You need to be realistic about it. And I think sometimes our religious ambitions get in the way of healing."[37]

There is, of course, a fine line between how "Everything is in God's hands" fatalism provides reassurance and peace of mind and how "I can't do anything about it" fatalism foments fear. So there is no way to quantify just how many people avoid cancer screening because of "I have no control" fear. We can't even be sure how many of those who avoid screening do so out of fear at all, and how many do so for all the other reasons discussed earlier. So we can't accurately quantify just how many people are harmed, in what ways, by their choice to avoid screening because of fear of cancer.

But cancer screening for breast, colon, lung, and cervical cancer, and for those at higher risk for prostate and ovarian cancer, is recommended because it can save lives. Some of the tens of thousands of people who have the risk factors that make such screening warranted but are too afraid to face that screening suffer the harms involved with finding cancer later, when some forms of it are harder to treat. Some of those people suffer the side effects of the more aggressive treatment their more advanced cancer requires. Some die because they were too afraid to face the disease in the first place. These individuals made the right choice for themselves in the context of their own lives, but taken as a whole, that population is yet another tragic consequence of our sometimes excessive fear of cancer.

This harm is even greater among those who are already symptomatic but choose not to go in for medical attention because they are too afraid of cancer to confirm that they have it. That's our next focus.

Chapter 10

delayed diagnosis

When Fear Scares Us Out of Doing Enough

Yeah, ignorance is bliss until the day
The things you ignored all come into focus.
—Jeff Rosenstock, "Wave Goodnight to Me"

There is always danger for those who are afraid.
—George Bernard Shaw

Recall the tragic story from chapter 3, of the woman who came in to see Dr. David Nathan with oozing reeking sores on her breast from a cancer so advanced there was nothing to do but ease her pain. She had clearly had the disease for weeks, if not months, but had only just come in to be examined because, as she told Dr. Nathan, "I couldn't face it. I couldn't allow myself to think that I had cancer."

Now consider the case of an Indian man described in a *British Medical Journal* article rather uncomfortably titled "Auto Amputation of Penis Due to Advanced Carcinoma Penis."[1] The man came in for medical attention for severe ulcers on his penis that he said had developed nearly a year earlier. It was squamous cell skin cancer, far too advanced to be treatable. His penis essentially fell off, and he died 15 days later. Bizarre as that sounds, the case is not unique. Skin cancer in the penis is rare, but delay in seeking care when it strikes is actually common. (The phenomenon has been studied. Warning: the papers cited here include medical photos.)[2] Delay going to a doctor after symptoms appear averages three months. The main reason patients give is embarrassment. Another, however, is fear of being diagnosed with cancer.

As these disparate stories suggest, regardless of the type of cancer, delayed diagnosis due to fear of cancer is not uncommon. And no one, not even the most educated among us, is immune to this fear.

> He had had trouble urinating for several months, not uncommon for a man in his seventies. It was annoying, the constant urge to go but not much success when he tried. Still, he had "assiduously avoided any medical care." Why? "Because the symptoms and signs of an enlarged prostate gland and prostate cancer are similar. My deepest fear was that I had prostate cancer."

Some people delay coming in for care because they don't realize that their early symptoms might indicate cancer. But this man certainly did. He was Dr. Vincent DeVita Jr., director of the Yale Cancer Center, formerly physician in chief at the Memorial Sloan Kettering Cancer Center, president of the American Cancer Society, and between 1980 and 1988, director of the National Cancer Institute and the National Cancer Program. No one understood better the importance of early diagnosis. Yet Dr. DeVita failed to do what he and the organizations he had led for decades had always preached—see a doctor as soon as the first sign of cancer appears—because of his fear of this form of the disease he had heroically battled all his professional life.

Dr. DeVita offers his story as a cautionary tale in his book *The Death of Cancer*.[3] Not until a knee injury required an operation and his postsurgical recovery was complicated by urine retention did he finally agree to see someone for his condition. He still refused to have a PSA test, knowing its limitations, but agreed to a digital rectal exam. When his doctor reported, "It feels normal," Dr. DeVita recalls, "I nearly cried with relief." But when he then needed a minor operation to reduce his enlarged prostate and went to his regular physician for the checkup and bloodwork prior to surgery, his doctor ran a PSA test—without telling Dr. DeVita or discussing it with him. The PSA level was high.

"You might assume that with my background," Dr. DeVita writes, "I would know exactly what to do and whom to go to. You might assume that I wouldn't be completely bowled over, to the point of numbness, by my diagnosis. But you would be wrong . . . For close to a week, I lived in a daze. What repetitively went through my head were the various scenarios that would take place leading to my death." This top expert, fully aware that even some aggressive prostate cancers can be managed by surgery and radiation, went straight to where we all go emotionally when we hear that we have cancer, no matter the details—the worst possible outcome. Death.

Dr. DeVita's story ends happily, but not without cautionary elements that harken back to topics discussed in earlier chapters, about the harms of false positives, and the harm that can arise as we look ever more closely for any sign of cancer. The former head of the National Cancer Institute was a victim of both.

> At Memorial Sloan Kettering Cancer Center in New York (the hospital he had helped run), Dr. DeVita underwent a scan with the most advanced MRI technology, which indicated that the cancer might have spread to his lymph nodes and bones, truly life-threatening conditions. Finally, he had a prostatectomy, but after his prostate was removed, inspection of the tissue found no indication of such spread. The super-sensitive and still experimental MRI had produced a frightening false positive. A more extensive pathological examination of his now-removed prostate found that the original Gleason score of 9—high risk—had been overly alarming. It was only a 7, far less threatening, a medium grade that might have warranted only active surveillance. This was not formally overdiagnosis, but it was close.
>
> Dr. DeVita didn't get all that good news until a week after his surgery, a week during which, he writes, he was "paralyzed with anxiety," reading mystery novels as a way of "disengaging my mind from worry." More than worry, the side effects of his surgery included "all the postoperative complications you can get. My wound opened and had to be packed daily. I developed deep vein thrombosis and had to go on anti-coagulation medicine, and I went into atrial flutter, a cardiac arrhythmia that required electrical cardioversion to normalize."

In other words, he nearly died, not from the prostate cancer but from the treatment, for a cancer that wasn't as bad as his scan and biopsy had suggested, a cancer that might not have needed such treatment, a cancer that had been growing in Dr. DeVita for months after he became aware of possible symptoms but before he even had it looked at it in the first place. Had it not been for that delayed diagnosis, a delay caused in part by fear, he might have been spared some of the suffering his treatment caused.

As with cancer screening, fear cuts both ways. It leads most people to seek attention for potential cancer symptoms right away. But for a sizable minority, like the woman who came to Dr. Nathan's office, or the man in India, or Dr. DeVita, it causes them to delay seeking medical attention when symptoms arise. No matter the common belief that finding cancer as early as possible is always best; for these people, the thought that they *might* have cancer is simply too frightening to face—so frightening that it literally keeps them away from care that could save their lives.

The problem of "delayed presentation," as researchers call it, has many causes, and fear is only one, and not the biggest. The primary reason people don't come in for medical attention when cancer symptoms first show up is lack of knowledge about what some of those symptoms could mean. Lumps in the breast or the throat or testicles, sure. Bloody urine or stool, sure. But heartburn? Fatigue? Bloating (in women)? Those common signs aren't as obvious.

Another reason for delayed presentation is that some symptoms that could indicate cancer—fever, cough, headaches—are often signs of more mundane health problems. If you have persistent heartburn, headaches, or a nagging cough, you probably won't go to an oncologist first. And your general practitioner may not think "cancer" first either, initially diagnosing those symptoms as something else. That causes what is called "practitioner delay," the time between when the patient is examined and when cancer is finally diagnosed, or the time between diagnosis and treatment.

(A few reliable sources listing the early symptoms that could indicate cancer include "Symptoms of Cancer," the National Cancer Institute, https://www.cancer.gov/about-cancer/diagnosis-staging/symptoms; and "Signs and Symptoms of Cancer," Cancer Research UK, https://www.cancerresearchuk.org/about-cancer/cancer-symptoms#accordion_symptoms.)

But an ample body of research has found that fear alone keeps a lot of people from seeking medical attention for a condition they're so afraid of they don't want to know they have it. Even when people do understand that their symptoms might be cancer—and in many cases, *especially* when they *know* their symptoms might be cancer—they put off seeking care to avoid the ominous diagnosis that would confirm it. And the research is starkly clear on what that means: more suffering, and more death, than had those people been diagnosed sooner.

The same caveat from the previous chapter applies here, about the difficulty of generalizing research findings about why some people don't screen. Studies have found that delayed presentation is more common with some types of cancers than others, that some types of people delay more than others, and that the delay is longer for some types of cancer than others. Average length of delay varies widely, from just a couple weeks up to several years. So what follows is an overview of the general trends this research has revealed.

- A review of 113 studies done from 1966 through 2003 determined, "Fear that a symptom was indicative of cancer, or fear of investigation, of treatment, or of powerlessness were also found to be factors in increasing time to presentation for upper and lower gastrointestinal cancers, urological cancers, gynaecological cancers, and lung cancer."[4]
- Another review, of colorectal cancer research, reported, "Fear that symptoms were indicative of cancer, fear of investigations related to diagnosis of cancer, and fear of powerlessness made patients consult less quickly, although, for some, fear that a symptom might be a sign of cancer brought about more rapid presentation."[5]
- One small literature review, of 24 studies regarding various types of cancer, reported that "delay was found to be seven times higher in patients who reported stress in the period prior to diagnosis," and that "some women delayed going for medical care after symptoms arose because of past experience of a member of the family who had a painful death and they feared the same experience. One patient refused the referral (after a positive mammogram) until terminally ill."[6]
- Among 18 surveys of cancer patients in the UK, "Approximately a third of all participants (30%) reported that 'worry about what the doctor might find' might put them off going to the doctor. 22% said 'I would be too scared.'"[7]
- A meta-analysis of 38 studies on delayed presentation of breast cancer reported that 20%–30% of women delayed

coming in for medical attention for least three months after symptoms appeared, and "that women who delay are more likely to express explicit fears about the consequences of diagnosis and treatment of the disease."[8]

· Of 40 studies on delay after development of symptoms of prostate, testicle, or penis cancer, "fear and anxiety were associated with delayed help-seeking in seven studies."[9]

· A literature review of 32 research projects conducted between 1985 and 2004 reported that in half, fear was found to contribute to delayed presentation, either fear of the suffering caused by cancer or fear that cancer was incurable.[10] Eight of those studies reported that delays were caused by fear of cancer in people who had "previous negative experiences" with cancer, seeing the disease kill a family member or friend, like this woman: "I did feel frightened because it was only a few months ago we lost my father with cancer, and not very much was done for him, he was just sort of sent home and left to get on with it, and I could just imagine myself—same sort of thing happening to me."[11]

· A study titled "Association of Cancer Worry and Perceived Risk with Doctor Avoidance" reported that "29.4% of respondents aged 50 . . . avoid[ed] visiting their doctor even when they suspected they should." Why? Fear of learning they had cancer. The study found that "people who worried about getting cancer [were] more likely to report avoiding their doctor." When asked what it was about cancer that scared them the most, participants often responded with some version of "incurability," the false but still common belief that cancer always kills.[12]

· Finally, in a 2018 survey in the UK, one person in four said that even after symptoms showed up that could be cancer, they would delay seeking medical care because, as one person put it, "I would be worried about what the doctor might find."[13]

Delayed presentation is more likely, and the delays are longer, among those with less education and lower incomes, and among certain ethnic, cultural, and racial groups. As with screening, these people generally have a greater sense of fatalism, of powerlessness, a sense that when some big challenge comes along, they can't do anything about it. Feeling power-less makes facing a cancer diagnosis even more frightening.

- A survey of British citizens in 2010 reported that "lower socioeconomic status respondents were more fatalistic, less positive about the value of early detection and more fearful of reporting symptoms." When presented with the statement "If I had a symptom that I thought might be cancer, I would be too frightened to seek medical advice," 10% agreed or strongly agreed, and the researchers found that "lower SES correlated to more of this feeling." People who rated highest on measures of fatalism were 25% more likely than the average population to fear seeking medical care and a potential cancer diagnosis.[14]
- A survey of 1,999 British cancer patients found that delay was greatest in those of lower SES (29% vs. 20% of those at the top of the income and educational ladder).
- A 2005 survey of 4,319 US citizens with either lung or colorectal cancer found that the more fatalistic they were, the more advanced their cancer was when it was finally diagnosed, a sign that their fear had played a role in delaying their diagnosis and diminishing their chances of more effective treatment. Patients with the highest fatalism scores were 30% more likely to have stage 4 cancer than those with the lowest fatalism scores. The survey revealed some telling differences in fatalism among different groups. Mean scores were 10.5 for whites, 10.9 for Asians, and 11.3 for Hispanics, and Black women had slightly higher mean fatalism scores than Black men (10.9 vs. 10.5). Those with lower educational attainment had higher fatalism scores (11.8 for those without a high school diploma, 10.9 for high school graduates, and 9.5 for college graduates). Patients with lower income, the other key characteristic of lower SES, had higher fatalism scores than patients with higher income (11.3 for those earning less than $20,000 per year, and 9.8 for patients with annual income above $60,000). For all these groups, as fatalism rose, so did the likelihood that the person's cancer was more advanced by the time they had it diagnosed.[15]

- A study about screening avoidance among Latina citizens in the United States who had immigrated from Central or South American countries reported that fatalism led to both screening avoidance and delay in seeking care. The women "did not want to go to the doctor for fear that they will be told they will die. Because informants believed that breast cancer is fatal, they anticipated that knowledge of a breast cancer diagnosis would render them terribly hopeless."[16]
- Among Black women in the San Francisco area studied in 1997, "Holding fatalistic beliefs about getting breast cancer or dying . . . negatively influenced help seeking intention."[17]

There is also evidence that religious fatalism—not a sense of "I am powerless to do anything about it" but rather the faith that "my fate is in the hands of a higher power"—contributes to delay. As with screening avoidance, this cause of delay results from the conflict between one's reassuring faith and their fear of a dread disease, between following one's beliefs in the omnipotence of God on the one hand, and on the other, seeking medical care for the most feared disease of all, cancer. Imagine the terrible choice facing someone who deeply believes that their fate is in God's hands but learns they may have cancer, and the only way to save their life is with medical treatment. Putting off a diagnosis avoids facing that frightening choice. The daughter of a Christian Science believer captures this frightening dilemma as she describes the choices her mother struggled with in facing breast cancer:

I get upset and frustrated when I think of what my mother put herself and the rest of us through at the end of her life. She knew she had the cancer for years. She waited and tried to "heal" it until the tumor was as big as her breast, then decided she would have it and the breast removed because it looked like it might break open and that happened to another lady in the church and it smelled awful. So, she had that operation but refused any further treatment, and eventually the cancer metastasized to her spine, causing enormous pain. She was finally so disoriented that I was able to get her to the hospital. I was told that the cancer had metastasized to her brain.[18]

Below are other research findings regarding the influence of religion on people's decision to delay seeing a doctor for cancer symptoms:

- Muslim women in Indonesia told researchers that they delayed seeking medical attention for breast cancer symptoms, in some cases for up to two years. (The median delay was seven months. Four study participants had delayed for between two and fifteen years.) The women all gave essentially the same explanation: "This cancer is my destiny; I just have to be patient, accept my condition and try to seek a treatment, but only God can heal."[19]
- In a study of 129 Black women, "an association was found between disclosing a breast symptom to God only and delay in seeking medical care." This was particularly true for women who were older, less educated, and unmarried.[20] Another study found the same thing with ovarian cancer; the more religious the women were, the more likely they had later stage cancer when finally diagnosed: "There was a twofold increase in the odds of stage III–IV disease for women who reported attending religious services more than once a week, those who considered themselves very religious/spiritual, and those who prayed many times a day."[21]
- A 2018 study of whether religious belief contributed to delayed diagnosis of colon cancer found that, for both whites and Blacks (in the Chicago area), the higher people scored on the God Locus of Health Control Scale, the more advanced their cancer was when finally diagnosed. Those with high scores expressed beliefs like these:

"If my cancer worsens, it is up to God to determine whether I will feel better again."
"Most things that affect my cancer happen because of God."
"God is directly responsible for my cancer getting better or worse."
"Whatever happens is God's will."
"Whether or not my cancer improves is up to God."
"God is in control of my cancer."[22]

The basic truism about cancer—early diagnosis maximizes the chance of a healthy outcome—is undeniable. Delayed presentation leading to delayed diagnosis undoubtedly causes much harm. Just how much, however, is impossible to quantify, for many reasons. First, different kinds of cancer and their various subtypes progress at different rates. Some interval breast cancers, for example, grow so quickly that they may not be there at all at the time of one mammogram but already be at Stage 3 or 4 by the next one. Delayed presentation is a greater risk for people with such cancers. For people with more slow-growing types of disease, delay is less likely to cause as much harm.

Second, nearly all research looking into this question considers only mortality, so a lot of harm from delayed presentation is simply missed. Certainly, delays in seeking care sometimes lead to deaths that might have been avoided. More often, however, delayed presentation leads to serious physical and/or psychological damage, from either the more advanced disease or the more aggressive treatments advanced disease often requires.

Third, even quantifying this harm based only on the metric of mortality is problematic. Rates of cancer mortality are commonly measured by comparing how many patients lived another 5 or 10 years after diagnosis, and then dividing that number into the total number of people diagnosed. But screening that identifies overdiagnosed disease inflates both the numerator and the denominator in that equation, not to mention the problem of lead-time bias. Screening produces earlier diagnoses of many cancers that never would have harmed the patient, and many of those who delay coming in for a diagnosis have learned they may have cancer from screening. So the "survival time" metric is also an imprecise measure of the harm of delayed presentation.

Fortunately, a massive review of 177 studies involving various cancers, done around the world over several decades, has taken all of these difficulties into account. In "Is Increased Time to Diagnosis and Treatment in Symptomatic Cancer Associated with Poorer Outcomes?" researchers considered these factors and reached a measured conclusion: "We believe that it is reasonable to assume that efforts to expedite the diagnosis of symptomatic cancer are likely to have benefits for patients in terms of earlier-stage diagnosis, improved survival and improved quality of life. The amount of benefit varies between cancers; at present, there is more evidence for breast, colorectal, head and neck, testicular and melanoma, with evidence from a smaller number of studies for pancreatic, prostate and bladder cancers." That literature review also found several studies about lung cancer suggesting that patient delay leads to worse outcomes for that disease.[23]

In addition to that review, a paper titled "The Size of the Prize for Earlier Diagnosis of Cancer in England" estimated that 5,000 to 10,000 deaths from breast, colorectal, and lung cancer (that occur within five years of diagnosis) could be avoided every year if patient delay were reduced.[24] That's 8%–16% of 63,200 total deaths from those cancers each year in England.

Applying those same percentages to the United States and considering overall cancer incidence and mortality, reducing delayed diagnosis could save between 27,000 and 54,000 lives annually. The two countries can't be compared, of course, so these figures can be taken as only a crude guide. And fear of cancer is only one of the reasons people delay seeking care once symptoms arise—and not the largest reason. So it is impossible to quantify with any precision just how many lives would be saved or how much harm from aggressive treatment would be avoided if fear of cancer didn't keep people from seeking care as soon as their symptoms indicated that they should.

But it is clear that thousands of people, probably tens of thousands, delay seeking medical attention for symptoms that might be cancer because they are afraid of finding out they have "the big C." This fear is so powerful that it leads to irrational behavior and great harm, precisely the "cancer*phobia*" Dr. Crile was talking about back in 1955. The economic cost of that harm to the health care system is staggering.

Part Three

=====

the costs to society

===

the stunning economic cost of our sometimes excessive fear of cancer

===

At least 25% of the money Americans spend on health care is wasted.
—Joseph Califano Jr., US Secretary of Health Education and Welfare, 1977–79

In the cases below, the stories are hypothetical. The numbers are not.

Charlotte was 53 when a small ghostlike spot on her mammogram was diagnosed as low-grade DCIS. Her doctor reassured her that this tiny growth was highly unlikely to progress or cause any symptoms and that it even might disappear on its own. Officially, Charlotte's doctor told her, all he could recommend was surgery to remove the growth. But unofficially he suggested the option of just monitoring her condition with regular checkups. As do most women in such circumstances, Charlotte chose surgery, to have her breast removed, followed by chemotherapy and breast reconstruction. The costs of her screening, biopsy, surgery, chemotherapy, and reconstruction came to roughly $60,000. There were more than 40,000 women like Charlotte in the United States in 2017.

Ray was 61 when his annual physical produced a PSA score of 5 and his prostate cancer cascade began. Two years later he was cancer free, but his prostate gland had been surgically removed, and as a result he had lost his ability to control his urination and to maintain an erection, despite surgical insertion of a device to restore his erectile function. This was the price Ray was paying for surgery to remove a low-grade cancer his doctors had told him would probably never cause any symptoms, much less kill him.

The full costs of Ray's "fear-ectomy" came to nearly $40,000. There were more than 10,000 Rays in the United States in 2017.

Harold was 67 when, after years of heavy smoking, he finally faced his fears and had a CT scan of his chest and then a biopsy of the suspicious growth the scan had spotted. His doctor told Harold he had lung cancer but quickly reassured him that it was only stage 1, a small growth that had not spread and that, based on the kind of cells it contained, was almost certainly so slow growing that it would never cause any symptoms for the rest of Harold's expected lifetime. He was offered the option of surgery, but given Harold's age, obesity, and diabetes, his doctor warned that the risks of surgery were high, so he recommended ongoing active surveillance and surgery only later if the tumor grew. But to Harold the fear of cancer outweighed the fear of surgery, so he had the affected lobe of his lung removed anyway. The one-year cost for his care, which included a second hospitalization and then occupational therapy for the stroke he suffered as a result of the lobectomy, came to roughly $130,000.

There were roughly 10,000 Harolds in the United States in 2017.

Overscreening, Overdiagnosis, Overtreatment

The health care system in the United States is often criticized for being the costliest in the world, spending twice what the average developed nation does and yet trailing countries that spend far less in key health metrics like life expectancy. Overscreening for and overdiagnosis and overtreatment of essentially nonthreatening cancer are unquestionably part of that problem. Roughly $9.2 billion was spent screening people below or above the USPSTF recommended ages for such exams, recommendations based on whom screening is more likely to help or harm. More than $5 billion was spent treating overdiagnosed disease with care that was far more aggressive than clinical conditions required. The National Cancer Institute calculates that as of 2020, $207 billion was being spent on all cancer care in the United States annually. Treatment of overdiagnosed cancer was roughly 3% of that total. Fear of cancer drove much of that spending.

Surprisingly, there hasn't been much research on the costs to the health care system of overscreening, overdiagnosis and overtreatment. But the few studies that have been done make clear just how enormous that cost is.

- A study of Medicare-aged men in 2006 found that PSA screening and associated diagnostic procedures (biopsy, pathology analysis, and hospitalization due to biopsy complications, but not treatment) cost Medicare $420 million. The authors wrote, "Particularly notable was the cost of screening among men 75 years and older, the group least likely to benefit from the practice: annual expenditures for screening this population were $145 million, or approximately one-third of total Medicare spending on prostate cancer screening."[1]
- An analysis of men 70 and older in the years 2004 to 2007 reported that the three-year cost to Medicare for prostate cancer screening *and* treatment only for localized cancer, which is most often overdiagnosed, was $1.2 billion.[2]
- A study in the journal *Health Affairs* found that for women aged 40–59 in the years 2011–13, false-positive mammograms and breast cancer overdiagnosis cost private insurance companies an estimated $4 billion a year.[3] The study, "The Cost of Breast Cancer Screening in the Medicare Population," reported that for women 75 and older in 2006–7 (who were recommended for screening at that time but aren't now), "the annual costs to Medicare for breast cancer screening–related procedures and subsequent treatment were $410.6 million and $498.5 million, respectively."[4]

These studies, now out of date since they were done years ago and cancer treatment and medical costs have changed, offer an ominous first glimpse of the big picture, which this chapter now dives into in greater detail. This analysis estimates the costs to both Medicare and commercial insurance for the screening exams, biopsies, and main treatments for the five overdiagnosed cancers examined in part two, as well as the costs of the principal side effects of those treatments. Multiplying those costs by the estimated number of scans and procedures done each year provides a rough estimate of the massive economic impact of our sometimes excessive fear of cancer on the health care system.

When studies couldn't be found that calculated these costs, this analysis establishes what Medicare would pay for the various procedures being considered. Then, to calculate what private insurance pays, it relies on a review of 19 studies by the Kaiser Family Foundation, which estimated that (very roughly) commercial insurance pays 85% more than Medicare (99% more for hospital services and 43% more for physician services).[5] This percentage difference is referred to as "the Kaiser factor." The Kaiser meta-analysis considered studies from 2010 to 2017.

"Overscreening" is defined as cancer screening by anyone outside the USPSTF recommended A and B groups who is asymptomatic and has no additional risk factors. A reminder: this book relies on the USPSTF guidelines, which are produced by unpaid neutral experts. Their recommended age ranges are generally narrower than those from medical associations and cancer advocacy groups, which have unique interests in encouraging more screening.

Before proceeding, some *big* caveats are necessary. The estimates that follow can only be general. There are myriad screening technologies, numerous biopsy techniques, and a vast range of surgical and other treatments for all these cancers and for their side effects. These variables all have different costs. Averaging them together as done here sacrifices a great deal of precision. In addition, the health care billing systems in the United States are almost unfathomably complex. Billing for any single procedure often consists of charges for various aspects: the doctor's fee, the hospital fee, the anesthesiologist fee, as well as inpatient hospital costs, outpatient hospital costs, additional physicians' services, and more. Different doctors and hospitals in different parts of the country charge different fees for the same procedures. Some accept what insurance pays as full payment; some add a charge. Medicare compensates hospitals at a different rate than nonhospital ambulatory surgical care centers for the same procedures. So the estimates below are admittedly crude, intended only to provide the most general idea of what our outdated fear of cancer costs the health care system.

Another caveat: The research used in this analysis reports on the frequency and costs for various screening exams and procedures at different times going back several years. The result is that some of the estimated totals are for different years, which means that they don't express those costs for any single year, certainly not the year in which you're reading this. (In all cases, dollar figures are converted to 2020 values.) Also, this research reflects medical practice from several years ago, and the way screening and treatment are done has changed in many ways. This analysis therefore examines a range of screening approaches and medical procedures for each form of cancer, noting how often each technique is used to achieve a rough estimate of how many of these tests and procedures are done. (The assumptions used to make these estimates are described in each section below.)

The most critical caveat of all is that these estimates are intentionally conservative and undoubtedly low compared to current reality. They only adjust dollar values to 2020 based on inflation, but medical costs have risen much more. They do not include all the additional fees that surgeries involve, like fees for the initial visit to the doctor, the presurgical consultations with a cancer specialist or surgeon, some diagnostic procedures, pathology reviews of biopsy samples, medications the patient has to take before various procedures, or follow-up visits to doctors after surgery or treatment. They don't include expenses like the medications thyroidectomy patients require, daily, for the rest of their lives, or the diapers that men have to wear for the rest of their lives after prostatectomies. And they don't include all the out-of-pocket expenses paid by patients.

So these admittedly very rough estimates are not comprehensive, are imprecise, and are certainly much lower than the actual full current costs. As the three health care economics experts from the Agency for Healthcare Research and Quality who peer reviewed this chapter put it, "the error bars around them are wide." But those reviewers agreed that the following figures provide a reasonably accurate general picture that is no less dramatic for a lack of precision. The cost to our health care system of overscreening, overdiagnosis, and overtreatment of some cancers, driven significantly by our fear of the disease, is enormous.

(One final note about what follows: In the interest of transparency, the calculations used to reach each estimate are explained, but the data may seem overwhelming. There are a lot of numbers. Later in the chapter, table 11.1 summarizes the estimates and provides a simpler, clearer view of the big picture.)

Breast Cancer

Overscreening

As of May 2023, the USPSTF recommended mammography every other year for women between ages 50 and 74 with no additional breast cancer risk factors, like family history. According to the CDC, in 2018 roughly 15.6 million asymptomatic women *under* 50 and 5.7 million over 74—a total of 21.3 million—reported that they had screened for breast cancer over the past two years anyway, despite the USPSTF finding that for women of those ages mammography is more likely to harm them than help. Dividing that biennial figure in half establishes the gross estimated number of women who overscreened *annually*: 7.8 million women under 50 and 2.9 million 75 and older, as of 2018.

But some of the women too young or old to meet USPSTF screening guidelines may have had additional risk factors warranting screening. To be conservative, those figures are reduced by 10%. So it is estimated that a net 7 million under 50 and 2.6 million over 74, a total of 9.6 million women with no breast cancer risk factors, overscreened per year as of 2018.

Assuming that half of the mammograms done in 2020 were done with 2D technology and half were done with 3D imaging (a conservative assumption—the rate of more costly 3D was probably higher), Medicare paid roughly $157 for a mammogram, the median between different payments for 2D and 3D technology. Based on the Kaiser factor, that commercial insurance pays roughly 85% more than Medicare, that makes the median commercial insurance payment for a screening mammogram $290.

For the 7 million asymptomatic women with no other risk factors and below the USPSTF recommended age range for screening who screened anyway in 2018, the cost to the commercial health insurance industry of *initial* mammography was $2 billion. For the 5.2 million women over 74 with no other risk factors who screen, the cost to Medicare for their initial mammograms was $408 million. The total cost to the health care system of just the initial overscreening mammograms—conservatively—was roughly $2.4 billion in 2018.

But we're not done. Remember, one mammogram in eight produces a worrisome false positive and requires a follow-up screen. An additional 1.2 million follow-up mammograms were triggered by false-positive results from the initial overscreening. Roughly two-thirds—800,000—were done on women under 50 who were mostly covered by private insurance, and one-third—400,000—were done on women over 74, mostly covered by Medicare. Follow-up mammograms are a different procedure than the initial scan, for which Medicare pays $155, and commercial insurance pays $255. The cost of these follow-up scans in 2018 was roughly $204 million to private insurance and $62 million to Medicare, adding a total of another $266 million in cost to the health care system.

But we're still not done. Roughly one false-positive mammogram in four leads to a biopsy.[6] That means that 300,000 biopsies were done on women who fell outside the USPSTF recommendation for mammography and had no additional risk factors but screened anyway. Roughly 200,000 were done on women under 50, mostly covered by private insurance, which paid $1,310, and 100,000 were done on women over 74, covered by Medicare, which paid $710. The cost of follow-up biopsies triggered by what turned out to be false positives was $262 million to commercial insurance and $71 million to Medicare, adding to the total by another $333 million.

That brings the total estimated annual cost of overscreening for breast cancer in the United States in 2018 to $2.5 billion by commercial insurance and $541 million by Medicare, <u>a total cost of roughly $3 billion</u>.

Overdiagnosis, Overtreatment

As reported in chapter 4, in 2017, 58,200 women had some type of surgery for DCIS, and it was conservatively estimated that only half of them—29,100—had surgeries to remove the low- and intermediate-grade disease most likely to be overdiagnosed.[7] An analysis of a major database of health care claims (the Truven Healthcare MarketScan) averaged the costs in the years 2010–12 for the various treatments of stage 0 breast cancer, including various types of surgery, chemotherapy or radiation follow-up treatment, medications, and additional hospital or doctor's office visits. (The study did not include costs for breast reconstruction, which are estimated separately below.) That analysis reported that treatment of women 18–64 for stage 0 breast cancer, like low-grade DCIS cases, cost the private insurance sector $60,600 per patient (in the first year).[8] Adjusted downward by the Kaiser factor of 85%, that means Medicare paid roughly $32,800 to treat women for a cancer that clinically did not require that treatment. Converting that to 2020 dollars, private insurance paid $64,000 per patient, and Medicare paid $34,600.

About 40% of DCIS cases occur in women of Medicare age.[9] So of our population of 29,100 surgeries for low- and intermediate-grade DCIS cases, 11,600 were covered by Medicare, and 17,500 were covered by private insurance.

The cost to the health care system of the initial surgical treatment of low-grade stage 0 DCIS, then—based on the 2017 population—was $1.1 billion to commercial insurance and $401 million to Medicare, a total of roughly $1.5 billion annually.

Side Effects

But again, we're not done. These surgeries have many side effects and sometimes follow-up procedures, often including breast reconstruction following unilateral or bilateral mastectomy. A study of trends in breast reconstruction reported that as of 2012, 63% of women who had mastectomies or double mastectomies for DCIS had breast reconstruction surgery.[10] So of the 8,730 women estimated in chapter 4 who had full breast removal surgery for the intermediate and lower grades of the disease, roughly 5,500 had some type of breast reconstruction. Another study reported that roughly 50% of all reconstructions—2,750—were done on women in age groups mostly covered by private insurance, and roughly 20%—1,100—were done on older women, mostly covered by Medicare.[11] (Those two rates don't add up to 100 because that study reported that some women who underwent postmastectomy reconstruction were uninsured.)

Breast reconstruction is done in many different ways and billed at widely variable rates. It is impossible to make anything close to a precise estimate of how much this surgery costs the US health care system. Based on information from the Alliance in Reconstructive Surgery Foundation, Medicare data for such procedures, several studies and reports, and a half dozen interviews with health care providers in this field, a crude and very conservative estimate of the average cost of breast reconstruction following mastectomies is $15,000 for Medicare and $27,000 for patients covered by private insurance.[12] That means that (based on utilization rates from 2010–12, but in 2020 dollars) Medicare paid roughly $17 million, and private insurance paid $74 million, for a total annual cost to the health care system of $91 million per year for this one aspect of overtreatment of DCIS.

That brings the total cost to the health care system of over*treatment* of low- and intermediate-grade DCIS in 2017 to $1.2 billion to commercial insurance and $418 million to Medicare, a total of roughly $1.6 billion annually.

Added to the cost of over*screening* (based on rates from 2018), the fear of breast cancer cost private insurance $3.7 billion and Medicare $960 million, a total annual cost for the US health care system of roughly $4.7 billion.

Prostate Cancer
Overscreening
PSA screening is not recommended by the USPSTF for men with no family history or additional risk factors, so all PSA screening could be considered overscreening: chosen by asymptomatic men with no other risk factors or, often, their doctor, out of worry about prostate cancer, even though studies find that on a population level, PSA screening does more harm than good. But the USPSTF does say that men 55–69 years old should talk with their doctors about whether to test. So this analysis calculates costs for two separate populations: overscreening by the 3.9 million men under 50 and the 6.2 million 70 or older who, according to the CDC, had PSA tests in 2018. (Note: The age 50 cutoff for those younger than screening recommendations used for these calculations is slightly different than the age 55 recommended by the USPSTF because the CDC supplied the overscreening data for this book and relied on a database that divided age groups at age 50, not 55. This analysis could not find data on how many men between 50 and 55 overscreened, another imprecision that makes these estimates conservative.)

The costs for the roughly 11.5 million men within the 55–69 age range who chose to have a PSA test in 2018, even though that test was not recommended by the USPSTF, are estimated separately, in italics.

As of 2020 private insurance paid roughly $50 per test, and Medicare paid $26.[13] So, mixing the number of tests done in 2018 and the rate charged for them in 2020, for that period, commercial insurance paid roughly $195 million, and Medicare paid around $161 million, a total of $356 million to the health care system, for PSA tests on people above or below the ages at which the USPSTF recommends only that men talk to their doctors about a test.

Commercial insurance paid roughly $575 million for PSA tests on the 11.5 million men from 55 to 69 who chose to have a test though it was not recommended.

(Both of these estimates are conservatively low since PSA tests that produce elevated scores are almost always followed by a second test, and those follow-ups are not counted here.)

But the PSA test is just the first step of the cascade. A positive result (confirmed not only by a second test but also by a digital rectal exam, another billable procedure not included in these calculations) often triggers a biopsy. The average prostate biopsy cost private insurance an estimated $3,500 and Medicare $2,020 in the years 2014–2015: $3,815 and $2,200 in 2020 dollars.[14] An estimated 265,860 prostate biopsies are done in the United States each year (21 per urologist × 12,660 practicing urologists), almost all of which are triggered by an initial PSA screen.[15] Roughly half, 132,930, are done on men outside the 55–69 age range, and half of *those*—66,465—are on men below the recommended age, with the other 66,465 performed on men 70 and older, above the Medicare age. So these biopsies cost private insurers $254 million per year, and Medicare $146 million, a total of $376 million to the health care system.

The health care system paid an additional $503 million for the 132,500 biopsies triggered in men between 50 and 69 by a PSA test that they elected to have, though it was not recommended.

Overscreening involves yet more cost. Recall from chapter 5 that approximately 5% of biopsies cause infections that need follow-up treatment requiring hospitalization. (Many more biopsies result in the need for follow-up treatment that doesn't require hospitalization. Those costs are not included here.) So roughly 3,300 men on private insurance and 3,300 on Medicare suffered a medical cascade that began with a PSA screen and led to a postbiopsy infection needing hospitalization for between 1 and 14 days. A meta-analysis of 18 studies from 2008 to 2015 reported that the median hospitalization cost of treating a sepsis infection after a prostate biopsy over that period was roughly $14,000: $15,820 in 2020 dollars.[16] Applying the Kaiser factor, private insurers paid $23,800, and Medicare paid $13,000 per patient for the costs of treating serious postbiopsy infections in men who had PSA tests despite not meeting

USPSTF guidelines: $79 million for private insurance and $43 million for Medicare, a total to the health care system of another $122 million.

Another 132,500 men within the suggested age range who chose PSA tests also had biopsies, and 5% of them—6,625—suffered infection needing hospitalization, paid for principally by private insurance, a total of $158 million.

That brings the total cost of overscreening for prostate cancer— just for those younger than 50 or older than 69—to $528 million per year for private insurers and $350 million for Medicare, <u>a total to the health care system of roughly $880 million per year</u>.

If we include all costs for men aged 55-69—$1.2 billion—the total cost for PSA overscreening to the US health care system is at least $2.1 billion per year.

Overdiagnosis, Overtreatment

There are several ways to treat prostate cancer—active surveillance (which includes ongoing biopsies), various types of surgery to remove the prostate, or different ways to use radiation to kill the gland and the cancer cells it contains. These procedures have such radically different costs that this analysis separates them into general categories. A study found that in 2015, 25,140 men in the United States were treated for low-risk overdiagnosed prostate cancer. Of those men, 3,965 chose active surveillance, 11,061 underwent radical prostatectomy, and 11,114 had radiotherapy (either external beam radiation or brachytherapy). Half the men in each treatment group were under or over the Medicare age of 65.[17]

According to a paper titled "Cost-Effectiveness of Active Surveillance, Radical Prostatectomy and External Beam Radiotherapy for Localized Prostate Cancer," in 2017 the Medicare cost for active surveillance was $12,143; for radical prostatectomy, $17,781; and for external beam radiotherapy treatment, $29,238.[18] Multiplying those figures by the Kaiser factor, private insurance paid $22,465 for active surveillance, $32,895 for radical prostatectomy, and $54,090 for radiotherapy treatment.

Multiplying those costs by the number of men who chose each option, total annual costs to private insurance (crudely, for those mixed years) was an estimated $45 million for active surveillance, $182 million for radical prostatectomy, and $301 million for radiotherapy. Medicare paid $24 million for active surveillance, $98 million for radical prostatectomy, and $163 million for radiotherapy.

Adding those totals together and updating from 2017 to 2020 dollars, the surgical treatment of overdiagnosed prostate cancer cost private insurers at least $560 million and Medicare $302 million, a total cost to the health care system of $862 million.

Side Effects

The side effects of prostate surgery are common and significant, principally erectile dysfunction (ED) and urinary incontinence. This analysis does not consider the costs of incontinence diapers or oral medication for ED, but among the roughly two-thirds of men who undergo surgery or radiation to remove their prostates and suffer ED, many choose vacuum pumps (average cost $300–$500), penile injections (average cost $6,000/year), or surgically implanted devices (average cost $17,500) to treat their symptoms.[19] Nearly two-thirds of the 22,200 men (in 2015) who had surgery or radiation—14,740—suffered ED. If only half of those men—7,370—chose some sort of treatment beyond medication, and those men chose equally among these three options, $1 million was spent on pumps, $15 million was spent on penile injections, and $43 million was spent on penile inserts: a total of $58 million on just the ED side effects of treatment of low-grade prostate cancer. There are wide variations in just how much Medicare and private insurance pay for each of these treatments, so it's impossible to tease out separate values for each. So let's crudely assign one-third of this cost to Medicare and two-thirds to private insurance. That means the cost of treating just some of the side effects of prostate surgery was $39 million for private insurance and $19 million for Medicare.

That brings the total estimated annual cost for the overscreening and overtreatment of overdiagnosed prostate cancer for men outside the 55–69 age range to $1.1 billion for commercial insurance and $671 million for Medicare, <u>a total cost to the health care system of roughly $1.8 billion</u>.

After adding the $1.2 billion spent on PSA tests for men between 50 and 69 though such screening is also not recommended for them, <u>the total rises to $3 billion.</u>

(This estimate of overtreatment costs is imprecise because the number of men choosing active surveillance vs. surgery or radiation has shifted since 2015, the most recent numbers available.)

Thyroid Cancer
Overscreening

The United States has no formal program of screening for thyroid cancer, so overscreening for that disease is not quantified. As noted in chapter 6, the American Thyroid Association (ATA) does not recommend screening, and the USPSTF strongly recommends against it. But screening does occur, either targeted or incidental. Sometimes doctors use ultrasound specifically looking for thyroid cancer, and sometimes tiny thyroid growths too small to feel are detected incidentally by a CT or MRI scan of the head and neck or chest for other conditions. Most of these are investigated further, with either ultrasound or needle biopsy, although as of 2015 the ATA recommended against a biopsy for any lump less than 1 centimeter, about the width of a pencil.

So though screening occurs, at significant cost, that cost can't be estimated with any precision. But we can roughly quantify the economic impact of the overtreatment of overdiagnosed disease, and those costs alone are enormous.

Overdiagnosis, Overtreatment

As reported in chapter 6, an estimated 30,150 total thyroidectomies are done on papillary micro tumors in the United States annually. These are almost all overdiagnosed, highly unlikely to cause the patient any harm. Research has estimated the cost of this treatment. One study, of Medicare-aged patients between 1995 and 2005, reported "Cumulative costs were $17,669/patient the first year."[20] Another, published in 2014, modeled the entire United States population in 2013 and estimated that the total first-year costs per overdiagnosed patient, regardless of age, was $21,000.[21] Another study, published that year but analyzing people of all ages between 2005 and 2009, put the mean cost of thyroidectomies for low-risk papillary thyroid cancer at $19,365.[22] These studies assumed that most patients received follow-up radiation treatment. That puts the general cost of surgical treatment for overdiagnosed thyroid cancer between 1995 and 2013 at, quite crudely, $20,000. Taking the mid-point of the years analyzed by those studies—2004—and adjusting dollar values to 2020, the average cost of such treatment was an estimated $27,400.

In 2021, 20% of the 30,150 total thyroidectomies for overdiagnosed papillary thyroid cancer—6,030—were done on patients of

Medicare age, so using the single cost figure of $27,400, overtreatment of thyroid cancer costs private insurance an estimated $661 million and Medicare $165 million per year, <u>a total cost to the health care system of roughly $826 million.</u>

Side Effects

The most serious side effects of thyroidectomy and subsequent radiation treatment include partial or total vocal cord paralysis and death, but these are rare. Far more common are hypoparathyroidism symptoms, including fatigue, bone and muscle pain, weight gain, and sensitivity to cold. But aside from the medication thyroidectomy patients have to take for the rest of their lives to replace their thyroid hormone, these don't have readily quantifiable health care costs at the population level. So even though the side effects of overtreatment of nonthreatening thyroid cancers certainly have costs, they can't be reliably estimated.

Lung Cancer
Overscreening

In 2015, 1.8 million people who did not meet the criteria for low-dose computed tomography (LDCT) lung cancer screening screened anyway.[23] For this analysis, that figure has to be adjusted, because LDCT lung cancer screening is still new, and participation rates have risen slowly in the last several years. Among those meeting the qualifications in the recommendations, participation increased from 3.3% in 2016 to 5% in 2018.[24] Assuming the same increase among those who do *not* meet current recommendations, and assuming the same growth in the two years after 2018, the annual overscreened population in 2020 was an estimated 1.9 million.

Based on the rates calculated in chapter 7, 25% of those people (475,000) had a suspicious initial reading, and 90% of *them* (427,500) went on to have at least one additional scan. That raises the total number of scans on people who did not meet the risk criteria for such screening to 2.3 million. (It is assumed that all these follow-up scans were CT, although an unknown number used more costly PET technology.)

As of 2018 Medicare paid $295 for an LDCT scan. Private insurance paid roughly $545.[25] The average age of a person undergoing these scans is 65, so it's assumed that half the scans were done on people with Medicare coverage, and half were done on people with private insurance. Adjusted by 3% to 2020 dollars, that's an annual total cost of $646 million paid by private health insurance and $349 million paid by Medicare per year—a total of $995 million—on lung cancer scans of people that don't meet the risk criteria for such screening.

But the overscreening costs don't stop there. Positive initial findings usually prompt follow-up tests, including various invasive biopsy procedures (needles through the chest wall, endoscopes down the throat). A study by Bernardo Goulart and colleagues, "Lung Cancer Screening with Low-Dose Tomography: Costs, National Expenditures, and Cost-Effectiveness," which was based on costs in 2009, estimated that Medicare coverage for these procedures was roughly $1,265 and private coverage payment was roughly $2,300.[26] But not all positive findings trigger these follow-up tests, so to be conservative, it's assumed that they were done on only two-thirds of the 475,000 patients who had an initial positive finding—317,000. Again assuming that half were covered by Medicare and half by private insurance, this aspect of overdiagnosed lung cancer alone cost private insurance $360 million and Medicare $198 million in 2009. Adjusting by 39% to 2020 dollar values, that means that in 2020, follow-up tests initiated by overscreening cost private insurance $500 million and Medicare $275 million, another $775 million.

Based on the number of people overscreening in 2020, then, between the scans and the diagnostic tests that those scans trigger (but conservatively not including the costs of side effects from those biopsies and diagnostic tests, which range from minor to life threatening), **the total annual cost of lung cancer overscreening in 2020 was roughly $1.2 billion for private insurance and $610 million for Medicare, a total cost to the health care system of $1.8 billion.**

Overdiagnosis, Overtreatment

A total of 2.2 million people in the United States, including those who met the recommendations and those who didn't, were screened for lung cancer by LDCT in 2015, when the rate of participation was roughly 3.3% of those eligible.[27] As noted above, utilization among the eligible rose to 5% by 2018. Assuming the same rate of increase until 2020, a total of 2.3 million people, eligible or not, were screened that year. Of those screened, 25% of them (575,000) had a finding of something suspicious, 5% of *them*

(28,750) actually had cancer, and 18.5% of *them*, roughly 5,300, were overdiagnosed with a localized and slow- or non-growing cancer that was unlikely to cause symptoms in their lifetime.[28]

Nearly all of those with overdiagnosed lung cancer underwent surgery. Across the various complex surgical procedures, very crudely, Goulart et al. reported (reflecting costs in 2009) that the average cost per patient for surgical treatment of localized lung cancer (stage 1 and 2) was $72,000 for Medicare and $133,000 for the private health insurance system.[29] Assuming half these surgeries were on people under Medicare age, as of 2009 surgeries for overdiagnosed lung cancer in the United States cost the private health insurance system $352 million and Medicare $191 million per year, a total of $543 million. Factoring in inflation, that brings the 2020 costs for surgeries on overdiagnosed lung cancers to an estimated $489 million per year for private insurance and $265 million for Medicare, a total of $754 million.

Side Effects

There are substantial costs from the serious side effects these surgeries sometimes cause. As discussed in chapter 7, roughly 3% to 5% of lung cancer surgery patients (counting only those who were overdiagnosed—5,300) suffer some sort of serious side effect (heart attack, stroke, hemorrhage) and second surgery.[30] Taking the median, 4%, means that 212 people suffered these effects: 106 of Medicare age, and 106 on private insurance.

Goulart et al. reported that the per patient cost of these serious complications (in 2009) was $21,000 to private insurance and $11,500 to Medicare, so total costs for treatment of these side effects was roughly $1.2 million to Medicare and $2.2 million to private insurance.[31] Adjusting only for inflation, that brings the costs for the side effects of surgery for overdiagnosed lung cancer to an estimated $3 million for private insurance and $1.5 million per year for Medicare, a total of $4.5 million. (This is another conservatively low cost estimate, since it does not include costs for the more common but less serious "intermediate" complications, which Goulart et al. estimate cost $6,000 per patient in 2009.)[32]

So the cost of treating people for lung cancers detected by LDCT screening that were overdiagnosed (based on 2020 dollars but using medical fees charged back in 2009) was $492 million for private insurance and $267 million for Medicare.

Adding these figures together, the total cost of overscreening and overtreatment for overdiagnosed lung cancer is an estimated $1.7 billion for private insurance and $877 million for Medicare, <u>a total cost to the health care system of $2.6 billion per year</u>.

Colon Cancer
Overscreening

As established in chapter 8, the CDC reported (in research done for this book) that in 2018, 1.3 million asymptomatic people with no risk factors and not in the age groups for which colonoscopy is recommended had colonoscopies anyway. Screening colonoscopies that find nothing are billed at one rate, and therapeutic colonoscopies, which involve removal of a polyp, are billed at a higher rate. To estimate the cost of overscreening requires quantifying each group. In 2021, Aasma Shaukat and colleagues reported that in a sample of 2.6 million patients aged 50–89, 4 in 10 colonoscopies detected adenomous polyps, which are almost always removed. Based on those figures, this analysis estimates 40% of colonoscopies that start out as "screening" end up as "therapeutic."[33]

So in the overscreened population, 780,000 were screening colonoscopies, and 520,000 were billed as therapeutic. Based on a 2005 study of colonoscopy participation, which reported that roughly 30% of these procedures are performed on people over 65, roughly 546,000 *screening* exams were covered by private insurance and 234,000 by Medicare, while 364,000 *therapeutic* exams were covered by private insurance, and 156,000 were billed to Medicare.[34]

The American College of Gastroenterology reports that in 2021, Medicare paid roughly $1,000 for a screening colonoscopy and $1,300 for a therapeutic exam, involving removal of one or more polyps.[35] With the Kaiser factor added, that comes to $1,850 or $2,405 for the two different procedures when covered by private insurance. So private insurance paid $1 billion per year for screening exams and $875 million for therapeutic exams, and Medicare paid $234 million per year for screening colonoscopies and $203 million for therapeutic procedures.

That comes to a staggering total cost to the health care system of $2.3 billion for colonoscopies for people outside the recommended age range. (This is yet another conservative estimate because it doesn't include the other types of screening used by people worried enough about cancer that they used those tools despite falling outside the age groups recommended for such testing.)

Overdiagnosis, Overtreatment, Side Effects
The huge gap between the number of polyps detected and the actual colon cancer mortality rate suggests that overdiagnosis and overtreatment may be occurring at some unknown rate among the 15.3 million people who screen and are within the recommended age range. But we can't estimate how many overdiagnosed cases actually occur. Nonetheless, even if the overdiagnosis/overtreatment rate is low, the cost to treat the harm they cause in tens of thousands of people must be in the hundreds of millions of dollars.

Summary

Adding things up, the rough and conservatively estimated cost to the health care system of overscreening, overdiagnosis, and overtreatment of these five cancers is staggering (table 11.1). The total annual cost to the health care system for just the clinically unnecessary *treatment* of overdiagnosed cancers is conservatively $3.7 billion to private insurance and $1.6 billion to Medicare, a total of $5.3 billion.

But that is just for cancer *treatment*. To take full measure of what our fear of cancer costs the health care system, we must add the phenomenal amount spent on overscreening by those so worried about cancer that they screen even though research has shown that screening is more likely to cause them harm than provide benefit. That comes to another $7.3 billion for private insurance and $1.9 billion for Medicare, a total just for overscreening of $9.2 billion.

These admittedly crude and purposefully conservative calculations find that the overscreening, overdiagnosis, and overtreatment that is largely driven by our fear of cancer costs private insurance at least $11 billion and Medicare at least $3.4 billion, <u>a total annual cost to the US health care system of at least $14.4 billion</u>.

But the economic costs to the health care system of our fear of cancer don't stop there.

Underscreening and Delayed Diagnosis

It is impossible to quantify how many people for whom screening is recommended avoid those initial exams or the follow-up tests suggested

TABLE 11.1.

Conservative Annual Cost of Overscreening, Overdiagnosis, and Overtreatment of Five Cancers, United States

TYPE OF CANCER	PRIVATE INSURANCE ($)	MEDICARE ($)	TOTAL ($)
BREAST			
Overscreening	2.5 billion	541 million	3 billion
Overtreatment	2 billion	750 million	2.8 billion
Total cost	**4.5 billion**	**1.3 billion**	**5.8 billion**
PROSTATE			
Overscreening on men younger or older than 50–69 (CDC data)	528 million	350 million	880 million
Overscreening on men 50–69 (CDC data)	1.2 billion	Data not available	1.2 billion
Total overscreening cost			2.1 billion
Overtreatment	599 million	321 million	920 million
Total overscreening and overtreatment cost	**2.3 billion**	**670 million**	**3 billion**
THYROID			
Overtreatment	607 million	152 million	759 million
LUNG			
Overscreening	1.2 billion	610 million	1.8 billion
Overtreatment	492 million	267 million	759 million
Total	**1.7 billion**	**877 million**	**2.6 billion**
COLON			
Overscreening	1.9 billion	437 million	2.3 billion
ALL FIVE CANCERS			
Overscreening	7.3 billion	1.9 billion	9.2 billion
Overtreatment	3.7 billion	1.5 billion	5.2 billion
Total	**11 billion**	**3.4 billion**	**14.4 billion**

after suspicious initial findings, because they're worried about finding out they have cancer. It's also impossible to know how many people with symptoms that may be cancer delay seeking health care because they're worried the doctor's visit will confirm that they have this dreaded disease. So the cost of this version of cancerphobia can't be quantified. But it certainly costs the health care system hundreds of millions of dollars, because it means that many cancers are being found at later stages that require more aggressive—and more expensive—treatment.

For some sobering numeric perspective, consider what these delays mean in lives lost:

- The American College of Radiology estimates that if everyone eligible for lung cancer screening had an LDCT exam, 30,000–60,000 lives might be saved.[36] Some of those lives are lost to fear of screening.
- The USPSTF reports that colon cancer screening saves 22 people per 1,000 screened.[37] That would come to a stunning 772,000 lives saved if everyone who should screen did. Some of those lives are lost to fear of screening.
- According to the USPSTF, breast cancer screening saves 9 lives per 1,000 people *over the lifetime* of all people screened, roughly 2 people per 1,000 *over ten years* of screening.[38] A modest benefit, certainly, but if everyone recommended for biennial breast cancer screening followed those recommendations, 39,000 lives might be saved over 10 years, 117,900 over the lifetime of all the women who don't screen. The lives of some women who fear cancer so much that they delay or avoid mammograms are being lost to fear of screening.

Even if those missed screenings or delayed presentation of symptoms to a health care professional don't lead to death, many certainly lead to cases that require more extensive, aggressive, and costly care. So though these expenses can't be quantified, given that late stage cancer treatment is one of the costliest forms of all health care, it is surely safe to say that this version of cancerphobia has significant economic consequences.

Lost Productivity

The economic cost to society of overscreening, overdiagnosis, and overtreatment of some cancers goes far beyond the direct health care costs. A person being scanned isn't at work. A person undergoing surgery, or recovering from surgery, isn't at work. A person suffering psychosocial impacts of false-positive screening results, or from the numerous physical side effects of treatment, is less productive. The dollar value of this lost productivity is enormous.

First, consider screening. Between the time spent getting to the exam, the screen itself, and time to get back to work or home, mammography takes at least a few hours. About 7.8 million exams are done per year in the United States on women of working age that can be considered overscreening, motivated to a great degree by fear of cancer. Conservatively estimating an average of three hours per test, that comes to 2.9 million lost days of work.

We will estimate, conservatively, that an LDCT lung cancer–screening procedure takes a minimum of four hours. If roughly 1.9 million LDCT lung cancer exams in the United States per year are performed on people who don't meet the recommendations for such screening, and half of those people are 65 or younger (assuming those at 65 retire, which is not the case and thus a conservative element in our estimates), that's another 475,000 lost work days. Furthermore, 29,300 people under 65 had a needle biopsy of the lung after an LDCT scan, another procedure that takes at least half a day, which adds another 14,650 lost days of work.

So a total of roughly 3.4 million work days are lost to the US economy by screening people for breast and lung cancer whose fear overrides the evidence that such screening is more likely to harm them than help.

Now let's move on to those who have surgery for an overdiagnosed breast cancer: 29,100 women had surgeries to remove the low- or intermediate-grade disease most likely to be overdiagnosed. Recovery from this surgery averages at least one month off the job.[39] At 22 work days per month, that's 640,000 lost days of work. For overdiagnosed prostate cancer, 25,140 people a year have surgery, and the average time off work after this surgery is 3–4 weeks, which means 18 lost days of work per person, a total of 453,000.[40] Roughly 30,000 people a year have total thyroidectomies for overdiagnosed cancers, as estimated in chapter 6. The average patient takes two weeks off work following such surgery.[41] That's 300,000 lost work days. An estimated 5,300 people had surgery for overdiagnosed lung cancer, but half of these people were over 65, so for the calculation of lost work, the number reduces to 2,650. It's further assumed that half of *them* had minimally invasive surgery and lost only one week of work—6,500 missed work days—and that the other half had open chest surgery, recovery from which can take two months or more, so a minimum of 57,200 more work days were lost.

Roughly, then, 1.5 million work days are lost to the US economy because of surgery performed on people whose cancer was overdiagnosed, surgery that was not clinically necessary.

Adding to the time lost to screening, fear of cancer and the overscreening, overdiagnosis, and overtreatment it produces costs the economy roughly 4.9 million lost work days. The Bureau of Labor Statistics reports that the average salary per day in the United States in 2020 was $350.[42] **That means that overscreening and the resulting overdiagnosis and overtreatment of nonthreatening cancer cost the economy $1.7 billion a year in lost productivity.**

========

Taken together, these metrics present a staggering reality. Overscreening for cancer, and the overdiagnosis and overtreatment of essentially nonthreatening cancers, costs the US economy on the order of $16.2 billion a year in health care spending and lost productivity alone. And remember, because these estimates are admittedly imprecise, the many assumptions on which they are based have all been chosen to err—if at all—on the low side.

Fear of cancer, and the outdated beliefs about the disease that are part of that fear, are significant drivers of these costs. People who screen despite recommendations that screening is more likely to harm them than help do so largely because they are afraid of cancer. People who choose aggressive and risky treatments for diseases they are told will probably never cause any symptoms do so principally because they are afraid of cancer. The health care providers who promote these choices in part because they are practicing defensive medicine are responding to our fears. The health care businesses that promote screening with little or no warning of its harms are taking advantage of our fear.

We all pay these costs, through our health insurance bills and our taxes. But the cost to society of our outdated and sometimes excessive fear of cancer goes much further still.

environmentalism's contribution to our fear of cancer

We cannot wish this world away: our task, then, is to sift through it vigilantly to discriminate bona fide carcinogens from innocent and useful bystanders. This is easier said than done.

—Siddhartha Mukherjee, *The Emperor of All Maladies*

I never met Jimmie Anderson. I only saw that poignant photo of him, with his slightly embarrassed young-boy-posing-for-a-picture grin, the photo that Anne, his mom, kept on the living room wall of her modest home. She would smile that sad smile of hers whenever she talked about Jimmie. Her pain was still sharp years after her young son died of leukemia when he was 12.

Jimmie wasn't the only one. Leukemia had killed several other kids in that same Woburn, Massachusetts, neighborhood. Anne saw a possible connection and marked the deaths on a map. They were all within a mile or two of her home. Was something in the environment the cause? she wondered. She took her concern to local officials, but they wouldn't take her seriously. Her pastor did, though, and through his church I got a call suggesting that what was going on deserved coverage on the news.

I was the environment beat reporter at a TV station in Boston, and to be honest, even though the story involved the sadness of dying children, the call was exciting. In the late seventies fear of environmental carcinogens was enormous. It was widely accepted that, as Rachel Carson had written in chapter 4 of *Silent Spring*, we were living in "a sea of carcinogens," in a "world filled with cancer-producing agents" that "pervaded our surroundings."[1] Here was a gripping story about that fear, with real victims—kids!—and stubborn officials who wouldn't take a grieving mother's concerns seriously.

Years later I had the privilege of escorting Anne to the premiere of *A Civil Action*, the movie about the investigation of one of the first "cancer clusters" in US history—the phrase had barely been heard of back then—and the trial of two companies accused of dumping chemicals that had contaminated the neighborhood's well water. By the time the movie came out, researchers had established that the water was the likely cause of the leukemia, one of only a few instances to this day in which a conclusive link was established between environmental contamination and a cluster of cancer cases. But that link hadn't been made at the time of the trial. One of the companies was acquitted, and the other one settled with the families that brought the suit.

As the movie ended, the lights came up in the theater, and the stars bowed to applause and moved toward their after-premiere parties. Anne and I sat toward the back, off to the side. I asked her if she wanted to stay. She was, after all, the person who had started all this, a pioneer in citizen environmentalism, the true star of the story. "I'm not much for parties," she said. "I think I'll just head home." She was wearing that same sad smile.

Cancer clusters. Hazardous waste. A Superfund site. These phrases all joined the common lexicon as fear of environmental carcinogens erupted in the seventies and eighties, fostered by the burgeoning environmental movement bringing these perils to public awareness and magnified by a news media that avidly dramatized that movement's alarms (*mea culpa*). The word "carcinogens" appeared 100 times more frequently in books published in 1980 than in 1950.[2]

Those environmentalist alarms perfectly tapped several psychological elements of what we fear. Remember from chapter 2 that we are more worried by a threat if it feels imposed on us (by modern technologies), if we can't detect it with our own senses (like invisible odorless tasteless substances in our air, water, and food), if it involves great pain and suffering (cancer), and if it isn't natural (anything human-made). These psychological "fear factors" fuel our worries about pesticides and plastics, fluoride and food coloring, radiation and flame retardants, PCBs and BPA, phthalates, PFAS, and a long list of industrial chemicals that have been the targets of the environmental movement's passionate campaign of alarm. That campaign has played a major role in producing the widespread belief that environmental carcinogens are a major cause of cancer.

This fear, however, flies in the face of the evidence that exogenous substances cause only a minor percentage of all cancers. Just how many is intensely disputed, and a precise number is impossible to establish with reliable scientific certainty, but it's believed to range from just a few percent up to as high as 15%–20%. No matter where the number falls on that range, it is undoubtedly worthy of our concern, and we should be grateful to the advocates who sounded (and still sound) the alarm. But even if it falls at the high end, it's still far fewer cases than most people assume. (For more on the dispute, see "How Many Cancers Are Caused by the Environment?" in *Scientific American*.)[3]

Fear of environmental carcinogens is a central element in our modern cancer*phobia*—a fear that exceeds the actual danger. A 2019 National Cancer Institute survey found that 70% of Americans either strongly or somewhat agreed that "it seems like everything causes cancer."[4] That common *mis*belief has dramatic consequences for society in several ways.

Pesticides, Herbicides, and Insecticides

You probably wouldn't know it by its formal name (much less be able to pronounce that name), dichlorodiphenyltrichloroethane. But by its abbreviation, DDT is the well-known poster child for our general fear of environmental carcinogens, especially the human-made chemicals that kill insects, weeds, and other unwanted species—*pesticides*. (Fear of these substances has become so engrained in our beliefs that *Merriam-Webster's Collegiate Thesaurus* lists "pesticide," "insecticide," and "herbicide" as near synonyms for cancer.) The fight to ban DDT, which started back in the late fifties, like the current fight to ban the weedkiller Roundup (glyphosate; more on that in the next chapter), exemplifies how our fear of anything that *might* cause cancer, no matter how weak the evidence might be, produces enormous resistance to a wide range of products, processes, projects, and even entire technologies that offer significant benefits—benefits that are sometimes not realized because of that fear.

DDT was so good at killing mosquitoes that Paul Müller, the Swiss scientist who discovered its insecticidal properties, won the 1948 Nobel Prize—for *medicine*. By the fifties it had replaced a natural pesticide, pyrethrum—basically crushed chrysanthemum petals—and saved millions of lives from malaria. But alarms had been raised as early as the forties that its uncontrolled use in agriculture threatened beneficial insects, as well as birds, fish, and maybe even people. An effort to ban it in one county in New York drew Rachel Carson's attention, and it became the highlight of *Silent Spring*, which raised concern about DDT's potential carcinogenicity, though Carson cautiously never actually called for an outright ban.

The fight against the unrestricted use of pesticides, and DDT in particular, was a major initial focus of the environmental movement as it was starting. The highly regarded Environmental Defense Fund was created exclusively to end the use of this one product. Legal battles were fought over DDT for years—environmentalists trying to ban it for its dangers to ecological and human health, the chemical and agriculture industries defending it for its benefits to farmers, and public health experts defending its value in disease control. A series of partial bans through the sixties culminated in a near total prohibition in the United States in 1973. A global ban took effect in 2004. But its benefits were still recognized. In 2006 the World Health Organization allowed its continued indoor application for disease control where malaria is a big problem and other solutions don't work as well. DDT is also still legal to use in the United States for limited control of disease-carrying insects.

A central aspect of the concern about DDT was its suspected carcinogenicity. Yet no reliable evidence back then supported that fear, and even today, despite multiple studies, the cautious International Agency for Research on Cancer rates it only a 2A ("*probably* carcinogenic to humans") based only on animal tests, while the US Centers for Disease Control and Prevention says, "Some studies in humans linked DDT levels in the body with breast cancer, but other studies have not made this link. Other studies in humans have linked exposure to DDT/DDE with having lymphoma, leukemia, and pancreatic cancer. *No definitive association with these cancers has been made*" (my emphasis).[5] Newer science suggests that DDT *might* have other harmful health effects on humans, but not cancer.

As the environmental movement fought to have DDT banned, many in the public health community noted the lack of evidence that DDT was carcinogenic to humans as they fought to preserve its use as an antimosquito insecticide that could reduce the death toll from malaria, one of the major human killers on the planet. Those fighting in favor of a ban denied that such restrictions would cost any lives, though some evidence suggests that malaria mortality did in fact rise in some places after the bans took effect.[6]

The story of DDT is summarized here not to take sides in the dispute but to illustrate how our deep fear of suspected environmental carcinogens, a fear shaped as much by our values and emotions as by an unbiased consideration of the evidence, shapes societal choices about many products and technologies that provide society significant benefits, including benefits to human and environmental health. DDT is just one example. Here are a few more.

Fluoride

In 1989, a year after hosting the Winter Olympics and shining in the eyes of the world as a modern metropolis, the city of Calgary, in Alberta, Canada, finally decided to add fluoride to their drinking water to prevent tooth decay. That was after voting against it in 1957, 1961, and 1971, in each instance because some citizens, backed by some environmental groups, feared that it caused cancer. The Calgary campaigners also tried to fire up public concern by claiming that the fluoridation of public drinking water, imposed by public officials, would infringe on individual liberty." An *imposed* cancer risk!

Fluoride was in the Calgary water supply only briefly. In 2011 the fears won out again, and the city stopped adding the decay-preventing substance to public drinking water. In 2016 a study by the University of Calgary found what most public health officials would have predicted, a significant increase in tooth decay in Calgary's kids.[7] The same thing happened in Juneau, Alaska. Fluoridation was stopped in 2007, and in 2012 kids there were 25% more likely to have cavities.[8]

These natural experiments help illustrate why fluoridation of drinking water has been called one of the greatest public health achievements in the last century, for the huge improvement it has provided in dental health. But does it cause cancer? It's well established that high levels of fluoride can cause fluorosis, white spots on the teeth that have only aesthetic impact. It's also suspected that at high levels, it can cause osteoporosis, or brittle bones. A few studies have linked high levels to neurotoxic effects, while the bulk of the research has found no such effect. One federal study in the United States reported "equivocal evidence of carcinogenic activity of sodium fluoride in male rats based on the occurrence of a small number of osteosarcomas (bone cancer) in treated animals."[9] But there was no similar effect in female rats. Essentially no solid evidence establishes a solid association between fluoride consumption and cancer.

Yet, since fluoridation of public drinking water began in the forties, it has triggered fierce resistance, largely because it has been associated with cancer. And as a result of that fear, a fear not supported by the bulk of the evidence, 27% of the US population on community drinking water systems does not receive the health benefit of fluoridated water.[10]

Nuclear Power

On March 11, 2011, one of the most powerful earthquakes to ever hit the coast of Japan sent a wall of water washing inland, flooding, among other buildings, the Fukushima-Daiichi nuclear power plant. With the reactors off as a precaution and auxiliary generators unable to pump cooling water over the hot nuclear fuel in three reactors, that fuel melted, leading to hydrogen gas explosions and the release of radioactive material into the air. The accident cost many lives, but the fatalities weren't from radiation. They were cause by the panicked evacuation of the area, when no one knew just how high the radiation exposure might get. That evacuation caused between 1,000 and 1,600 deaths. Most of the victims were elderly.[11] Based on hindsight and careful study of how much radioactive material was actually released, experts predict that radiation from the Fukushima-Daiichi accident is highly unlikely to ever lead to a single death from cancer. They say the doses released were too low to increase the rate of any disease associated with ionizing radiation above normal morbidity and mortality rates for those diseases.[12] But the Fukushima-Daiichi accident reignited society's deep fear of nuclear power—and the cancer that nuclear accidents are assumed to cause—that goes back to the fifties and sixties. As a result, even as environmentalism helps lead the enormous effort against anthropogenic climate change, the fear of nuclear radiation branded into the public psyche by that movement is impeding progress in that fight. In the fearful aftermath of Fukushima, Japan shut down all its nuclear power plants, which were producing 25% of the country's electricity at the time. In terms of greenhouse gas emissions that cause climate change, nuclear energy is "clean." It emits none of those pollutants. But Japan had to keep the lights on and its economy running, so it replaced its nuclear energy with power from coal, oil, and natural gas—fuels that do. Fukushima also led Germany to immediately close several plants. Nuclear was providing 22% of Germany's electricity at that time, and it was replaced by burning coal. In the wake of Fukushima, more than a dozen other nations also decided to phase out nuclear power, citing fear of radiation as a principal reason. Greenhouse gas emissions from the fossil-fueled energy generation rose in all those locations.

Fear of radiation and opposition to nuclear power has been a cornerstone of environmentalism since it began. The nascent environmental movement was actually born of this fear, not fear of chemicals. In *Silent Spring* Carson writes of how the risk of uncontrolled use of pesticides could be as bad as the threat of nuclear fallout from weapons tests. Political activist Ralph Nader reportedly said, "Nuclear power must be dealt with irrationally . . . nuclear plants are carcinogens. Let's get that story out." Environmentalists turned positive public attitudes toward nuclear power in the early seventies to deeply fearful by the end of the decade, when the fictional movie *The China Syndrome*, about a nuclear plant meltdown, was released just 12 days before the actual meltdown at Three Mile Island nuclear plant in Pennsylvania. That accident also helped sear deep fear of nuclear power into public hearts, even after it was understood that the small amounts of radioactive material released killed no one.[13]

A key effect of the fear-driven campaign against nuclear power was to dramatically raise the cost to build and operate nuclear plants, which are required to have vastly more complex and expensive safety systems than any industrial facility. That cost dramatically disadvantages nuclear power in the energy marketplace. Fear-based opposition to nuclear power has also made it a hot political issue, shaping public policy. In many jurisdictions trying to reduce greenhouse gas emissions, nuclear power does not enjoy the economic incentives that solar, wind, and hydro power do in "clean" energy policy.

Our fear of nuclear radiation is so deep that we have all but entirely ignored the evidence from the longest-running public health study ever, the Life Span Study (LSS), of the survivors of the atomic bombs dropped on Japan, described in chapter 7. That research has taught us that even at the very highest doses, much higher even than what was released by Fukushima or the Chernobyl accident, ionizing radiation is a remarkably weak carcinogen and causes no genetic damage passed from those exposed to their offspring.[14] But journalists who report with great drama about radiation risk issues rarely include any of this critical reassuring information. As a result, all we hear are the alarms sounded by nuclear power opponents that fuel our fear. And driven by that fear, we pressure policy makers to close existing nuclear power plants; as of 2021 12 had closed in the United States since 2012, and 7 more were due to close by 2025.[15] A large portion of the power they used to produce is now generated from fossil fuels.

(Intriguingly, as the effects of climate change begin to be felt, fear of that truly existential threat is finally trumping some of the cancer-related fear of nuclear power. As of 2023, Japan is starting to bring nuclear energy back, to meet its goal of carbon neutrality by 2050. Other nations are as well, in part because of fossil fuel energy shortages caused by the war in Ukraine and in part to fight climate change. Facing the threat of power shortages and failure to meet commitments to reduce greenhouse gas emissions, the state of California in 2021 provided funding to keep the Diablo Canyon plant open, reversing an earlier decision by its owners—in the face of fierce environmental pressure—to close.)

From Smart Meters to Cell Phone Towers to Power Lines

Fear of *any kind of radiation,* the foundation for which is our fear of cancer, goes beyond fear of nuclear energy, from which the term "radiophobia" first arose. In 2010, when the Pacific Gas and Electric company proposed installing smart meters on homes in liberal Marin County outside San Francisco, a surprising opposition began. Surprising because these devices allow communication via radio signals between the power company and individual users, facilitating more efficient use of energy, which reduces both local air pollution and greenhouse gas emissions. Smart meters also reduce energy bills.

The residents of Marin County objected to these energy-saving devices, however, because they receive and transmit radio signals—*radiation.* Never mind that this is RF (radio frequency) radiation, just wide waves of radio energy, totally unlike the ionizing radiation from nuclear power that can break atoms apart and cause mutations in DNA. Never mind the solid scientific evidence that these low-frequency, low-power radio waves are far too weak to damage DNA in a way that would lead to cancer. Never mind that these radio waves are nearly identical in wavelength to the remote-control devices, portable phones, and Wi-Fi systems in the homes and offices of the very people opposing smart meters. Smart meters use radiation, and the very word radiation—no matter what kind—is associated with cancer. That scared a lot of people into opposing smart meters, and still does.[16]

The same thing still happens in some places with the installation of cell phone towers. Cancer-related fear of radiation leads to opposition based on claims about cancer risk, which amounts to outright science denialism of the massive evidence that these installations do not raise that threat.[17] Fear of radiation even includes cell phones themselves. Suspicion that radiation from cell phones might cause cancer was sparked when a Baltimore doctor claimed in 1992 that radiation from his wife's cell phone caused her brain cancer, on little more evidence than that the tumor occurred on the same side of her head as the ear where she held her phone.[18] That sparked massive international research, on which the IARC based an interpretation that cell phone radiation might *possibly* be carcinogenic (a rating of 2B—the lowest of its four ratings). Yet dozens of large multinational multiyear epidemiological follow-up studies have found no evidence in the real word for such an effect.[19] (The original Baltimore lawsuit the doctor brought against cell phone manufacturers, and several like it, failed for lack of evidence.)

Despite all the reassuring evidence, however, the cities of San Francisco and Berkeley, California, passed laws requiring that cell phones have labels on the package warning of exposure to radiation. The San Francisco law was struck down in court. The Berkeley law stands. The label doesn't inform, doesn't explain *why* people should worry. It just raises alarm because, well, *radiation!* These issues are largely playing out the way the cancer scare about power lines did in the eighties, and still does in some places. Some research initially suggested a possible link between elevated cancer rates and proximity to these high-power transmission wires—any wires, in fact. Dramatic headlines and TV stories (again, *mea culpa*) warned ominously about this new potential cancer risk. Ultimately careful science showed no such link, and the fear died down, but not before huge battles ensued over siting new power lines. These battles grew so prevalent that Congress had to include a section in the Energy Policy Act of 2005 giving the federal government power to supersede state authority if public opposition causes states to fail to site power lines needed for the interstate power grid.[20]

Radiation, fluoride, and DDT are just a few examples of products and technologies that are opposed, principally by environmentalists, for fear that they cause cancer. That threat has been used by some environmental groups to frighten people about genetically modified food, plastics, chlorination of public drinking water, food coloring, high fructose corn syrup, artificial turf, fracking, and a host of other modern products and processes.[21] Indeed for anything that *any* group wants to oppose, including "not in my backyard" (NIMBY) neighbors who don't want to look at wind turbines or live near any kind of waste disposal facility, linking it with cancer is a common tactic.

Let's be clear. Some substances we are involuntarily exposed to in our air, water, and food *do* lead to cancer if we are exposed to high enough doses for a long enough period or at critical ages (vital qualifiers that are usually overlooked by the public and the news media). Concern about potential carcinogens is entirely reasonable. We should applaud responsible advocates who help protect society against such threats. But to see how that reasonable fear turns into a phobia—a fear that exceeds the actual danger—consider the work of a leading campaigner against environmental carcinogens, the Environmental Working Group. EWG gets a lot of media attention (news and social) when from time to time it publishes a report about how many suspected carcinogens we have in our bodies, as in a 2016 news release titled "The Pollution in People. Cancer-Causing Chemicals in Americans' Bodies." "We found that up to 420 known or likely carcinogens have been measured in a diverse array of populations," the group ominously warned.[22]

EWG acknowledged in that release that "the mere presence of a carcinogen in the body is not necessarily a serious health threat," and that only "a small subset of the chemicals inventoried for this report (nine of the more than 400 carcinogens) were measured at levels high enough to pose non-trivial cancer risks in most Americans." But then it essentially dismissed its own cautious caveat: "But it is clear that current exposures are a real risk—not only for chemicals found at levels above government standards." Essentially that says, "Worry about all regulated chemicals," even though those regulations are based on careful research that has found that those substances do not cause cancer at the doses to which we're exposed.

EWG is hardly alone in sounding persistent alarms about environmental carcinogens. Many scientists in various fields have become well-established advocates warning that a large fraction of cancer is caused by substances we're exposed to in the environment. When two of the world's leading experts on the biology of cancer published a study in 2015 saying that two-thirds of cancers arise as a result of natural mutations that occur as we age, those other scientists lashed out, arguing that environmental carcinogens play a much bigger role.[23] (There is an enlightening back-and-forth between the two authors of the main study and their critics in *Science* magazine.)[24]

The reason for noting this argument and the work of EWG is not to take sides but to illustrate how the environmental movement and the scientists aligned with it have, since the fifties and sixties, helped embed in the zeitgeist a fear that "everything causes cancer," a phobia that conflicts with the evidence. Their alarms have certainly been abetted by a news media that regularly reports about new findings that "X might cause cancer," or "Y *is associated* with cancer," warnings with lots of drama, personalized with a putative victim (even better if the victim is a child, like Jimmie), but usually failing to include critical information that would help put things in perspective. (Again, *mea culpa*. I failed at this too often during my years as an environmental journalist.)

There is no hard and fast answer to the question of just how many cancers are caused by environmental agents, rather than by aging, lifestyles choices, and genetics. "The environment" is way too broad and complex to tease out specifics. Most cancer experts agree that the percentage is low and that the common fear that "everything out there causes cancer" is excessive. But consider how that fear has driven federal government policy and spending. Far more is invested in managing the threat of cancer than on any other cause of death. And then consider how fear of cancer affects consumer spending, the law, and research into various health threats, areas we turn to next. The costs to society of our sometimes excessive fear of cancer are indeed broad.

other societal impacts of our fear of cancer

Worry gives a small thing a big shadow.
—Swedish proverb

Awareness of and worry about cancer is woven through every part of our lives. It's in the decisions we make about what to eat, what to buy, what to wear. It's in the news we read—about the latest celebrity stricken with cancer, the newest potential cure, or the latest potential carcinogen or cancer cluster. Cruelly, it's in the personal experiences that too often touch us all, when family or friends or colleagues struggle with or succumb to the disease. In the marketplace, the courts and other branches of government, in medicine, science, music, film, literature, sports, entertainment, and in so many other aspects of society, the C-word, the Big C, casts a nearly inescapable shadow of concern over our lives, influencing the choices we make as individuals and jointly as a society, choices with consequences both good and bad.

Government

Since 1937, when Congress passed the first National Cancer Act, establishing the National Cancer Institute with an annual budget of $700,000 ($12.8 million today), the US government has spent roughly $158 billion (not adjusted for inflation) on cancer research through the National Cancer Institute, as well as hundreds of billions more on cancer risk reduction through dozens of federal agencies. Nothing close to that amount has been spent protecting the public from any other cause of death. The reason for that massively disproportionate investment in this one health threat was specified plainly in the Statement of Purpose in the

2nd National Cancer Act, in 1971: "Cancer is the disease which is *the major health concern of Americans today*" (my emphasis). Not the leading cause of death, but the most feared. President Richard Nixon, who signed that law, once observed, "People react to fear, not love—they don't teach that in Sunday School, but it's true."

That enormous investment has accomplished a great deal. It's a big part of why cancer mortality is declining. Cancer research and government programs to reduce our exposure to environmental and occupational carcinogens have saved tens of thousands of lives and spared many more from great suffering. But consider the impact on our overall health of spending more on what *scares* us the most rather than on what actually *harms* us the most. Over the decades since World War II, had we invested in risk-reduction policies for protection from all major causes of death *in proportion to lives they each claim*, it is fair to suggest that more lives would have almost certainly been saved.

Consider one example of this disproportionate spending. The National Institutes of Health (NIH) has 26 divisions that investigate all the major diseases we face. Yet there is a clear star among them: the National Cancer Institute (NCI), by far the largest component of the NIH. One measure of its preeminence is that the NCI is the only institute with a director appointed directly by the president. A clearer indication is the money it gets. In 2020 the NCI budget was $6.4 billion, funding a staff of 3,500. (Several other NIH institutes also work on cancer, spending about $900 million more.) Compare that to the $3 billion budget of the National Heart, Lung, and Blood Institute (NHLBI), with a staff of 960. The NHLBI is responsible for the nation's research program on heart disease, the leading cause of death in the United States. Heart disease killed 696,962 people in 2020, roughly 7% more than cancer, which killed 602,350. Nonetheless, the NHLBI budget is half that of the NCI, and in fact only $2 billion of the NHLBI total budget goes toward work on cardiovascular disease. The NHLBI also researches lung diseases like asthma and chronic obstructive pulmonary disease, itself the fourth leading cause of death in the country. So very crudely, $2 billion goes to the disease that kills the most, and $6.4 billion goes to the disease that, though a major killer, scares us the most.

Certainly cancer and heart disease pose very different research challenges, and the budgets of the two institutes appropriately reflect that. But a fair question can be asked: If overall spending within the NIH was more proportional to the mortality threat of these diseases, might more lives be saved?

Our emotional relationship with cancer also shapes spending within the NCI (table 13.1). The spending doesn't sync with the mortality. Breast cancer, one of our most feared cancers (and a passionate focus of the women's movement) but only the fourth leading cancer cause of death, gets more research spending than the two leading cancer killers, lung and colorectal, combined.

To be fair, these numbers reflect more than just our fears. Each disease poses unique research challenges, and the allocation of resources has to match those demands. But it's clear that higher concern about some types of cancer strongly influences how the NCI spends its money. So another fair question can be asked: If spending within the NCI itself was proportional to the mortality of each type of cancer, might more lives be saved?

The disproportionately high investment in cancer research is only one indicator of how fear of the disease shapes our government's use of tax dollars to protect us. Tens of billions of dollars are spent by dozens of federal and state agencies trying to reduce the chance that we'll get cancer. Consider the list of the departments and agencies working on cancer at the federal level. There is nothing like this effort to protect us from any other major cause of death.

TABLE 13.1.

National Cancer Institute Research Spending vs. Incidence and Mortality per Cancer, 2017

CANCER TYPE, IN ORDER OF SPENDING	SPENDING ($)	INCIDENCE	MORTALITY	RANK AMONG CANCER CAUSES OF DEATH
Breast	545 million	252,710	41,070	4
Lung	321 million	222,500	155,870	1
Prostate	233 million	161,360	26,730	5
Colorectal	208 million	135,430	50,260	2
Pancreatic	172 million	53,670	43,090	3

Source: *American Cancer Society*, Cancer Facts and Figures 2017, *https://www .cancer.org/content/dam/cancer-org/research/cancer-facts-and-statistics/annual -cancer-facts-and-figures/2017/cancer-facts-and-figures-2017.pdf.*

DEPARTMENT OF HEALTH AND HUMAN SERVICES

Centers for Disease Control and Prevention
National Comprehensive Cancer Control Program
National Program of Cancer Registries
National Breast and Cervical Cancer Early Detection Program
Colorectal Cancer Control Program

Food and Drug Administration
Foods Program (chemicals and pesticides in food)
Center for Devices and Radiological Health
Center for Tobacco Products
Oncology Center for Excellence (cancer care product approvals)
Center for Drug Evaluation and Research
Center for Food Safety and Applied Nutrition

Agency for Toxic Substances and Disease Registry
Health-related aspects of the Superfund law regulating hazardous
    waste sites

Centers for Medicare and Medicaid Services
Government insurance coverage of cancer health care services

National Institutes of Health
National Cancer Institute (including the Surveillance, Epidemiology,
    and End Results [SEER] Program, a massive database that tracks
    cancer statistics)
National Institute of Environmental Health Sciences (environmen-
    tal carcinogens)
National Toxicology Program (studies and identifies carcinogens)

Agency for Healthcare Research and Quality
Health care research

Health Resources and Services Administration

THE ENVIRONMENTAL PROTECTION AGENCY
Dozens of programs. Of the 33 laws under which the EPA operates,
    18 deal specifically with environmental carcinogens.

DEPARTMENT OF LABOR
Occupational Safety and Health Administration
Regulation of substances "posting potential cancer risk to workers"

Mine Safety and Health Administration
Office of Workers' Compensation Programs

DEPARTMENT OF ENERGY
Office of Nuclear Energy
Office of Environmental Management

DEPARTMENT OF DEFENSE
Cancer research and environmental clean-up of contaminated military
    sites

DEPARTMENT OF AGRICULTURE
Pesticide regulation and food safety

DEPARTMENT OF VETERANS AFFAIRS
Cancer care and research

NUCLEAR REGULATORY COMMISSION
Radiation issues from nuclear energy

FEDERAL COMMUNICATIONS COMMISSION
Cell phone radiation

CONSUMER PRODUCT SAFETY COMMISSION
Carcinogens in consumer products

FEDERAL TRADE COMMISSION
False cancer claims by businesses

**CHEMICAL SAFETY AND HAZARD INVESTIGATION
BOARD**
Accidents

These government agencies, and more, participate in the Cancer Cabinet, a program created as part of the Biden administration's renewed Cancer Moonshot initiative. In announcing the enhanced focus of the government's efforts on cancer, President Biden said, "The goal is . . . to end cancer as we know it." An unquestionably admirable, and familiar, goal. But there is no Heart Disease Moonshot, no Heart Disease Cabinet.

It's impossible to calculate with any precision the total amount of federal spending on cancer risk reduction, because many programs that reduce the threat of cancer, like the EPA's Superfund law or the Nuclear Regulatory Commission's work to prevent nuclear power plant accidents, also target other dangers. The money devoted specifically to cancer risk can't be teased out of those budgets. But it is certainly safe to say that annual federal spending on cancer prevention is tens if not hundreds of billion dollars.

We should cheer and support that spending by all those agencies and programs. It has increased cancer screening, reduced smoking, encouraged healthier diets and lifestyles, and eliminated many carcinogens from our food, water, and air. It's a big part of why a diagnosis of cancer is no longer the automatic death sentence we used to assume, and why the cancer mortality rate in the United States has dropped 30% from 1991 to 2020, saving 100,000 more lives per year over that period.[1] The largest single component in that decline, according to most experts, is the steep declines in the number of people who smoke, reducing lung cancer deaths 51% from 1990 to 2017 among men and 26% from 2002 to 2017 among women, according to the American Cancer Society.[2] There have also been dramatic declines with other cancers.

- The mortality rate for breast cancer dropped 40% from 1989 to 2017.
- The mortality rate for prostate cancer dropped 52% from 1993 to 2017.
- The mortality rate for colorectal cancer dropped 53% from 1980 to 2017 among men, and by 57% from 1969 to 2017 among women.[3]

But the disparity between what our governments, federal and state, spend to protect us from cancer and what they spend to protect us from anything else has real consequences. As we consider the impact of our fear of cancer on society, it is fair to suggest that a more proportional investment based on the actual mortality rate of the various risks we face would almost certainly save more lives.

Consider as an example just one area of environmental protection, particulate air pollution. These tiny particles, produced from the burning of fossil fuels, agricultural activity, and other sources, burrow deep into our lungs and contribute to heart attacks, strokes, and other health problems. According to a 2019 report, particulate air pollution caused 107,000 deaths per year in the United States (as of 2011).[4] Environmental carcinogens, on the other hand, cause between a few percent up to as many as roughly 20% of all cancers. (Recall the earlier discussion of how controversial this number is.) Assuming every one of those cancers is fatal, that's a range of between 18,000 and as many as 120,000 deaths per year: at the higher end, roughly the same number of deaths as caused by particulate pollution. But the EPA spends much more time and energy, and money, to reduce our risk from environmental carcinogens than from particulate air pollution, largely in response to our deep fear of cancer.

Of course, it's not just the federal government we turn to for protection. Many states have their own regulations and programs (and cumulatively spend billions more) to reduce cancer risk. One of the most well known is California's Proposition 65, a law proposed by citizens' petition that passed by a 2-1 majority in 1986. As with all government programs to reduce cancer risk, Prop 65 has done a great deal of good, but it also provides a clear example of how our fear of cancer leads to government actions that many experts believe exceed the actual threat. Prop 65—officially the Safe Drinking Water and Toxic Enforcement Act—does two things. It prohibits businesses from polluting drinking water with industrial chemicals that might cause cancer, birth defects, or other reproductive harm, but it is more well known for requiring businesses to warn

⚠ **WARNING:** This product can expose you to chemicals including [name of one or more chemicals], which is [are] known to the State of California to cause cancer. For more information go to www.P65Warnings.ca.gov.

FIGURE 13.1
Label used in California to warn about the presence
of carcinogenic substances in products.
State of California

⚠**WARNING:** [Name of one or more exposure source(s)] on this property can expose you to chemicals including [name of one or more chemicals], which is [are] known to the State of California to cause cancer. Talk to your landlord or the building owner about how and when you could be exposed to these chemicals in your building. For more information go to www.P65Warnings.ca.gov/apartments.

FIGURE 13.2
Warning used in California to warn about the presence of carcinogenic substances in apartment buildings.
State of California

consumers about products that contain anything that might cause cancer. Anything. As I was writing this section, I picked up a small part for an outdoor hose faucet I was repairing. It carried a Prop 65 warning label.

But it's not just products that require warnings. Any building that has anything inside that might cause cancer has to have a warning at the front door. Stores, office buildings, banks, gas stations, parking garages, bars and restaurants, doctor's offices and hospitals, even places like Disneyland bear these warning labels. Every apartment building in California must warn occupants and visitors of "Prop 65" risk.

The language of the law says its purpose is "to facilitate the notification of the public of potentially harmful substances, so informed decisions may be made by consumers on the basis of disclosure." But these warnings offer no specific information or details that would empower people to make truly informed choices. They are designed to scare, to tap our cancerphobia about environmental carcinogens. The idea is that if companies have to post these frightening labels, they'll get rid of the risky substance instead. And some have. But a bar can't get rid of alcohol. Gas stations can't get rid of gasoline. Hospitals can't get rid of x-ray machines. An apartment building can't guarantee that nobody inside smokes cigarettes and exposes others to secondhand smoke. So labels warning about the presence of an unspecified carcinogen are everywhere. They are so ubiquitous that many believe they are ignored. The California attorney general argued in one court case, "It really does not serve the public interest to have the almost entirety of the state of California swamped in a sea of generic warning signs."[5]

Prop 65 is also widely seen to be excessive in the way decisions are made about just what qualifies as a carcinogen that requires the warning. The law qualifies anything as a carcinogen if it could cause at least one extra case of cancer in 100,000 people over a 70-year lifetime, an exceedingly protective standard far beyond that used for nearly any other health threat. To make sure substances are judged objectively, Prop 65 requires that chemicals should be listed as carcinogens only if they "have been *clearly shown* through scientifically valid testing according to generally accepted principles to *cause* cancer" (my emphases), yet the toxicology and epidemiology the law relies on, as powerful as they are, struggle to reliably determine things at Prop 65's required level of certainty.

Instead, the California Carcinogen Identification Committee (CCIC) ends up making judgment calls about what to include, and fear of cancer informs those judgments. Their list of chemicals that meet the standard *"clearly shown* to cause cancer" is far longer than that of any other agency in the world identifying human carcinogens. It includes dozens of chemicals about which other agencies are far more equivocal. The US National Toxicology Program, for example, lists 56 known human carcinogens and another 200 substances that are "reasonably anticipated to be a human carcinogen." The International Agency for Research on Cancer (IARC), widely recognized as highly precautionary, lists 121 substances as *known* to cause cancer in humans, 89 that *probably* do, and 315 substances that are *possibly* carcinogenic, a total of 511. All those *probably* and *possibly* carcinogenic substances, which don't meet the legal standard of "clearly shown," are on the Prop 65 list anyway—along with hundreds more, a total of nearly 900.

Prop 65 and the super-precautionary CCIC are only doing what California voters want. It's just one example of how passionately we press government to protect us from anything that might cause cancer. But consider the potentially harmful consequences of this excessive fear. The ubiquitous Prop 65 warning labels create a positive feedback loop, reinforcing "everything out there causes cancer" cancerphobia (and its offspring, chemophobia and radiophobia), which fuels public fear and rejection of many useful products that pose minimal or no risk, and leads to pressure on government to focus on this one threat, leaving less time and money to protect us from other major causes of death.

Cancer in Court
Regulatory agencies aren't the only part of government influenced by our sometimes excessive fear of cancer. It shows up in court too. Juries award

enormous damages to plaintiffs who claim that some suspected carcinogen made them sick, claims that are sometimes based on highly speculative scientific evidence. Those awards caution corporations to be more responsible, and that's a huge benefit to society. But these verdicts have other consequences. First, they reinforce "everything out there causes cancer" thinking. More significantly, they establish a mechanism by which society determines what is or isn't a carcinogen that is far from scientifically objective. Instead, the subjective judgment of 12 regular citizen jurors who carry their fears about cancer into deliberations means that some products or even whole technologies that might provide great benefit to society don't—not because they pose an actual cancer threat but largely because of our cancerphobia.

These cases often fall under what is known as toxic torts law. (The trial chronicled in *A Civil Action*, prompted by the work of Anne Anderson, whom we met in the previous chapter, helped establish this body of law). The law asks juries of lay citizens with no scientific expertise to make sense of complicated technical evidence about whether some suspect substance is or is not carcinogenic, as well as whether, at the doses the plaintiff was allegedly exposed to, it actually caused their illness. Twelve regular citizens listen to experts present research from toxicology, epidemiology, molecular biology, genetics, the hydrogeology of how underground pollutants move, the fate and transport of chemicals in the air and the body, and lots of medical testimony about the cancer the substance supposedly caused. Often these jurors have no more than a high school diploma or basic undergraduate college degrees. (Plaintiff's attorneys try to select such jurors.) The lawyers for both sides are of course not out to establish what is scientifically true. They are out to win, so the expert testimony they present about complicated science is twisted and manipulated, and the jurors are left to sort out the conflicting *opinions* of the experts on each side, some of whom say X *is* a carcinogen, some of whom say it isn't, some of whom say the plaintiff's cancer probably *was* caused by the substance, while others say it almost surely wasn't.

In some cases, like those involving asbestos or benzene, the evidence is clear that the chemical does cause cancer and that the exposure was high and clearly caused the plaintiff's disease. (Worse, in some cases, the company on trial knew about the risk and covered it up.) But in many others, like those alleging cancer risk from the pesticide glyphosate (trade name Roundup) or from Johnson & Johnson's talcum powder,* the science of whether the material is actually harmful is flimsy.

Flimsy is enough, however, because the cases take place in civil court, where the standard for a finding of liability is "more likely than not," sometimes referred to as the 51% standard of proof. The jury doesn't have to find beyond a reasonable doubt that the chemical is a carcinogen or that it caused the plaintiff's cancer. They only have to find that it is *more likely than not* that the substance is guilty as charged. A substance charged with causing cancer is a long way toward guilty in most jurors' minds before the testimony even begins.

The common fear that cancer is often caused by environmental agents imposed on an unsuspecting public by unscrupulous greedy corporations is the inescapable emotional context in which jurors' make those judgments. These emotions contribute to verdicts that are hardly objective analyses of the substance on trial, and to damage awards that run into the hundreds or even billions of dollars. Now consider the costs of those judgments not just for the defendants, but for society as well. The case of glyphosate is an informative example.

In 2016 a jury awarded groundskeeper Dewayne Johnson $289.2 million after finding that it was more likely than not that his exposure to glyphosate caused his non-Hodgkins lymphoma. The trial judge subsequently reduced the award to $78.5 million, and an appeals court lowered it further, to $20.5 million, but not until juries in two subsequent cases ordered Monsanto—the manufacturer of Roundup, which contains glyphosate—and then its new owner, Bayer AG, to pay more than $2 billion in damages. Eager lawyers filed hundreds more suits, with similar outcomes, and Bayer AG proposed a $10.9 billion fund to settle all of them—a settlement a judge later refused to accept, suspicious of "shenanigans" by the company. Bayer AG lost two appeals to get the US Supreme Court to throw out lower court rulings.

Interestingly, while all this was going on, a California judge ruled in a Prop 65 case that there wasn't enough evidence to call glyphosate a "known" carcinogen, finding that it didn't need a warning label. Judge William Shubb wrote in his ruling in June 2020, "Notwithstand-

---

* I was paid to consult the attorneys for Johnson & Johnson in the talcum powder litigation, on the risk-perception psychology of the issue in general. I offered no opinion on the scientific merits of the case, nor did I testify.

ing the IARC's determination that glyphosate is a 'probable carcinogen,' the statement that glyphosate is 'known to the state of California to cause cancer' is misleading." "Every regulator of which the court is aware, with the sole exception of the IARC, has found that glyphosate does not cause cancer or that there is insufficient evidence to show that it does."[6] (Even IARC, which rates glyphosate as "probably" carcinogenic, describes the evidence specifically associating it with non-Hodgkins lymphoma as "limited.") Judge Shubb was referring to rulings by the US EPA, the European Food Safety Authority, and other government agencies that read the same research IARC did but found that, at the tiny doses to which the public might be exposed, glyphosate is not a potential human carcinogen.

But it does have some environmental advantages. Glyphosate is one of the least toxic herbicides available, less toxic in fact than some herbicides approved as organic. It breaks down and loses its toxicity in just a couple of days after application, and it doesn't build up in groundwater, as many other weed-control products do. For 40 years it has been one of the most widely used herbicides in the world, replacing chemicals that are far more toxic to wildlife and people. It wasn't even a target of environmentalists until the midnineties, when Monsanto came up with a genetically modified Roundup Ready crop that could withstand glyphosate. That allowed farmers to use glyphosate to control weeds without harming the crop, corn, which allowed them to stop using greater quantities of more toxic herbicides. It also reduced the amount of farmland that had to be tilled to kill weeds, which reduced the environmental damage of soil loss. It diminished the greenhouse gas emissions of farm machinery that didn't have to operate as often. It increased commercial agricultural productivity, saving farmers time and money (and exposure to more toxic substances), and easing upward pressure on food costs for the public. But Roundup Ready seeds had been genetically modified, and environmentalists opposed that whole technology, largely on the grounds that genetically modified food is not "natural." That made glyphosate a target in a larger battle.

Despite the common opinion among national food safety regulators around the world that glyphosate is not carcinogenic at the doses to which most people are exposed, and despite its advantages over more toxic herbicides, because of the verdicts in the *Johnson v. Monsanto* and similar subsequent cases, glyphosate usage is now declining. (The decline is also the result of weeds developing resistance to glyphosate, so higher and more expensive doses are required, which reduces the economic advantage of Roundup Ready seeds for farmers.) Some jurisdictions have banned glyphosate, and in some cases more toxic substances are being used instead. Government research in the European Union recommended in 2021 that the ban on glyphosate should be lifted—based on the finding that it poses no cancer risk at the doses to which the public is exposed. (For a balanced summary of the science and the legal case against glyphosate, see "Cancer, Juries, and Scientific Certainty: The Monsanto Roundup Ruling Explained" on Snopes.)[7]

Clearly, toxic torts law makes for messy decision making about what is or isn't a carcinogen. But cancer fear shapes other court rulings as well. We can be held legally liable not just for causing someone's cancer but just for making them afraid they might get it. Dread of the disease is such an accepted part of our lives that just doing something that makes someone fear they *might* get cancer—not get it, just fear they might—is a tort, a legal harm for which the party causing the fear is liable in civil court.[8] Railroad workers exposed to asbestos on the job (mostly from train brakes) sued the Norfolk and Western Railway Company simply because they were afraid they *might* develop lung cancer in the future. Even though five of the six workers who sued smoked for as long as 30 years, they won. The lower courts and ultimately the Supreme Court ruled that asbestos was a known carcinogen, that the workers were exposed, and that they were *suffering from their fear*. The men, heavy smokers, were awarded a total of $5.8 million, just for being afraid that they might develop lung cancer from the on-the-job asbestos exposure. As Justice Ruth Bader Ginsburg wrote for the 5-4 majority in the *Norfolk and Western Railway Company v. Ayers* ruling, the fear of cancer "must necessarily have a most depressing effect upon the injured person . . . Like the sword of Damocles, he knows it is there, but not whether or when it will fall."[9] (Justice Ginsburg knew the fear of cancer intimately at the time of that ruling. She had survived colon cancer just three years before. Years later she survived lung cancer but ultimately died of pancreatic cancer.)

Cancerphobia shows up in court in still another way. The threat of medical malpractice lawsuits leads to "defensive medicine" and shapes the care that doctors provide. According to a survey of general practice doctors in 2009, 42% believed that patients in their own medical practice, *their own patients*, were receiving too much care. Six in ten of these primary care doctors believed that patients were also being overtreated by specialists. Nearly eight general practice doctors in ten said the biggest reason for providing more care than their patients needed was the fear of being sued if the patient thought their doctors hadn't done enough.[10] Defensive medicine plays a role in the aggressive care they recommend to patients diagnosed with essentially nonthreatening overdiagnosed cancers, and in their enthusiasm for cancer screening, even for patients for whom screening is not recommended. It also shapes how some doctors read the results of such screening.

A review of malpractice cases found that more than any other kind of mistake, doctors were sued for errors in diagnosis, and most of those cases involved misdiagnoses of cancer.[11] And not just any cancer. Another study found that the most common cause of all malpractice lawsuits against physicians is delayed diagnosis of breast cancer.[12]

The majority of these suits are brought against radiologists. Of the 48 breast cancer malpractice cases in New York from 2007 to 2017, for example, 32 were against radiologists.[13] The shadow of this threat hovers over radiologists as they interpret a mammogram, especially one with vague results. It's not hard to see how this affects their work. One obvious effect is more false positives and the harm they can cause. A 2011 survey of radiologists in three different regions of the United States found that among 124 who interpreted mammograms, roughly eight in ten expressed concern about the effect medical malpractice has on their judgments; over half said that worry either moderately or greatly increased how often they recommended breast biopsies; and, dramatically, roughly one in three radiologists had considered withdrawing from mammogram interpretation altogether because of malpractice concerns.[14]

The Cancer Advocacy Community

In 1913 the American Society for the Control of Cancer became the first civic advocacy organization working to educate the public about the disease. More than 250 such groups now work on cancer generally or on specific types of the disease, funding research, providing patient support and education, and advocating for more investment in cancer research and prevention. That's more organized advocacy than for heart disease, Alzheimer's, and stroke combined. At least 15 groups are working on breast cancer, 12 on lung cancer, 12 on prostate cancer, 8 on melanoma. Many of these groups have dozens of state and local affiliate organizations. This vast cancer advocacy complex is yet another reflection of how we fear this disease more than any other.

These groups do valuable and honorable work. Together they provide billions of dollars for cancer research and offer vital patient support and public education. Yet as they raise awareness about cancer, the very ubiquity of these organizations and their inescapable drumbeat of concern also reinforces fear of the disease. While most groups have become more cautious about using the most blatant appeals to fear, their activities ensure that cancer is as inescapable in the public arena as it is in our private lives. There are thousands of awareness and fund-raising campaigns, from the neighborhood level to national programs connected with professional sports leagues and major brands. There are 47 officially declared months or days for various cancers: National Cancer *Prevention* Month (February), National Cancer *Control* Month (April), National Cancer *Research* Month (May), National Cancer Survivors Day (June). November is the official month of pancreatic, lung, stomach, and carcinoid cancers, as well as the National Hockey League Hockey Fights Cancer Month. There are cancer license plates, cancer stamps, cancer Christmas ornaments, and all sorts of cancer awareness apparel, including a wide range of bracelets and ribbons. The pink ribbon for breast cancer spawned a veritable rainbow of ribbons and decorations for other types of the disease.

The honorable effort by all these groups to promote cancer awareness and concern is amplified by the intense competition among them for the enormous amount of money people donate to these organizations. Cancer is by far the leading recipient of public donations for work on any disease. One study reported that 190 of these groups together raised $6 billion in 2015.[15] Groups as big as the American Cancer Society ($728 million in contributions in 2018) and as small as Stupid Cancer, dedicated to helping young adults diagnosed with the disease ($2.5 million in 2018), compete for attention and donations with messages and activities that are as dramatic and emotional as possible.

Not only does this messaging contribute to the pervasive cloud of cancer awareness in society, but the competition among groups for donations siphons an enormous amount of money away from doing any direct good. Many of their publicity campaigns are marketing and fund raising for their organization. As just one example, the largest of the breast cancer advocacy groups, Susan G. Komen, reported public donations of $184.7 million in 2019. Thirty million dollars of what had been donated for research or patient education was spent on fund raising.[16]

Beyond the legitimate advocacy organizations, dozens of phony charities prey on our fear of cancer, taking in tens of millions of dollars that go not to patient advocacy or research but into the pockets of the charlatans who create these groups and the fund-raising companies they use. This includes the fake personal fund-raising campaigns that ask for donations for some poor stricken victim who claims to be suffering from cancer but isn't sick at all. Our deep fear of cancer makes us vulnerable to all these scams.

Coming from hundreds of organizations, the constant alarms from all these groups magnifies how often, and how poignantly, the public hears about the threat of cancer. That would be fine if their messages, particularly about screening, were more balanced. Few are. Overwhelmingly the "education" they provide emphasizes the benefits of screening while downplaying all the damage it can cause, or in many cases failing to mention that aspect of screening at all.

Information promoting screening often features moving first-person stories about how screening "saved my life." But hardly any cancer advocacy websites include first-person stories from the thousands of people suffering the serious side effects of screening. There are no stories from people whose screening led to discovery of an overdiagnosed cancer that frightened them into more aggressive treatment than they needed, and who are suffering serious side effects and regret their choices. There are no first-person testimonials by women living with post-mastectomy pain syndrome after a mammogram found a frightening but essentially non-threatening case of low-grade DCIS, leading them to choose a mastectomy. There are no first-person stories on the prostate cancer advocacy websites about men living with loss of erectile function or urinary leakage after a PSA test found low-grade prostate cancer, leading to a prostatectomy.

The author of a review of how breast cancer advocacy groups communicate put it this way: "Our concern is that what we are seeing in too many public awareness campaigns is unilateral advocacy of annual mammogram screening with no thorough going into it, while research shows the benefits of mammograms are less than many people believe and the potential harm greater . . . A greater emphasis should be placed on educating women about the choices they have and also the risks associated with being overdiagnosed and overtreated."[17] The same thing is true for prostate, lung, and other cancer-screening programs: advocacy groups trumpet the positives while barely mentioning or entirely ignoring the harms. Ostensibly these groups are devoted to helping people make fully informed decisions. But the imbalanced emphasis on the benefits of screening without adequate discussion of the possible harms is not full education. No matter how well intended, promoting screening without appropriate caution contributes to real harm.

Cancer Commerce

Our fear of cancer makes us ready prey for the many industries happily profiting from that concern. One is the "awareness" merchants, peddlers of the cancer ribbons, bracelets, keychains, clothes, and more. Most familiar is the vast array of pink products and pink branding spawned by the pink ribbon awareness campaign. That started, quite innocently and noncommercially, in the home of Charlotte Haley, whose grandmother, sister, and daughter had all had breast cancer. Inspired by the yellow ribbon for prisoners of war in Vietnam in the seventies and the red ribbon for AIDS in the eighties, working at her dining room table, Charlotte attached a peach-colored ribbon to a postcard people could send to the NCI to urge them to spend more on breast cancer prevention. The Estee Lauder company and the women's magazine *SELF* wanted to use Charlotte's ribbon, but she refused, wary of commercialization. Shrewdly, as it turns out.

Instead, the cosmetics firm and women's magazine came out with their own ribbon by changing the color to pink, and within a few years, pink products and pink branding as a new front in the war on cancer were so ubiquitous (newspapers printed on pink paper, police using pink handcuffs, the White House lit in pink light in 2015—there were even pink drill bits for fracking) that the whole pink campaign offended many in the breast cancer advocacy community and sparked a backlash, including the Think Before You Pink campaign of the group Breast Cancer Action.[18] Their complaint: that billions of dollars spent on these "pinkwashing" awareness campaigns don't go to research or patient care.

Besides diverting a huge amount of money (many pink products produce only private profits for companies that share none of their revenue with any breast cancer organizations), this omnipresent breast cancer advocacy contributes to overscreening and overdiagnosis, by supporting mammography with no mention of the harms it can lead to. As Gayle Sulik wrote in *Pink Ribbon Blues*, "How are women to assess the risks when every T-shirt, ad campaign, and pink ribbon comes fully equipped with the unequivocal message that 'Early detection saves lives'?"[19]

As noted earlier, pink is hardly the only color used to sell cancer awareness merchandise. A company whose very name plays on our fear of cancer, Choose Hope, sells 120 products—ribbons, bracelets, T-shirts, sweatshirts, tote bags, teddy bears, and more—in each of 28 different colors, boasting that 10% of its profits go to unspecified cancer research. Its website, on which the company says, "We're in Business to End Cancer," claims that nearly $1 million had been donated as of December 2020. This means that close to $10 million spent on these products went into the pockets of the parent company, Phoenix Reawakening, which also owns product lines under the trademarked names Together We Will Win, No One Fights Alone, Cancer Bites, I'm Stronger Than You Think, and Girls Fight Tough.

And then there is the commerce by companies, health clinics, and individuals peddling modern-day cancer quackery, taking advantage of our fear of cancer to sell products that not only fail to protect from or cure cancer as promised, but in some cases cause serious harm. This topic alone could fill a book, but a few glaring examples illustrate how easily our fear of cancer makes us vulnerable to the allure of anything that might protect us from the Big C.

Clark's Cure for All Cancers
Zoetron therapy
Quantum Xrroid Consciousness Interface machine
Electrohomeopathy
Antineoplastons

The marketplace is full of outrageous products that prey on our fear of getting cancer. You can buy "socks that prevent breast cancer" and a "breast cancer voodoo chicken foot protection charm." One supposed environmental carcinogen in particular is a target for these scams: dozens of devices claim to protect you from getting cancer caused by electromagnetic radiation. All of them are pure quackery. Remember, extensive research has established that radiation from power lines and wires, Wi-Fi signals, microwave ovens, cell phones, and cell phone towers does not cause cancer. Nonetheless, you can buy:

- DefenderShield organic bamboo EMF protection antiradiation blanket, $130
- Energetic bracelet, EMF protection 7.83 Hz, Mineral Collection resonance bracelet, $60
- EarthCalm Quantum Cell, cell phone radiation electromagnetic EMF protection (using "scalar resonance" technology), $129
- 5G electromagnetic radiation protective cap (conceptually just a tin foil helmet masquerading as a baseball hat), for anywhere between $25 and $89.
- EMF Protector Pyramid, made of "orgonite crystal," $49.95

"Orgone" was concocted by Austrian psychoanalyst Wilhelm Reich, who claimed to be able to protect people from cancer with "esoteric energy," "a hypothetical life force," or "the anti-entropic principle of the universe." Reich's orgone products and treatments were identified as frauds and banned from interstate commerce by the FDA in 1954, but you can still buy "orgonite crystals" with supposed magic cancer-protection properties, which are no more than plastic resin hardened with various flowers, crystals, and other decorative materials inside.

But obvious quackery is hardly the only type of cancerphobia commerce. We spend far more on mainstream products that falsely promise to reduce our risk of cancer.

Do you buy organic food? The Organic Trade Association reported that 82% of Americans have, and for most, the reason is health and safety, including a reduced risk of cancer from pesticides used in commercial agriculture.[20] The Pew Research Center estimates that "among those who bought organic food in the past month, 76% say a reason was to get healthier food."[21] We pay a premium for that supposed health benefit, an average 25 cents per dollar more for equivalent products, despite decades of research that has produced no evidence that organic food reduces cancer risk at all. (In fact, no firm research shows that it is healthier to eat either. Its main benefit is that organic is an approach to agriculture that some favor.) As the UK Food Standards Agency put it, "Consumers may also choose to buy organic food because they believe that it is safer and more nutritious than other food. However, the balance of the current scientific evidence does not support this view."[22] While there *is* evidence that farm workers may be at greater risk of some cancers from the high doses of pesticides to which they are exposed in commercial agriculture, no robust evidence shows that consumers are from the practically nonexistent levels of pesticides in the final products we eat and drink.[23]

So Americans spend nearly $50 billion on food they incorrectly believe provides them health and safety benefits. That's $12.5 billion more than had they bought the nonorganic version of the same products. Part of that spending is driven by fear of pesticides, and much of that fear is really our fear of cancer.

Do you take vitamins and other health supplements? Nearly 8 in 10 Americans do.[24] We spend $50 billion a year on these products to improve our health, despite evidence that, except in a few specific circumstances, they have no benefit.[25] Millions of people take these products in part to reduce their risk of cancer, though the evidence here is clear as well: according to the US Preventive Services Task Force (USPSTF), "Limited evidence supports any benefit from vitamin and mineral supplementation for the prevention of cancer or cardiovascular disease (CVD)."[26] The World Cancer Research Fund International specifically warns "do not use dietary supplements for cancer prevention."[27] There is even evidence that high doses of some supplements—beta carotene and vitamin E—may increase the risk of some cancers.

A review by the American Institute for Cancer Research reported, "Randomised controlled trials of high-dose supplements have not consistently demonstrated the protective effects of micronutrients on cancer risk suggested by observational epidemiology. Furthermore, some trials have shown potential for unexpected adverse effects."[28] A literature review found, "Supplement use is fueled in part by the belief that nutritional supplements can ward off chronic disease, including cancer, although several expert committees and organizations have concluded that there is little to no scientific evidence that supplements reduce cancer risk. To the contrary, there is now evidence that high doses of some supplements increase cancer risk."[29]

Yet the marketplace is full of vitamins and supplements that offer protection from cancer: antioxidants, turmeric, omega-3 fatty acids, selenium, vitamin D, resveratrol (the substance in red wine once thought to help with longevity), aloe, Cansema paste and other "black salves," goldenseal, soursop, shark cartilage, and others. You can still get laetrile, a substance derived from peach and apricot pits debunked as a cancer cure in the seventies. Today it is marketed as protection from developing cancer under names like amygdalin and vitamin B17 (there is no such thing), or as apricot pits. Peddlers of dozens of these pills, oils, and salves, with names like Fungustum, CancerGene, Carcinogex, and Men's Prosta-Life, have been prosecuted by the FDA for falsely advertising nonexistent cancer-protective properties.

The marketplace is also busy with popular figures hawking these products, like Dr. Joe Mercola, the Health Ranger Store, Dr. Oz, and the Food Babe, "snake oil salesmen," according to former US senator Claire McCaskill; "unscrupulous marketers taking advantage of our desire" for safety, according to C. Lee Peeler, vice president of the Council of Better Business Bureaus. Under the appealing mantle of "natural" and "alternative" foods and medicines, they recommend supplements and other substances that claim to protect you against cancer, when the science says they don't. These products and hucksters are preying on and profiting from our cancerphobia.

There are also dozens of books offering diets and lifestyles that promise to *prevent* cancer—not just reduce the likelihood that you will develop cancer, which reputable books note can be achieved with good diet and exercise (along with not smoking and minimal alcohol consumption)—*prevent* cancer entirely, a false promise no book or product can keep.

Do you try to avoid "chemicals"? Hundreds of everyday products profit from our chemophobia, preying on "the naturalistic fallacy," our instinctive assumption that anything natural is less risky than anything synthetic. Organic food is just one category. Many other foods, while not claiming to meet the legal standards of organic, boast that they are "all natural" or "green" or contain "no artificial colors/flavors/ingredients." There are "natural" household cleaners and detergents, soaps, shampoos, personal hygiene products, and cosmetics. There are products—car seats, strollers, blankets, strap-on infant carriers—that claim to protect children from the toxic risks associated with various ingredients in plastics. A foundation of the fear that these products play to is our fear of cancer.

It may sound almost sacrilegious to criticize these products. Either they actually do protect us from some risk or they don't, but we feel safer buying them. But commerce preying on the naturalistic fallacy causes hidden harm. Natural is not always safer, synthetic is not always danger-ous, and our fear of the risks from food coloring, plastics, artificial sweet-eners, and many other substances is in most cases wildly overblown. The misrepresentation of risk does harm.

Because of chemophobia—a first cousin of cancerphobia—we waste money on many of these products, buying ourselves only a false sense of safety. Further, the ubiquity of products claiming to protect us from the supposed harm of synthetic chemicals reinforces the mistaken belief that "everything out there causes cancer," which is the foundation for many of the other effects of cancerphobia described in this chapter.

The Cancer Industry

Thousands of hospitals, clinics, physician practices, small and enormous companies, and hundreds of thousands of people make their living work-ing in cancer care. For these businesses and professionals, including the most well-respected hospitals and other institutions helping reduce the terrible toll of cancer, our fear of the disease and our unquestioning be-lief in the benefit of screening are immensely profitable, and the allure of those profits encourages many in the cancer industry to tap our fears in ways that do great harm.

The market for providing cancer care and treatment is incredibly lu-crative; the NIH estimated that medical expenditures on cancer treat-ment in 2020 would be as high as $207 billion.[30] Four times as much is spent caring for the average cancer patient as for the average noncancer patient.[31] So the competition for these patients is intense, which helps ex-plain why the nonprofit organization Truth in Advertising reported: "The amount spent by designated U.S. cancer centers on advertising soared 320 percent, from $54 million in 2005 to $173 million in 2014."[32]

Advertising is one thing. Misleading advertising about cancer care is another. An investigation by Truth in Advertising found that the market-ing materials of the top 50 cancer centers, including several of the most prestigious hospitals in the country, misleadingly featured hopeful testi-monials from patients who survived but whose cases were highly unusual, a fact the advertising fails to mention. These unusual success stories de-ceitfully play on people's hopes and fears to make money. As a researcher in the field of ethical medical advertising, Yael Schenker, put it, "Clearly the concern is that imbalanced or misleading advertising content may drive inappropriate decisions about cancer care."[33] A study in the *Annals of Internal Medicine* found, "Clinical advertisements by cancer centers frequently promote cancer therapy with emotional appeals that evoke hope and fear while rarely providing information about risks, benefits, costs, or insurance availability."[34] The Federal Trade Commission said as much when it issued a consent order against the Cancer Treatment Centers of America in 1996, ordering the business to stop misleading potential patients/customers by using only highly unusual patient success stories in its advertising.[35] The consent order expired in 2016. As of 2022, Cancer Treatment Centers of America was still engaged in the same misleading advertising, merely adding the vague caveat that "no two cases are alike" as a heading on the patient testimonials web page.

Several questionable practices are common in the industry that supplies screening and diagnostic equipment for cancer. Small wonder. The overall global market for these technologies was $169.1 billion in 2020.[36]

- The global colonoscopy equipment market was worth $36 billion in 2020.[37] The market value for just the bowel preparation medicines for these exams was $1.6 billion, and the market for stool sample testing for colorectal cancer was worth another $1 billion in 2020.[38]
- The North America breast cancer–screening market (mostly US) was worth roughly $2.1 billion in 2020, with the breast biopsy market alone worth nearly $1 billion.[39]
- The global prostate cancer diagnostic market was estimated to be worth $2.8 billion 2019.[40]
- The global lung cancer–screening market was estimated to be worth $36 billion by 2023.[41] The US share was predicted to be $1.2 billion.
- The US market for the assessment of biopsy samples from solid tumors was estimated to be worth $8.2 billion in 2019.[42]

All these markets are predicted to grow at healthy rates. The public is hungry for any new screening or diagnostic technology that claims it can find cancer better (earlier, more accurately), so companies in this field—screening equipment manufacturers like Hologic, General Electric HealthCare, Boston Scientific, Fujifilm, and Medtronic; tumor analysis equipment makers like Abbott Labs and Thermo Fisher—regularly roll out updated versions of their equipment.

As this book is coming out, a major new field of cancer-screening technology—blood tests that can detect molecules indicating the presence of several types of cancer—is coming to market with huge fanfare. Like so many screening technologies before them, these so-called MCED tests—multi cancer early detection tests—have gotten regulatory approval though they have not been thoroughly investigated by randomized control trials to establish both their benefits and their potential harms, cautions raised by the National Cancer Institute itself.[43] And like all other screening technologies, while these tests may be able to detect cancer, they can't predict what that cancer may go on to do, so they may be yet another potential contributor to overdiagnosis.

Hospitals, clinics, and physician practices that compete for lucrative customers in the health care marketplace spend millions buying the latest technology and millions more marketing it. That draws customers not only for screening and diagnosis but the far more profitable care and treatment that often follows. Overscreening is just the beginning of the medical and *revenue* cascade.

With billions of dollars at stake, every company, hospital, clinic, or doctor making money from screening and the cancer care it triggers has a direct financial incentive to promote more of it, engaging in practices that raise serious questions of potential conflict between the financial interests of the company, hospital, or doctor, and the interests of the patients. The rollout of 3D mammography beginning in 2011 is just one cautionary example of how economic incentives contribute to the harms of overdiagnosis and overtreatment.

First, a description of the technology: 2D mammography takes only two images of a breast, one from the top and one from the side; 3D takes a series of images from various angles and then uses a computer process called tomosynthesis to combine those perspectives into a clearer and more detailed image. (The addition of artificial intelligence to help interpret these results is another technology just coming online as of 2023.) Three-dimensional mammography reduces the number of false positives by as much as one-third, an important improvement. Some research suggests that it may find roughly one more cancer per thousand screens than 2D, particular in denser breasts, although a study of 29,000 Norwegian women reported that 3D found no more confirmed cancers than 2D.[44]

But remember, the ultimate goal of any cancer screening is not just to find cancers but to save lives, and the USPSTF reports that there is no reliable evidence showing that 3D saves more lives than 2D.[45] The American Cancer Society and the Susan G. Komen breast cancer advocacy group agree. A study called the Tomosynthesis Mammographic Imaging Screening Trial (TMIST) is under way to compare the two technologies.[46] It will compare mortality outcomes, and it will also help resolve whether 3D mammography adds to the problem of breast cancer overdiagnosis by finding even more tiny cancers, many of which would never cause any symptoms. But the study won't be done for several years. Fully aware of the public's desire for the latest and greatest technology in the fight against cancer, in 2011 the FDA approved 3D mammography even before research had clarified whether this technology does more harm than good, only on the basis that 3D is "safe and effective," not necessarily better at saving lives. Use of the technology has spread quickly. Now consider how this plays out in the real world, of real people, worried about breast cancer.

Terry was somber as she told her husband there was something they needed to talk about. She said she'd felt a small lump in her right breast. She was worried. They hugged, and her husband reassured her that she had gone through this before—felt a lump, had a diagnostic mammogram, gotten the all clear. That helped her keep her fear in check for the week until she could see her doctor, who felt the lump and prescribed a mammogram. Terry made an appointment at a major well-respected hospital. When she got there, there was no discussion of which technology would be used.

Following the screening, her general practitioner reassured Terry that nothing of concern had been found. But Terry, still worried, wanted a second opinion from the breast cancer specialist she had seen before at a major Boston teaching hospital. The diagnosis was the same—no sign of cancer. Terry asked whether her screening had been with 2D or 3D mammography, and whether that made a difference. "Three D" the specialist said. "But it really doesn't make much difference. People think newer is better, so that's the way things have been going for a few years, and it's what we recommend, mostly because it's what people seem to want, and because it can spot things a little more clearly so it reduces callbacks. But other than that there really isn't much evidence it makes a difference."

Though Terry had long worried about the health effects of radiation, and she knew that 3D mammography exposed her to slightly more than 2D, she was smiling as they left the doctor's office. As they drove home, she told her husband, "I feel better that they used the new test."

The FDA reported that as of 2016, the United States had 2,444 3D-equipped mammography centers, and by mid-2018, there were 4,074. That's despite the cost for these machines starting at roughly $500,000. But expensive as they are, 3D machines are lucrative investments. They produce more revenue per test, an additional $56 per test for doctors and $25 per test for hospitals for patients covered by Medicare, and $103 more for doctors and $46 more for hospitals for each patient with private insurance, plus the much larger revenues from the cancer patients that screening often produces, a significant number of whom don't have a disease that clinically warrants the costly care they fearfully choose.[47]

So there is a lot of money to be made by the companies selling this technology and by the health care providers using it. That encourages those businesses to engage in practices that appear to put profit ahead of patient welfare, hyping the benefits of 3D technology but playing down or often entirely failing to mention its limitations and potential harms. Examples cited by journalist Liz Szabo of *Kaiser Health News* in a 2019 investigation, "A Million-Dollar Juggernaut Pushes 3D Mammograms," included:

- "Influential journal articles [touting the benefits of 3D mammography]—those cited hundreds of times by other researchers—were written by doctors with financial ties to the 3D industry." (Research by doctors with financial ties to the companies developing 3D mammography, particularly Hologic, provided much of the evidence on which the FDA based its approval of the technology.)
- "In the past six years, 3D equipment manufacturers—including Hologic, GE Healthcare, Siemens Medical Solutions USA and Fujifilm Medical Systems USA—paid doctors and teaching hospitals more than more than $9.2 million related to 3D mammograms, for research, speaking fees, consulting, travel, meals or drinks."
- "Hologic (the leading manufacturer of 3D screening technology) gave educational grants to the American Society of Breast

Surgeons, a medical association that recently recommended 3D mammograms as its preferred screening method."
- Manufacturers paid celebrities like Cheryl Crow and Kristin Chenoweth to urge women to demand what advertisements call "the better mammogram."[48]

There is nothing wrong with a for-profit company promoting its products. Szabo quotes Hologic as arguing that "it would be 'irresponsible and unethical' to withhold technology that detects more breast cancers, given that definitive clinical trials can take many years." But it is also misleading—irresponsible and unethical—to promise that 3D mammography can save more lives when no reliable research supports that promise, while ignoring or minimizing the risks this technology also poses. Szabo quotes Dr. Otis Brawley, professor at Johns Hopkins University: "It's unethical to push a product before you know it helps people." Dr. Alex Krist, vice chair of the USPSTF, is quoted as saying that "by steering women toward 3D mammograms before all the evidence is in, 'we could potentially hurt women'"—by increasing overdiagnosis and overtreatment. (If this sounds familiar, it should. There are many similarities here to the way mammography—and the PSA test and MCED tests just coming to market—were approved: regulatory approval before careful research confirmed a benefit and identified possible harms, eager companies hyping their technologies, doctors and hospitals competing in the medical marketplace by offering the latest technology, all driven by the public's blind belief in the benefits of, and demand for, early detection, and their ignorance of its potential harms.)

The 3D mammography story is just one example of how the cancer industry promotes the screening from which it profits, hyping its benefits and hiding its harms. Another is the plethora of free prostate cancer-screening programs offered by hospitals, clinics, and urology practices, including some of the most prominent cancer centers in the United States, health care providers fully aware of the limitations of the PSA test. The screenings are advertised with grave warnings about the prevalence of prostate cancer and praise for the benefits of early detection, enticing men to "take control of their health." Unsurprisingly, most of the marketing makes little or no mention of the imprecision of the test or the harms that PSA tests so often lead to. These free clinics are opposed by the

American Academy of Family Physicians, the American Urological Association, and the USPSTF. Yet they are common. Why? In a word: money.

As one industry insider described them (in Brawley's book *How We Do Harm*), free prostate cancer screenings draw lucrative customers to hospitals, clinics, and physician practices, since participants in screening usually go to the same facility for all the medical care PSA testing often triggers: expensive biopsies, surgeries, and other treatments. As Dr. Brawley told me in an interview in December 2019, "PSA is a huge part of the business plan of most of the hospitals in America."

Other companies that directly profit from the harmful side effects of PSA-triggered overtreatment also promote screening. Recall that as many as one-third of men who undergo prostate surgery end up with long-lasting urinary incontinence. In 2009 and 2010 Kimberly-Clark, maker of Depends Underwear for Men adult diapers, partnered with the prostate cancer advocacy organization Zero, donating $250,000 "to help fund education for patients, and to fund *free screenings* for those at risk and cancer research" (my emphasis). PSA screening creates diaper consumer customers for Kimberly-Clark. Partnering with an advocacy group to promote free screenings (a group that also plays down the potential harms of PSA screening—there is no mention of overdiagnosis or overtreatment on Zero's web page describing PSA testing) hardly erases the questionable morality here.

Dozens of companies do the same sort of thing, partnering with cancer advocacy organizations to keep awareness of and concern about cancer high. That is certainly honorable in some ways. But companies know that these seemingly well-intentioned relationships also help increase demand for their products and services, by turning the public's fears into their profits.

———

Considering the long list and wide range of harms described in this chapter, we need to once again step back and acknowledge the other edge of the sword. The immense government research program driven by our fear of cancer has helped reduce cancer mortality in the United States by nearly a third and helped make as many as two-thirds of all cancers treatable as chronic diseases or curable outright. That fear has helped drive enormous environmental quality improvements that have saved millions of lives. Concern about cancer has led to the range of government and private programs working on cancer *prevention* that help us avoid developing the disease in the first place. Fear of cancer has driven government regulation, backed up by court rulings, that together have made industries far more responsible about the safety of their products, reducing the use of toxic ingredients and the amount of toxic waste they produce, and improving worker safety—though much more remains to be done in all these areas.

We should also celebrate that we have responded to the threat of cancer with our instinct for altruism, donating our time and money to a robust advocacy community, which provides billions of dollars to research, offers education to help people avoid developing cancer, and provides enormous support to those who do. And for all its profiteering in the capitalist free market, the cancer industry has given us the tools and products that have helped us make remarkable progress against a formerly invincible enemy.

So as with all chapters in this book, this one closes with the recognition that fear of cancer, even the sometimes excessive fear called cancerphobia, does not only harm but great good. This leads us to the next chapter, an optimistic examination of the progress being made to reduce some of the harms discussed throughout this book. As we can't yet entirely cure the disease, we certainly can't entirely cure cancerphobia. Our fears of the disease are as intrinsic to our nature as cancer itself is to our biology. But a lot of work is being done to reduce the overdiagnosis and overtreatment our fear can lead to, and perhaps most important, to help society modernize our emotional relationship with the Emperor of All Maladies and develop a more proportionate fear of a disease that is no longer the threat most of us still mistakenly assume it to be.

Part Four

reducing
the costs

combating cancerphobia

I will use those dietary regimens which will benefit my patients according to my best ability and judgment, and will do no harm or injustice to them.
   —The Hippocratic oath, classical version

I will apply, for the benefit of the sick, all measures [that] are required, avoiding those twin traps of overtreatment and therapeutic nihilism.
   —The Hippocratic oath, modern version

On a dreary London day in January 1948, Dr. John Ryle stood in the Maudsley psychiatric hospital before a group of distinguished physicians and named a new psychological condition: "nosophobia"—fear of disease. Dr. Ryle meant fear of any disease, but he focused much of his talk on "the special case of Cancer Phobia. Cancer phobia without cancer is far commoner than cancer phobia with cancer." He argued that this fear was so widespread that it "is to be thought of both as an individual and, by reason of its prevalence, as a social problem." And he argued that this fear had real costs: "My concern today," he said, are "fears which scarcely one of us escapes, which may be trivial and transitory, but which may also assist the perpetuation of much unhappiness and physical and mental illness."[1]

This was nearly a decade before oncologist George Crile Jr. used the term "cancerphobia" in his campaign to warn that fear of cancer was doing great harm, in some ways more than the disease itself. As Crile would some years later, Ryle optimistically proposed in 1948 that this disease could be treated—not cured entirely, but treated. He prescribed public education to take some of the fear out of the C-word itself. "We would do our patients and the public a real service if we were to remind them more often, firstly, that cancer in its early stages is today more readily recognized and eradicable than ever before, and, secondly, that even when intractable it is by no means always a painful disease."[2]

Years later Crile agreed that education could treat cancerphobia but not cure it. "There is no technical way," he wrote, "that man's fears can be permanently allayed." But he then spent years doing what Ryle prescribed, not only warning of the harms from our fear of cancer—"Fear of cancer has been beaten into [us] until this fear has become almost as great an enemy as cancer itself"—but educating people about the disease, at a time when cancer was still talked about only in whispers, to help "develop a positive philosophy toward cancer, a philosophy which does not fear cancer, but which meets the issue squarely."[3]

In the late forties and fifties, when our fear of cancer was beginning to explode, the suggestion of doctors Ryle and Crile that we can in some ways be too afraid of cancer met fierce resistance from both the medical community and a frightened public. But their call to recognize cancerphobia and temper its harms is now resonating with a growing group of pioneers leading a wide range of efforts to moderate our fear of this dreaded disease and reduce the enormous damage that fear does to us as individuals and as a society.

Wait and Watch

Tom is one of the most irrepressibly positive people I'm lucky enough to know, which is remarkable given that he lost his mother to colon cancer when he was 7, his father to heart trouble at 19, his oldest brother to prostate cancer when Tom was 50, and then his other brother to suicide three weeks later. It's also remarkable given that several years ago, Tom was diagnosed with prostate cancer.

"I kept track whenever I had a blood test of all of my various levels, cholesterol, all those things, going back to '78, '79. I just sort of monitor that stuff. So off and on the PSA kicks up and kicks down, up and down. Then it kicked up, and stayed up, and kicked up again. So this urologist I worked with said let's do a biopsy. It hurt like #@$!

"I remember sitting in my house when the doctor called and said you have prostate cancer, and it's low but you should come in so we can talk about what we're gonna do. That acts on your head. It was like, holy #*~%! I was already under a lot of stress, planning my wedding, planning a new house. All kinds of stress . . . and now it went from here to THERE!

"But I had to sort of say 'Be cool. Let's see what happens. Let's find out what the deal is.'" That was more easily said than done, Tom admitted. But the adversity of his early life had forged skills he was now able to tap.

"One of the things I used to do when I was in my twenties was whitewater canoeing. One of the things I learned was if you go faster than the current, your canoe will swamp, because you cut across the waves and water splashes into your boat. If you go the same speed as the current, you have no control of your boat. So you have to go slower than the current. You have to backpaddle, paddle against the way the river wants to take you. So I use that metaphor a lot. I just say, 'I'm backpaddling in my life right now. I'm slowing myself down. Slow the world down here.' The imagery in my brain was 'Just slow down' and stay in control in that way. Stay on top of the water, not under it."

Control. A feeling of empowerment. A feeling that you can *do* something to fight back against the fear that wants to flip your boat.

Tom saw his doctor a week later. "I said, since it's the lowest level, I'd like to do the active surveillance. I think I'll wait a bit. There are always people that want to jump right in and take the damn thing out. I know a lot of people who have prostate cancer and they're fine, and some people have done stuff, and some haven't. So I said, let me just pause for—that's my backpaddling—let me just pause and not jump because that could be worse."

Active surveillance (AS), or watchful waiting (WW), is fighting the urge to have what we perceive as the monster of cancer cut out of our body as soon as possible and instead choosing to just wait and carefully monitor our condition; as inadequate as that choice feels for many facing the fear of cancer, just a few years ago, most people were never even given that less aggressive option, for two reasons. First, only with the advent of more perceptive screening technologies have we recently come to understand that many of the tiny tumors we can now find are slow- or non-growing (or even regress and disappear) and pose *little or no threat*. Second, we have only recently come to understand that, for some types of disease, the mortality rates from surgery and watchful waiting are the same. That evidence allows doctors to confidently prescribe a wait-and-see approach to appropriate patients.

Before we had that evidence, professional societies that set formal standards of practice were reluctant to recommend AS or WW as treatment options, which meant that a doctor who suggested that choice risked a malpractice lawsuit if the patient agreed and the cancer later became life-threatening. Now, however, doctors can recommend various versions of AS or WW, with more or less frequent and more or less invasive monitoring tests depending on the clinical specifics of each case, not only because they feel it's the right thing for the patient, but because it's now professionally safe for them to do.

A growing number of doctors, recognizing the harm that overdiagnosis and overtreatment are doing, are offering these less aggressive options as ways of minimizing that harm. Some doctors actively encourage patients toward these options, and a growing number of patients are choosing them. One leading example is prostate cancer. Doctors have known for decades that prostate cancers are often slow growing and essentially nonthreatening, but before the advent of PSA testing, nearly all urologists prescribed surgery. In the late nineties, however, as the PSA test started to discover thousands of indolent cancers for which men were having surgery anyway—often suffering serious side effects—physicians began researching options that would allow them to honor their professional oath to do no harm.

Researchers learned that survival rates for men diagnosed with low-risk prostate cancer are similarly high, above 90%, whether they opt for AS, WW, or more aggressive treatment. (A big study confirming that was published in March 2023.)[4] Those findings gave doctors the confidence to add wait and monitor as a treatment option. It is now a sanctioned form of care for some patients in the professional guidelines of the American Urological Association.[5] First proposed in 2002, the use of watchful waiting and active surveillance has grown significantly since.[6] Only 7 out of 100 men diagnosed with low-risk prostate cancer between 1990 and 2009 chose it. According to one study, that had jumped to 40 in 100 for the period between 2010 and 2013.[7] The men more likely to choose it were 62 and older, for whom aggressive treatment was less likely to significantly extend their lives.[8]

As the number of men opting for AS or WW rose, the rate of men with low-risk prostate cancer choosing radical prostatectomy or radiation

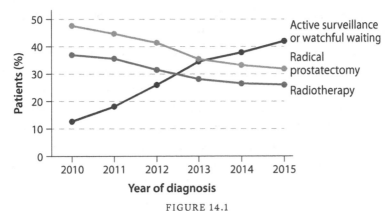

FIGURE 14.1

Treatment choices of men with low-risk prostate cancer, 2010–2015.
*Courtesy of Dr. Brandon Mahal, from B. A. Mahal, S. Butler, I. Franco, D. Spratt,
T. R. Rebbeck, A. V. D'Amico, and P. L. Nguyen, "Use of Active Surveillance or
Watchful Waiting for Low-Risk Prostate Cancer and Management Trends across
Risk Groups in the United States, 2010–2015," JAMA 33212, no. 7 (2019): 704–6*

dropped dramatically. Despite that, the mortality rate for the disease remained stable for that period.

Progress has also been made in offering active surveillance to some
thyroid cancer patients. In the early nineties Akira Miyauchi of Kuma
Hospital in Kobe, Japan, recognized that many thyroid cancers were such
a negligible threat to his patients that they probably didn't require total
removal of the thyroid gland. This was nearly two decades before the concept of overdiagnosis was formalized in the medical community. Miyauchi
organized research at two cancer centers in Japan, comparing outcomes in patients who were offered either ongoing monitoring (regular
ultrasound checkups of their small low-risk papillary tumors) or surgery.[9]
Follow-up showed equally high survival rates for both. Based on that research, in 2011 the Japanese Association of Endocrine Surgeons adopted
AS as a standard of care option. With follow-up research confirming the
Japanese results, the American Thyroid Association adopted AS as a standard of care option in 2015.

A growing number of cancer centers in the United States have begun offering this option, and its acceptance by patients has surprised
endocrine surgeons. One of the first to provide patients this choice was
the Memorial Sloan Kettering Cancer Center in New York, where skeptical doctors expected acceptance by perhaps 25% of their patients who

qualified. As of late 2019 the hospital reported an acceptance rate of closer to 80%.[10] The rate in Japan is 88%.[11]

As was the case when this less aggressive form of treatment was introduced in Japan, however, many doctors in the United States remain skeptical that watchful monitoring is as good as surgery at saving lives. Some also remain reluctant to offer that option because they think patients who don't have surgery will worry more about having cancer. But that's not what Miyauchi found. A 2019 study of Japanese men found that among patients who were on active surveillance as of 2017, 60% said they were less worried about their cancer than when they were first diagnosed, and 83% of them agreed that, looking back, they had made the right choice.[12]

There is less progress with breast cancer. As of 2021 no professional standard of care recommendation had been made for AS or WW as a treatment option for low-grade DCIS, which is one significant reason that nearly everyone who gets that diagnosis—close to 60,000 women a year in the United States—opts for some type of surgery. A doctor who suggests "wait and monitor" to a patient—and some do—does so at risk of being taken to court. Recall that the most common cause for a medical malpractice suit is an alleged *mis*diagnosis of breast cancer.

Another reason that AS or WW is not being more widely offered for DCIS is that, as noted in chapter 4, resistance remains fierce among some in the breast cancer medical community to the very idea of overdiagnosis and overtreatment. That resistance has delayed research comparing AS or WW to surgery to see if there is any mortality difference between the two approaches, research that professionals in the prostate cancer and thyroid cancer fields have been able to do. Without that evidence, providers of health care for breast cancer, quite understandably, believe they must still err on the side of caution.

That research has finally begun. Randomized clinical trials in the United States and Europe are under way to compare the two treatment paths. But as mentioned in chapter 4, fear of cancer is making this work difficult. Many women don't want to sign up for a study and take the chance that they will be randomly assigned to the group that gets only surveillance as treatment, not surgery. Yet the evidence of overdiagnosis and overtreatment of low-risk DCIS has been strong for more than a decade, and a growing number of doctors don't want to wait for the results of that research, which remains several years away at best. Many want to offer women the less aggressive treatment regime now. Shelley

Hwang, vice chair of surgery at Duke Cancer Institute and principal investigator on one of the research trials, said in a roundtable discussion organized by the American Society of Clinical Oncologists, "It is important for women to have the freedom to choose what they feel is the best balance between treatment and treatment-related morbidity. We're not giving them the full range of options right now because often we're treating all patients as if they have a life-threatening illness."[13] Dr. Hwang and others are frustrated that the only option they can offer women with low-grade DCIS is likely to do them more harm than good. "Surgery and radiation are not without side effects," she said. Another researcher, Ann Partridge, professor at Harvard Medical School and medical oncologist at the Dana Farber Cancer Institute, said, "Patients are understandably in a state of distress when they are diagnosed with DCIS, and physicians sometimes treat the condition as if it were a medical emergency . . . We all have experienced patients in our practices who have been destroyed by their breast surgery, especially mastectomy."

Eliminate the C-word

As we've seen, controversies about the PSA test and mammography were getting plenty of attention in the 1990s and early 2000s. But in May 2010, formal recognition of the general problem of overdiagnosis in cancer took a big step forward, with publication in the prestigious *Journal of the National Cancer Institute* of "Overdiagnosis in Cancer," by H. Gilbert Welch and William Black.[14] That article triggered bitter resistance from many in the field of cancer care, but it also catalyzed a whole movement to study the problem, understand its causes, quantify its harms, and recommend solutions. A meeting at the National Cancer Institute in March 2012 helped that movement get organized, and among the many suggestions that came from that meeting, one was to simply remove the frightening words "cancer" or "carcinoma" from the diagnoses of diseases that pose negligible risk.

Attendees wrote:

> The words used to describe a disorder substantially affect choice of intervention. Thus, precancerous lesions that confer low risk for development of a malignant disorder or lesions that have low risk for development of metastatic disease should not include the term cancer. . . .

. . . Unfortunately, when patients hear the word cancer, most assume they have a disease that will progress, metastasize, and cause death. Many physicians think so as well, and act or advise their patients accordingly. However, since many tumors do not have the unrelenting capacity for progression and death, new guidance is needed to describe and label the heterogeneous diseases currently referred to as cancer. . . .

. . . The rationale for this change in approach is that indolent lesions with low malignant potential are common, and screening brings indolent lesions and their precursors to clinical attention, which leads to overdiagnosis and, if unrecognized, possible overtreatment.[15]

Change in the semantics of cancer diagnosis actually began years earlier. The first was in 1988, when stage 0 cervical carcinoma in situ was renamed cervical intraepithelial neoplasia (CIN). Neoplasia is defined as abnormal or uncontrolled cell growth. It is a medically accurate way of describing cells that have the visual characteristics Dr. Rudolf Virchow first identified as cancer back in the mid-1800s (chapter 1) but avoids reference to the C-word. Critically, while some neoplasias spread—metastasize—some never do. The change was made not to reduce fear of low-grade nonthreatening cancers, but to help doctors more accurately communicate among themselves so their treatment matched the disease. But it reduced the number of women having clinically unnecessary surgery. There are three grades of CIN, and after the name change, the lower two grades were more frequently treated with active surveillance rather than surgery, especially in women of child-bearing age, since surgery could affect a woman's fertility and increase the risk of preterm births.

Then, in 1998, Grade 1 carcinoma of the bladder was renamed papillary urothelial neoplasia of low malignant potential—quite a mouthful but scientifically accurate, and no sign of the scary C-word. This too was done for doctors, not patients, but again the effect of this new nomenclature was that more patients chose less aggressive treatment.[16]

The first change specifically to address fear of the C-word came in 2016, when a panel of thyroid cancer experts renamed non-invasive encapsulated follicular variant of papillary thyroid carcinoma (EFVPTC) as non-invasive follicular thyroid neoplasm with papillary-like nuclear features (NIFTP). (The history behind this change is described in chapter 5). Still a mouthful, but when a patient hears the diagnosis now, the word "carcinoma" is gone. The goal was quite purposefully to reduce harm caused by fear of cancer. The experts recommending the change wrote, "The reclassification will affect a large population of patients worldwide and *result in a significant reduction in psychological and clinical consequences associated with the diagnosis of cancer*" (my emphasis).[17]

It's too early to know if the change is having any effect on the treatment patients choose, but a study found that removing the C-word from a *hypothetical* diagnosis of low-risk thyroid cancer changed people's choices. One thousand people were presented with three similar diagnoses, with one word changed, to either "nodule," "cancer," or "tumor." Subjects were also given various possible outcomes—from good to bad—for each. Researchers reported that people were so averse to the word "cancer" that they "were willing to accept a worse prognosis to avoid their disease being labeled as cancer." Researchers concluded "Omitting the word *cancer* from the disease label of low-risk epithelial malignant neoplasms may reduce overtreatment."[18]

No changes have yet been made to eliminate the frightening words "cancer" or "carcinoma" from diagnoses of low-grade prostate cancer or DCIS, but the idea has been proposed—formally in the case of prostate cancer. In 2011 a panel of experts convened by the NIH Office of Disease Prevention recommended, "Because of the very favorable prognosis of low-risk prostate cancer, strong consideration should be given to removing the anxiety-provoking term 'cancer' for this condition." The experts specifically said that the change was proposed because "treatment of low-risk prostate cancer patients with radical prostatectomy or radiation therapy leads to side effects such as impotence and incontinence in a substantial number." They recommended that the change might encourage more men to opt for "active surveillance," which "has emerged as a viable option that should be offered to patients with low-risk prostate cancer." The experts made clear that overscreening with PSA had prompted their proposal, writing, "The natural history of prostate cancer has changed dramatically in the past three decades because of PSA screening."[19] Others have made the same proposal.

Yet the medical community resists the change. So in 2022, a decade after the idea was first formally proposed, a group of prominent experts, including two urologists, a pathologist, an epidemiologist, and a patient care advocate, authored an essay in the *Journal of Clinical Oncology*, "Low-Grade Prostate Cancer: Time to Stop Calling It Cancer," writing, "When a cancer-related death rate approaches 0%, even in the absence of treatment, consideration should be given to modifying the screening, diagnostic, management, and terminology paradigms." They note that changes *have* been made in the screening paradigm (PSA is no longer recommended), and the management paradigm (active surveillance or watchful waiting is recommended), but "no matter how much time a physician may spend downplaying the significance of a GS6 [Gleason score 6] diagnosis or emphasizing the phrase 'low-risk,' the words 'you have cancer' have a potent psychological effect on most men and their families . . . Even if GS6 is biologically inert, its labeling is not, as it has an important influence and tangible consequences on how patients, providers, and the general public react and respond."[20]

That is precisely the case for changing the name of low-risk DCIS. In 2009 another group of experts convened by the NIH Office of Disease Prevention proposed, "Because of the noninvasive nature of DCIS, coupled with its favorable prognosis, strong consideration should be given to remove the anxiety-producing term 'carcinoma' from the description of DCIS." They too noted that treatment of low-risk DCIS may be doing more harm than good. "DCIS has a high probability of long-term disease-free survival and . . . all current therapies have short- and long-term side effects."[21]

At the 2012 Overdiagnosis in Medicine conference at the NCI, proponents of renaming low-risk DCIS offered an alternative: indolent lesion of epithelial origin (IDLE). Other proposals include "high-grade dysplasia," "precursor lesion," and "ductal intraepithelial neoplasia." Whatever the change, research has suggested that taking the word "carcinoma" out of the DCIS diagnosis could reduce a lot of harm. Researchers gave 394 women three fictitious DCIS scenarios describing DCIS as either "noninvasive breast cancer," "breast lesions," or "abnormal cells," and after each scenario, they offered the women one of three treatment choices—surgery, medication, or watchful waiting. When DCIS was described as "noninvasive breast cancer," 47% chose surgery, but when it was described as "breast lesions," only 33% wanted surgery, and when it was called "abnormal cells," only 30% wanted surgery." No matter the order in which the women read the scenarios, after reading all three and then being given the option of changing their initial choice, more women switched from surgery to nonsurgery than the other way around.[22]

Another study in Australia found much the same thing. Women who saw DCIS described as "abnormal cells" were less eager for aggressive treatment than those who saw it described as "pre-invasive cancer cells" (as it currently is). The authors wrote, "In a hypothetical scenario, interest in watchful waiting for DCIS was high, and changing terminology impacted women's concern and treatment preferences. Removal of the cancer term from DCIS may assist in efforts towards reducing overtreatment."[23]

Those who practice marketing or public relations or study cognitive heuristics would laugh at how obvious this is. It is no mystery that wording matters, or that deeper fear motivates more protective choices. Yet the name changes for prostate cancer and DCIS have sparked heated opposition. Opponents argue that it might lead some people to avoid more aggressive treatment that would save their lives. They say we still don't understand those diseases well enough to know which types merit the less alarming language. That's a curious argument for prostate cancer, since that disease is understood well enough to know which cases are sufficiently low risk that AS or WW can be offered as an alternative to aggressive treatment. Why not just rename those, when medically appropriate? ask advocates of that change.

Beyond the argument about the medical details, resistance to new terminology for a DCIS diagnosis is certainly also a reflection of the deep passions connected with breast cancer and women's health in general. Though the arguments against the change for DCIS are couched in medical specifics, the intense and visceral nature of the resistance suggests a defensiveness against the implicit message, that mammography isn't doing as much good (saving as many lives) as most people think it is. That doesn't bode well for this change happening anytime soon. Even without those passions, the redefinition of some types of cervical cancer took 40 years. The change in thyroid cancer took 20. The fight over changing the diagnostic nomenclature of low-grade DCIS will probably take many more years, during which tens of thousands of women frightened by the word "carcinoma" will choose surgeries they don't clinically require.

As an example of the medical community's conservatism about changing the nomenclature for indolent, or nonthreatening, cancers, consider lobular carcinoma in situ (LCIS), another tiny abnormality in breast tissue that mammography can spot. It's essentially the same as DCIS—especially in its prognosis—but the suspicious cells are found in the linings of the milk-producing glands, not in the ducts that carry the milk to the nipple. Because research has found that LCIS is not immediately threatening (though it can raise the risk of breast cancer later in life), doctors are no longer treating it as a cancer, and they *can* prescribe ongoing surveillance as a treatment option. Some doctors informally call it a "pre-cancer." Yet it still has carcinoma in the formal name.

Imagine how confused and worried a woman might be who is diagnosed with LCIS and goes to the American Cancer Society web page to learn more: "Lobular carcinoma in situ (LCIS) is a type of breast change that is sometimes seen when a breast biopsy is done. In LCIS, cells that look like cancer cells are growing in the lining of the milk-producing glands (lobules) of the breast, but they don't invade through the wall of the lobules. And then it says, "LCIS is not considered cancer."[1] Yet the word "carcinoma" is still in the name. In the simple English a worried patient needs, is LCIS cancer or isn't it?

Those in favor of taking the C-word out of some diagnoses acknowledge that more research is needed to identify just which cases warrant the less frightening wording. But they say that we know much more now than before widespread screening revealed so many nonthreatening cancers, enough so that some wording can be confidently changed. As Otis Brawley observed in many interviews when he was chief medical officer of the American Cancer Society, "We need a 21st-century definition of cancer instead of a 19th-century definition of cancer, which is what we've been using."

Changing Screening Protocols

More radical than calls to change the semantics of what screening finds are proposals to fundamentally change screening programs altogether, so they find fewer of the nonthreatening cancers that scare people into more treatment than they clinically require. The harms of overdiagnosis are now so widely recognized that these proposals are being taken seriously by some medical leaders. Any suggestion of less cancer screening, however, strikes directly at the public's deep belief in this first line of defense against our most feared disease, and of course it threatens the billions of dollars at stake for the screening industry. So the war over proposals to limit screening, especially for mammography, will make the nomenclature battle look like a skirmish.

The recommendations vary depending on which screening is being considered, but in general, the idea is to make cancer screening more targeted to those at risk.

- Some propose further narrowing the age range for whom screening is recommended.
- Others suggest going further, adding factors beyond age, like ethnicity and race, to the characteristics on which recommendations are based. Several research groups are using artificial intelligence to improve predictions of who is at risk for which types of cancer. This might expand screening for some while contracting it for others.
- Another recommendation is to make screening less frequent; for example, every two or three years for mammography instead of every other year as the USPSTF recommends now. Adjustments like that have already been made to the recommended frequency for colorectal cancer screening.
- Some suggest alternative screening methods, when available. Research has established that the fecal immunochemical test (FIT; take a sample at home and mail it in for analysis) is just as good as colonoscopy at indicating the possible presence of precancerous or cancerous cells, and colonoscopies should only be done after a suspicious FIT finding, which occurs in just 5%–6% of those using that test. The rest avoid the colonoscopy, reducing the possibility that unnecessary removal of polyps could cause problems. Kaiser Permanente health care and the Veterans Health Administration are both recommending this to people between 50 and 75, which as of January 2021 was the recommended age group for colorectal screening.
- Another suggestion is to narrow not who screening looks *at* but what screening looks *for*. The idea is to focus the search on only the conditions we know are actually dangerous. The experts at the "Addressing Overdiagnosis" meeting at the NCI in 2012 said, "Screening guidelines should be revised to lower the chance of detection of minimal-risk . . . and inconsequential cancers with the same energy traditionally used to

increase the sensitivity of screening tests (the higher the sensitivity the less likely it is that the test will miss something and produce a false negative)." Some suggest that these tighter standards be applied not just to what the initial screenings find but to the way radiologists interpret the results of mammograms, and to the decisions doctors make about whether to recommend follow-up biopsies when anything suspicious is found.

· One proposal is to scale back general population-wide early detection screening like mammography and PSA testing—which looks for *cancers that are already there*—and focus more on *preventive screening* like colorectal screening and cervical testing—which removes suspicious tissue before it even becomes cancer. In "Time to Abandon Early Detection Cancer Screening," five experts propose: "Cancer screening remains promoted as a fundamental component of current and future cancer control despite constantly growing evidence that more harm than benefit is created for most commonly used tests. *The currently prevailing nudging of the population towards cancer screening tests with little effect and a doubtful benefit-harm balance should be stopped.* [my emphasis] People should be informed unpassionately and objectively, and informed nonparticipation should be an accepted choice. Consequently, high attendance for such screening needs to be abandoned as a quality indicator for health care."[24]

The authors of this controversial editorial argue that the majority of cancers found with early detection screening either need no treatment or can be treated after they become symptomatic, with no increase in mortality. They call population-wide early detection screening "a large scale medical experiment" that has taught us that not all cancers go on to metastasize and kill, and that we need to recognize that the firm belief that "early detection is always beneficial" is simply not true. They note that when population-wide screening for several cancers—neuroblastoma in children, x-rays for early detection of lung cancer, ovarian cancer detection with a blood test looking for a marker protein called CA 125—were found to be ineffective and causing more harm than good, those programs were terminated. They argue that that's where we are with population-wide mammography and PSA testing, lamenting that in these two areas, particularly mammography, the medical community stubbornly refuses to accept that evidence. "Over time, both the scientific and the health care community have been surprisingly unwilling to embrace accumulating evidence that wide population-based early detection screening for cancer has not fulfilled our expectations, and indeed induced considerable harm to a large population of healthy individuals."[25]

They stop short of proposing the elimination of population-wide mammography and PSA testing, however, aware of how deeply the public believes in such screening. They suggest greater transparency between doctor and patient about these screenings' limitations and their potential harms as well as their benefits. "This may be more realistic and respectful of people's wishes rather than making screening completely unavailable. Nevertheless, we still need to be honest to ourselves and to our patients about what screening can achieve and what (mostly) it cannot achieve."[26] In another commentary, "Population-Based Screening for Cancer: Hope and Hype," other leaders in the movement to rethink screening make a similar case, suggesting that in light of all the evidence, "Individualized data and patient values should be taken into account when making key decisions on whom to screen, when to initiate and cease screening, how often to screen, and what action to take for patients with abnormal findings."[27]

As radically as such proposals challenge popular sentiment, they are being carefully considered in some places. As noted in chapter 3, the issue of overdiagnosis and overtreatment has gotten sufficient attention that England, Switzerland, and France convened expert panels to review their national mammography programs, and the Swiss and French both proposed significant changes. The French panel, which included members of the public and experts from the social as well as medical sciences, initially proposed dramatically scaling back general population mammography. But that met such opposition, mostly from the medical community and the screening industry, that the proposals were tempered and, in France, now only suggest modifications to the government's mammography program:

- End screening for women 50 or younger who are at average risk.

- Provide complete and neutral information for men and women, the public, and doctors that acknowledges the limitations of mammography and the problem of overdiagnosis.
- Train doctors to do a better job of helping women making fully informed decisions about breast cancer screening.
- Regularly assess the impact of screening on not only mortality but quality of life, as well as costs.
- Consider screening based on risk, so women at low risk would be screened less or not at all, and those at higher risk would be screened more intensively.

The Swiss Medical Board recommendation in 2014 to entirely phase out population-wide mammography was based on a review of the evidence that found, "the absolute reduction in breast cancer mortality was low and that the adverse consequences of the screening—false-positive test results, overdiagnosis and overtreatment of patients, and high costs, including the expense of follow-up testing and procedures— were substantial." The panel said,

> It is easy to promote mammography screening if the majority of women believe that it prevents or reduces the risk of getting breast cancer and saves many lives through early detection of aggressive tumors. We would be in favor of mammography screening if these beliefs were valid. Unfortunately, they are not, and we believe that women need to be told so. From an ethical perspective, a public health program that does not clearly produce more benefits than harms is hard to justify. Providing clear, unbiased information, promoting appropriate care, and preventing overdiagnosis and overtreatment would be a better choice.[28]

As evidence that there is a long way to go in actually making these changes, however, the Swiss recommendations were met by the same response as in France: strong opposition from the medical community, the screening industry, and breast cancer advocacy organizations. As a result screening actually expanded in Switzerland. The panel that reviewed mammography in England rejected the very idea of weighing mammography's benefits against its harms: "Uncertainty about possible interaction between the benefits of screening and of contemporary treatments is not a reason for stopping breast screening."[29]

Better Screening Tools

The demand for ever-better screening produces enormous profits for the businesses that develop new versions of these tools, so research is constantly under way to create improved technologies. This could reduce overdiagnosis and overtreatment by improving the *sensitivity* of screening tools, so no cancers are missed, reducing false negatives, and their *specificity*, so only truly threatening disease is found, which would reduce false positives.

One technology being hailed as a huge advance is the "liquid biopsy" approach to screening, the MCED approach discussed earlier, just coming into use in 2021. Analysis of blood samples can identify tiny bits of DNA released into the bloodstream from cancerous cells. A simple and inexpensive blood test can identify not only whether a person has a cancer somewhere in the body, but even which of 12 organs the cancer is in. (This goes beyond the genetic testing that identifies whether a person is at greater risk of developing cancer in the first place, or the molecular testing that is now being used to guide treatment.)

Yet, though liquid biopsy dramatically increases the potential to find more cancers and broadens the types of cancer for which screening is available, as this is being written, it still can't tell us what we really need to know: not whether cancer is present but what it's likely to do. So more people may get the frightening news that they have some sort of cancer and launch more aggressive follow-up testing and treatment than they clinically require. On the other hand, since cancers in their earliest stages slough off fewer cells that get out into the bloodstream, liquid biopsy is more likely to find more developed cancers in their later clinical stages. Those types of disease are far more likely to be life-threatening and not overdiagnosed—the ones where detection truly saves lives.

Work is also under way to take the truly critical next step in cancer screening, developing methods that not only identify what the cancer is but what it is likely to do. Two multiyear research projects are looking at the DNA in precancerous growths (like the polyps removed in a colonoscopy or the preinvasive cells of DCIS), and then tracking the DNA in those growths over time to see what they do. The goal is a "Pre-Cancer Atlas" that can identify which cancers are faster or slower growing, which ones are likely to metastasize, and which ones are likely to remain in situ or regress and disappear on their own, never causing any harm. As Sudhir Srivastava, the head of the project at the National Cancer Institute's Division of Cancer Prevention, says, the idea is "to accurately assess how likely it is for a precancerous growth to progress to life-threatening disease."[30]

Tests that have *some* of this predictive ability are already available. The Oncotype DX test looks at 21 key genes in a specimen of breast tumor cells and provides a score rating the likelihood that a breast cancer will recur or spread, even after surgery. Doctors base recommendations for postsurgery chemotherapy on that score. But not all breast cancers are the same, and the Oncotype DX test does not completely predict the future behavior of DCIS. The experience with this one hopeful tool highlights the immense challenge researchers face in understanding cancer genetics well enough to diagnose the cases that will become threatening and those that won't, the true solution to overdiagnosis.

Removing Screening's Halo

Any proposal to limit screening, in any way, especially by recommending it for only those at higher risk, faces an enormous hurdle: educating the public that widespread cancer screening causes harm as well as benefit. That is a huge challenge. Screening is central to the public's emotional relationship with cancer. It gives people a feeling of power, of control, something they can do to combat their deep fear of an often deadly disease. Recall the words of medical historian Robert Aronowitz quoted earlier: "When you've oversold both the fear of cancer and the effectiveness of our prevention and treatment, even people harmed by the system will uphold it, saying, 'It's the only ritual we have, the only thing we can do to prevent ourselves from getting cancer.'"

The cancer advocacy community will have a particularly difficult time making this shift. For decades their goal has been to increase screening participation. They have praised it, encouraged it, lobbied to expand it. And they're not alone. The positive message about screening has been magnified by the marketing from hospitals and clinics that provide, and profit from, screening services. Entire government and academic programs exist with the sole purpose of increasing participation in screening. As a result, the promotion of screening is ubiquitous, and as discussed earlier, often unbalanced, extolling its benefits while offering little or no information about how modest its benefits may be (mammography) and no caution about its potential harms.

Consider, for example, *Breast Cancer Screening and Diagnosis* 2022, an information resource published by the National Comprehensive Cancer Network, a group of 32 of the top cancer centers in the United States.[31] It offers clear and helpful information about breast cancer and explains mammography and its benefits. Yet in its 51 pages there is not a whisper about the potential harm of mammography. The words "overdiagnosis" and "overtreatment" don't appear. The problems are not hinted at, not even in the five-page section "Risk Assessment for Screening." Nor are they alluded to in the "Questions to Ask" section, which begins with this text: "In shared decision making, you and your health care provider (HC) discuss the risk for developing breast cancer and agree to a screening schedule." If you rely on this guide, the discussion of risk includes nothing about the potential harm mammograms can sometimes lead to, only its benefits. This is from the most well-respected cancer hospitals in the country.

The situation is similar for prostate cancer. Research published in 2022 analyzed the communications from 607 US cancer centers that recommend prostate cancer screening. Four in ten failed to mention anything about the potential harms of that screening. And one in four failed to suggest that men discuss the pros and cons of screening with their doctors as recommended by the US Preventive Services Task Force (USP-STF). Major cancer centers accredited by the National Cancer Institute were twice as likely as non-NCI-accredited centers to fail to recommend shared decision making. And eight in ten of all 607 centers also failed to inform men that the USPSTF recommends that testing stop at age 70.[32]

As a result, faith in cancer screening remains almost religious, and the public knows practically nothing about screening's drawbacks and limitations. Recall from chapter 3 the findings that a large majority of people want cancer screening even when they are told it will do them no good and cause harm. Misleadingly imbalanced recommendations for screening that fail to alert people to potential harms are complicit in the harm that screening leads to.

But steadily, the message is starting to come from some in the medical community, the cancer advocacy community, and even the news media that screening is not all we've been led to believe. The evidence for over-diagnosis and overtreatment triggered by mass screening programs has convinced all but the most stubborn opponents that some of the ways we're trying to help people are hurting people too. The websites of most major cancer advocacy organizations now offer at least some information on the limitations and harms of screening, cautions that didn't used to be there.

- In the National Breast Cancer Coalition's "22 Myths and Truths" quiz, Myth 2 is "Mammograms can only help and not harm you," and the response is "FALSE. What's the risk? False-positive results may lead to unnecessary, intrusive surgical interventions, while false-negative results will not find cancerous tumors."[33]
- A Susan G. Komen web page on mammography promi-nently notes, "There are questions related to: How much benefit mammography offers" and offers links to "The over-diagnosis and over-treatment of ductal carcinoma in situ (DCIS) and small, slow-growing invasive breast cancers."[34] The site even summarizes the research ques-tioning whether mammography actually saves lives, and the ways it can cause harm.
- The American Cancer Society still heavily promotes screen-ing, but now includes cautions about mammography, though the page "Limitations of Mammograms" is buried several links inside on their website: When (if) you finally get to that link, the page goes into detail about the risk of false positives, overdiagnosis, and overtreatment.[35]
- The ACS also offers, buried deep inside its website, this caution about PSA testing: "If prostate cancer is found as a result of screening, it will probably be at an earlier, more treatable stage than if no screening were done. While this might make it seem like prostate cancer screening would always be a good thing, there are still issues surrounding screening that make it unclear if the benefits outweigh the risks for most men."[36]
- The Prostate Cancer Foundation website includes a page that acknowledges, "There is controversy about the risks and

benefits of prostate cancer screening," although it says nothing about the overdiagnosis and overtreatment the PSA test often leads to.[37] (One of the largest prostate cancer advocacy groups, Us Too, which has merged with the group ZERO Prostate Cancer, offers numerous testimonials about PSA testing but practically nothing about its limitations or harms.)

Some professional medical organizations, especially those that don't have a financial interest in screening as the American College of Radiology does, are paying more attention to the drawbacks of cancer screening.

- The influential American Academy of Family Physicians, whose advice shapes the care delivered by thousands of general practitioners, has carried numerous articles like one headlined "Don't Recommend Screening for Breast, Colorectal, Prostate, or Lung Cancers without Considering Life Expectancy and the Risks of Testing, Overdiagnosis, and Overtreatment."[38]
- The American College of Obstetricians and Gynecologists recommendations for mammography state: "Regular screening mammography starting at age 40 years reduces breast cancer mortality in average-risk women. Screening, however, also exposes women to potential harms, such as callbacks, anxiety, false-positive results, overdiagnosis and overtreatment."[39]
- The American Urological Association guidelines on PSA testing state: "The quality of evidence for the benefits of screening was moderate, and evidence for harm was high for men age 55 to 69 years. For men outside this age range, evidence was lacking for benefit, but the harms of screening, including over diagnosis and overtreatment, remained."[40]

Across the medical world, the limitations of screening are getting increasing attention. A flood of research is coming out on the issue of overdiagnosis. Influential journals like the *British Medical Journal*, *JAMA Internal Medicine*, the *New England Journal of Medicine*, and *Nature*, among others, have featured dozens of studies and commentaries on the issue. In 2017 the NIH newsletter published an article titled "To Screen or Not to Screen? The Benefits and Harms of Screening Tests."[41]

While those publications may not reach the general public, the news media do, and here too there is progress. Hundreds of stories have appeared in recent years about the harm of overdiagnosis. More and more those stories are making it clear that some cancer screening is not as beneficial as widely believed and often leads to real damage. The following headlines all ran in mainstream media outlets.

> "Prostate Cancer Screening Is No Longer Automatic; That's Turned Out to Be a Sensible Change"; "Debating the Value of PSA Prostate Screening"; "More Doctors Say Men Should Think Twice about Prostate Cancer Screening"; "Mammograms More Likely to Cause Unneeded Treatment than to Save Lives"; "The Case for Annual Mammograms Is More Complicated than Ever"; "Breast Cancer Screening Programme 'Does More Harm than Good'"; "Quandary with Mammograms: Get a Screening, or Just Skip It?"; "Screening for Lung Cancer Is a Controversial Idea"; "Colonoscopies Can Cause Greater Infection Risk"; "Are We Now Doing Too Much Cancer Screening?"[42]

The whole concept of overdiagnosis and overtreatment of cancer is getting more news media attention too:

> "'Overdiagnosis' in about 20% of Common Cancers"; "Breast Cancer and Mammograms: Study Suggests 'Widespread Overdiagnosis'"; "Debate over Early-Stage Cancer: To Treat or Not to Treat?"; "We Really Need to Rethink How We Diagnose and Treat Breast Cancer"; "Doubt Is Raised over Value of Surgery for Breast Lesion at Earliest Stage"; "Thousands of Australians Undergo Chemo after Being 'Overdiagnosed' with Cancer Each Year"; "What Is DCIS and Is This Type of Breast Cancer Overtreated?"; "When Treating Abnormal Breast Cells, Sometimes Less Is More"; "The Danger of DCIS, the Breast 'Cancer' That's Often Not."[43]

There has also been reporting on the idea of renaming certain low-risk cancers.

> "Doctors Debate Whether to Stop Calling Low-Risk Tumors 'Cancer'"; "'Cancer' or 'Weird Cells': Which Sounds Deadlier?"; "Doctors Should Stop Using the Word Cancer: Low-Risk Tumours Should Be

Renamed 'Indolent' Because the C-word Traumatises Patients,
Leading Expert Says."[44]

Even news coverage of the controversies over revised USPSTF recommendations for PSA and mammography have helped broaden public
awareness that screening might not be right for everyone. A content
analysis of the coverage of the controversies around changes to mammography recommendations found "shifts in the relative attention
given to mammography screening's risks and benefits, with consistent
and, in some cases, heightened attention to screening's risks during more
recent media events."[45]

The Overdiagnosis Movement

Many of the journal articles and news media coverage of the limitations
of screening and the prevalence of cancers that don't kill have been generated by what might be called the overdiagnosis movement, a growing
group of doctors, academics, journalists, and others trying to raise awareness of the issue and reduce the harm it causes.

In 1978, as mammography was just starting up, Dr. Anthony Miller
of the University of Toronto (who peer-reviewed chapters 4-8) challenged
the orthodoxy about screening in a paper, noting "Screening is not a
simple and direct approach to cancer control. [There is] differing awareness of the hidden costs of screening and of the excess morbidity that
screening can create. For example, screening leads to some diagnostic
procedures that otherwise would never be done."[46] In a 1991 article for a
textbook, he referred to this as "overdiagnosis."

The true pioneers of the overdiagnosis movement, though, were Drs.
William Black and H. Gilbert Welch. In 1993, with mammography finding more and more cases of DCIS, and PSA testing starting to spread, they
described in a paper how the misleading measures of lead-time bias and
length bias (see chapter 3) make breast cancer screening seem more effective at saving lives than it is, leading to discovery of "cases that would
regress, remain stable, or progress too slowly to become clinically apparent during the patient's lifetime. Some authors have described these
cases as of 'pseudo-disease' and consider this aspect of length bias separately, as a basis of overdiagnosis." They also presciently warn, "Mispercep-
tions of disease prevalence and therapeutic effectiveness can promote a
cycle of increasing medical interventions. The cycle usually begins with

some form of increased testing that lowers the threshold of detection, such as technical improvement in imaging tests, more frequent testing, or closer scrutiny of images. This immediately leads to a higher diagnostic yield of the disease and a spectrum of milder cases. These effects are almost always interpreted as indicating progress and provide immediate reinforcement for the increasing testing, despite the caveat that earlier detection is a double-edge sword."[47] (Later authors would call this the "popularity paradox," writing, "The greater the harm through overdiagnosis and overtreatment from screening, the more people there are who believe they owe their health, or even their life, to the programme."[48] A Google search in March 2023 of the phrase "screening saved my life" produced 176 million entries.

Black followed with the study "Overdiagnosis: An Underrecognized Cause of Confusion and Harm in Cancer Screening" in 2000, and in 2010 he and Welch authored the most widely read paper on the subject, "Overdiagnosis in Cancer," which has been cited nearly 1,500 times.[49] These pieces, along with many that focused on just the DCIS or PSA controversies (and others that looked at overdiagnosis and overtreatment of cervical cancer, melanoma, and neuroblastoma in children), helped increase awareness of the overdiagnosis and overtreatment issue in the medical community and in the general public.

Overdiagnosis is getting more attention in books. In 2008 Shannon Brownlee authored *Overtreated: Why Too Much Medicine Is Making Us Sicker and Poorer*.[50] In 2012, H. Gilbert Welch and Dartmouth colleagues Lisa Schwartz and Steve Woloshin wrote *Overdiagnosed: Making People Sick in the Pursuit of Health*; Otis Brawley authored *How We Do Harm: A Doctor Breaks Ranks about Being Sick in America*; Gayle Sulik wrote *Pink Ribbon Blues: How Breast Cancer Culture Undermines Women's Health*; and Anthony Horan published *How to Avoid the Over-Diagnosis and Over-Treatment of Prostate Cancer*.[51] In 2014 Richard Ablin and Ronald Piana published *The Great Prostate Hoax: How Big Medicine Hijacked the PSA Test and Caused a Public Health Disaster*.[52] In 2018 Renée Pellerin published *Conspiracy of Hope: The Truth about Breast Cancer Screening*.[53] According to Google's Ngram, between 1960 and 2019, the number of books using the word "overdiagnosis" increased 30 times.

In 2013 a few hundred doctors, researchers, and journalists working on the issue around the world convened at Dartmouth College in the first "Preventing Overdiagnosis: Winding Back the Harms of Too Much Medicine" conference, a partnership between Bond University in Australia, the Dartmouth Institute for Health Policy and Clinical Practice, the *British Medical Journal*, and *Consumer Reports* magazine. (The academic field of overdiagnosis that this conference helped coalesce looks at the problem of "too much medicine" across all of health care, not just cancer.)

These details may seem unimportant, but they are included here because the work of these academics and activists, and the dissemination of that work by prominent medical journals, has played a significant role in all the efforts to reduce overdiagnosis. Troublingly, though, in the hundreds of papers and posters presented at the annual Preventing Overdiagnosis conferences, and in the several hundred papers about the issue published in academic journals, the blame is laid on the medical industry, the cancer industry, the news media, lawyers, doctors who fail to adequately inform their patients, and the advocacy community. But very little research has been done to understand the role that the public's fear of cancer plays in the overscreening, overdiagnosis, and overtreatment problem. At the Preventing Overdiagnosis conferences I attended where I raised this aspect of the issue, there seemed to be a reluctance to say anything that sounded like blaming the patient for part of the problem. This means that across all the efforts to combat overscreening, overdiagnosis, and overtreatment, little is being done to deal with one of the underlying causes, people's sometimes excessive fear of a dread disease. Little organized research is trying to understand the psychological roots behind people's judgments and choices about cancer screening and what to do about a diagnosis of a low-risk type of cancer.

That understanding could help the overdiagnosis movement develop more effective tools to help people make more informed and healthier choices. But plenty of tools are already out there. And there are things you can do to keep the fear of cancer from overwhelming your ability to think things through so you can make the healthiest possible choices.

combating cancerphobia in yourself

To fear is one thing. To let fear grab you by the tail and swing you around is another.
—Katherine Patterson

I'm not afraid of storms, for I'm learning how to sail my ship.
—Louisa May Alcott

A thousand fearful images and dire suggestions glance along the mind when it is moody and discontented with itself. Command them to stand and show themselves, and you presently assert the power of reason over imagination.
—Sir Walter Scott

In chapter 4 we met Kathy as she learned she had DCIS. In chapter 5 we met Michael as learned he had low-grade prostate cancer. We met Tom in chapter 14 as he heard that same frightening diagnosis. They each reacted as nearly everyone does who hears "You have cancer": with fear first, and then, even as the shock is still wearing off, by trying to learn everything they could to gain a sense of control as they decided what to do.

As described in chapter 2, this fear first, critical thinking second reaction to danger is how the brain works. We can't help it. It is instinctive and protects us if the threat requires a quick reaction. But it can start us down the path to less-than-optimal choices if we let those initial emotions continue to dominate how we respond to the threat as time passes. Avoiding this pitfall is difficult because, as also explained in chapter 2, even after the initial shock is behind us and we've calmed down, emotion continues to have more influence on our thinking than rational objective reasoning. Think of it like a conversation in the mind between reason and emotion. Reason speaks quietly. Emotion shouts.

So if we want to make the best choice, the most thoughtful choice, the most informed choice, and avoid being swept away by the emotional current of our fear of cancer, we have to make a conscious effort to fight back against these cognitive instincts. We do so not just by getting more information, but by consciously working to give that information more weight as we make our choices. The challenge is not to ignore our emotions but to give reason a louder voice in the mental conversation. If we can consciously "command" our "fearful images and dire suggestions" about cancer "to stand and show themselves"; if we pause, even for just a moment, and step back and recognize how our emotions are making it harder to consider things objectively; if we can realize that sometimes we are so afraid, choices that feel safe actually make things worse, then we can "assert the power of reason" and use the facts and the evidence to make choices that feel right *and* that will do us the most good. That's the real challenge Kathy, Michael, and Tom faced—not just getting the information and the reassuring sense of empowerment and control it provides, but slowing down, "backpaddling against the current of our emotions," as Tom put it, so we can use that information wisely.

It would be insufficient for this book to suggest that we need to rethink our fear of cancer without offering at least a few specific suggestions about how we might do that in our personal lives as we face the choices this book considers. What follows, then, are a few key insights from cognitive psychology that can help us improve our critical thinking. Some may seem obvious, but they are key recommendations from leading experts about how to temper our emotions with reason to make the wisest and healthiest possible choices.

- Most important, don't jump to conclusions. (I warned you some of these would seem obvious.) In most cases, our first and almost instantaneous judgment—"Yes, I should screen" or *"Cut it out of my body!"*—though obviously not thoroughly thought through, will frame how you feel about anything you subsequently learn. As Nobel Prize–winning economist Daniel Kahneman puts it in his seminal book, *Thinking, Fast and Slow*, "If there is time to reflect, slowing down is likely to be a good idea."[1]

It's generally wise when facing any choice, but especially a heavily emotion-laden choice about your health and safety, to stop, even for just a moment, and think, not just feel, to paddle backward, to slow the decision-making process down. The first choice you make may feel right—and it may end up being the choice you finally make—but it will be more thoughtful if you don't let the loud voice of your emotions drown out your ability to think more analytically. Remember, despite all the adages that recommend going with your gut instinct first, that quick not-thought-through initial judgment can also get you into trouble. Decision-making about risk is a risk all by itself.

- We tend to seek, and believe, information that comes from sources we trust.

That reasonable instinct sometimes leads us to sources of information that tell us what we like to hear but aren't providing the most reliable, balanced information. Advertisers and marketers, from the best cancer centers to the most outrageous quack cure peddlers, prey on this instinct. Work hard to find sources that are both credible and neutral. Here is one approach: Imagine as you do your research that you are a journalist researching a story you will write for others. You're not just trying to learn about things for yourself, through the lenses of all your personal emotions and life circumstances. A good journalist needs to be more independent, neutral, curious, thorough, and reasonably skeptical.

The very first thing a cautious journalist looks for is bias. Does the source have some motivation for spinning the facts one way or another? Are they selling a product or service? Do they have a political interest, or an interest in some general cause, like promoting the benefits of screening and therefore playing down or ignoring its harms? Many health websites market themselves to certain audiences, like people seeking information about "natural medicine" or "alternative medicine." Information from these sources will be biased.

Most importantly, ask yourself: Does the source have a financial interest? Remember, the economic incentives are enormous for doctors, hospitals, and companies to promote screening and more treatment rather than less. You may not be getting complete and neutral information from these sources either, no matter how reputable they are. So be wary of bias, which is a warning that the information you'll be getting is not the whole picture, intended to emphasize one perspective, not to fully inform. (A good place to check for potentially biasing interests is in the "About Us" section on most websites, which provides an idea of the motivations of the site publisher.)

Journalists will also ask themselves whether a source seems knowledgeable and reputable. Is the source credible? What is their expertise? A lot of sites offering "natural" medicines, for example, are produced by people with very little or no real training in either Western or "alternative" medicine. They are often just hucksters. Again, don't just read the information they provide about the issue. Read the "About Us" section, which should tell you not only who the organization is, but its goals, history, leadership, and crucially, the level of expertise of those leaders.

It is also common to seek discussion groups about an issue we're interested in, to hear from people who have gone through what we're facing. But good journalists know that people who post the most and speak with the greatest passion are disproportionately people who had negative experiences. The people who had positive experiences contribute far less often to these conversations. That means these discussion groups can provide a distortedly negative picture of what you're trying to carefully think through.

- We tend to believe the information we want to believe. We see the facts the way we want to, based on our beliefs, the beliefs of the groups we identify with and want to be loyal to, our education, and our life circumstances. The *facts* become our *truth* only after passing through all those filters. As you gather more information, try to fairly consider facts that may conflict with how you feel. This can be difficult given that feelings have so much power in shaping our perceptions and judgments, especially matters about our safety and survival.
- Due to a cognitive trap called "primacy and recency," we give disproportionate weight to the first few things we read and the last few things we read, paying less attention to what comes in the middle. So make a mental or even a physical note of all the important points you want to remember. It's also a good idea

to go back and read things through more than once. You'll probably discover something relevant that you glossed over.

· We are disproportionately influenced by information that carries the most emotional power. This is why the websites of hospitals, clinics, and doctors that want your business, and advocacy groups trying to convince you to make a certain choice, prominently feature moving personal stories of outcomes that praise certain options over others, like testimonials from people convinced that "screening saved my life." In our fearful hunger for hope, we can't help being moved by these stories, but they are only the story of *one* person in the context of *their* life. And they are on the website for a reason, which has more to do with advocating a particular choice than neutrally informing yours. Beware being swayed by any information or marketing message with high emotional content.

· Remember the pitfall of "loss aversion," a mental filter that leads us to emotionally overweight anything associated with a negative outcome. This is why we're likely to feel, quite under-standably, that "a one in a million chance is still too high if that one could be me." One way to counteract loss aversion and consider statistics more objectively is by seeing them as though they applied to someone else, to the public you are writing for as a journalist, not to yourself. From that less personal perspec-tive, one in a million looks like a pretty small risk.

· Remember that certain inherent psychological characteris-tics related to cancer make it more frightening than other risks: there is the fear of anything that causes greater *pain and suffering*, there is *uncertainty*, the feeling that we have *no control*, that it has been *imposed* on us by *human-made* substances, and most of us know someone who has had it, or died of it, which makes it more likely we will imagine ourselves as that person. These are the emotional, psycho-logical "fearful images and dire suggestions" we need to "command to stand and show themselves." Try to be consciously aware of how these "fear factors" are fueling your worries. You can defuse their impact by consciously

being alert to their influence rather than letting them work
hidden in the background, clouding your critical thinking.

Awareness of these factors helps you use them as tools for decision
making. For example, knowing that a sense of control is important, consider how some choices, like screening, provide a comforting sense of
control. You might want to think about active surveillance or watchful
waiting for slow-growing cancers as a real way to take control. These approaches are not just sitting back and doing nothing. They *empower* you
to carefully, *actively* monitor things, on a rigorous schedule. Knowing that
pain and suffering is part of what makes cancer so frightening, don't consider only the pain and suffering from the disease, but also the pain and
suffering from the side effects of the treatment you're considering. Knowing that we worry more about cancer because it feels imposed on us, ask
yourself if your disease is mostly the result of exposure to human-made
substances (lung cancer from asbestos exposure), or if it's most likely just
the result of aging (prostate cancer) or voluntary lifestyle choices (lung
cancer from smoking). Remind yourself that while you may have known
people who have had the cancer you have, you may not have known all
the details of their experience, and your life and your medical circumstances are unique.

Tools to Help with Your Decisions

Here's another key point to remember as you consider the frightening
choices about whether to screen for cancer or what to do about a diagnosis
of a low-risk type of the disease: you're not alone. A lot of people have done
a lot of research to develop tools that can help you think through these
choices. Many are available through health care providers. Others are
available online. Research finds that these decision tools help users feel
more comfortable that they have thought things through more carefully.

As helpful as these tools can be, however, keep in mind two key warnings. Most tools should be used only in concert with a health care provider with expertise. Learning about things online is empowering and
important, but your ability to use Google doesn't make you a Google
doc(tor). The other caution is that while finding these tools may be easy,
some do a better job than others. The challenge is finding those that not
only provide reliable, thorough, and balanced information on both the

benefits *and the risks* of various options, but also walk you through making choices in the context of your emotions.

Deciding Whether to Screen

Dozens of tools can help you think through the choice about whether to screen. The simplest are "risk calculators," which let you enter your personal characteristics to see how high or low your risk of a particular cancer might be and to determine whether screening is right for you, at least based on key demographic and health characteristics. The Breast Cancer Surveillance Consortium offers a risk calculator for breast cancer.[2] The Cleveland Clinic offers one for prostate cancer.[3]

These calculators are helpful, but even more valuable are what are known as "decision aids." These describe the screening process itself, list the recommendations for who should screen, and explain how those recommendations were determined. Many even help you think through the emotional aspects of the choice you face, posing questions like "Do I want to know I have _____ cancer?" or "How do I feel about the possibility of getting a false positive?" Tools like these were developed as part of the shared decision-making movement in medicine in the nineties to empower patients to be more involved in their care.[4] National and international groups set standards for decision aids to make sure they're clear, accurate, thorough, and balanced.[5] Several states promote the use of these tools. Doctors aren't supposed to be reimbursed by Medicare for a lung cancer screening unless they can prove they had a shared decision-making conversation with their patient *and* provided at least one decision aid.

But as we've seen, the idea that screening is not right for everyone and that it can lead to harm from overdiagnosis and overtreatment is still relatively new in medicine, and it challenges the nearly blind belief in screening and that finding cancer as early as possible is always beneficial. As a result, many of these aids promote the benefits of screening but fail to mention the risks, an imbalance that will leave you less than fully informed. Sadly, that imbalance is common, at least among screening decision aids offered online. One study found that as of 2015, two-thirds of the online decision aids for cancer screening didn't provide a balanced description of screening's benefits *and* risks. That study looked at the websites of reputable and knowledgeable sources: the USPSTF, the American Cancer Society, the American College of Physicians, and the National Comprehensive Cancer Network—a coalition of the top cancer hos-

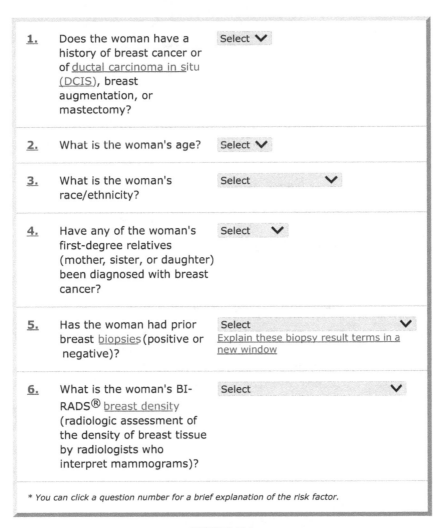

1.	Does the woman have a history of breast cancer or of ductal carcinoma in situ (DCIS), breast augmentation, or mastectomy?	Select ⌄
2.	What is the woman's age?	Select ⌄
3.	What is the woman's race/ethnicity?	Select ⌄
4.	Have any of the woman's first-degree relatives (mother, sister, or daughter) been diagnosed with breast cancer?	Select ⌄
5.	Has the woman had prior breast biopsies (positive or negative)?	Select ⌄ Explain these biopsy result terms in a new window
6.	What is the woman's BI-RADS® breast density (radiologic assessment of the density of breast tissue by radiologists who interpret mammograms)?	Select ⌄

You can click a question number for a brief explanation of the risk factor.

FIGURE 15.1

Breast Cancer Surveillance Consortium Risk Calculator V2.

Image courtesy of Breast Cancer Surveillance Consortium, https://tools.bcsc-scc.org /BC5yearRisk/; risk model tested in J. A. Tice, M. C. S. Bissell, D. L. Miglioretti, C. C. Gard, G. H. Rauscher, F. M. Dabbous, and K. Kerlikowske, "Validation of the Breast Cancer Surveillance Consortium Model of Breast Cancer Risk," Breast Cancer Research and Treatment *175 (2019): 519-23*

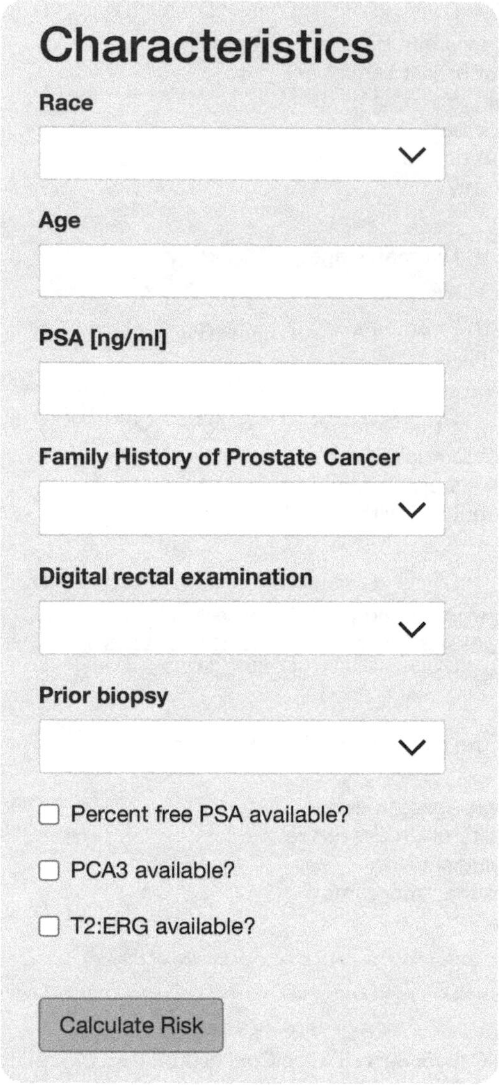

Characteristics

Race

[⌄]

Age

[   ]

PSA [ng/ml]

[   ]

Family History of Prostate Cancer

[⌄]

Digital rectal examination

[⌄]

Prior biopsy

[⌄]

☐ Percent free PSA available?

☐ PCA3 available?

☐ T2:ERG available?

[Calculate Risk]

FIGURE 15.2
Prostate Cancer Prevention Trial Risk Calculator Version 2.0.
Courtesy of Cleveland Clinic, https://riskcalc.org/PCPTRC/

pitals. Researchers found that the USPSTF site did a balanced job, but that the other three played up the benefits of screening and downplayed or entirely failed to discuss the risks.[6]

Another study, which reviewed 85 screening decision aids available through health care providers for prostate (36), breast (26), lung (10), colorectal (10), thyroid (1), and other cancers (2), found more encouraging results. As of 2017, roughly eight in ten of those tools made some reference to the concepts of overdiagnosis and overtreatment. One-third used those specific terms, explaining them with language like "What does overdiagnosis mean? This means a diagnosis of a breast cancer that, in hindsight, would not have caused harm," or describing overtreatment as "treatment for a slow-growing lung cancer that would not have caused problems even if you never got treatment." Two-thirds of these tools avoided the specific terms "overdiagnosis" and "overtreatment" but still alerted users to the problem with language like "A high PSA test may find a prostate cancer that is slow-growing and never would have caused you problems" or that screening could lead to "an unnecessary diagnosis (being diagnosed and treated for cancer that might not be harmful)." The review found that all the aids for lung cancer and nearly all of the aids for prostate cancer mentioned both benefits and harms of screening, but only six out of ten aids for breast or colorectal cancer screening included this critical balance. And only one decision aid out of three that discussed overdiagnosis and overtreatment in general then offered probabilities, putting the pros and cons of screening in clearer numeric perspective, as in the figure depicting the statistical pros and cons of lung cancer screening in chapter 7.[7] The Harding Center for Risk Literacy created one like it for breast cancer screening.

Researchers including Steve Woloshin, Gird Gigerenzer, Brian Zikmund-Fisher, Isaac Lipkus, and Ellen Peters have done a lot of work developing tools that help us with our innumeracy by making statistical information clearer and more useful. Research has confirmed that presenting numbers this way can help.

So if you are not presented with a decision aid by your health care provider, ask them to provide one.

From a review for this book of more than 100 decision aids for screening available online and intended for a general audience, a few stand out as clear, reliable, and balanced. Critically, they cite the recommended age ranges for screening from the neutral USPSTF, as opposed to those from cancer advocacy groups or medical organizations, which generally have wider ranges for when to start and stop. These tools also discuss screening's limitations and risks as well as its benefits. An online tool for PSA screening is available from medical publisher UpToDate.[8] The Australian Screening Mammography Decision Aid Trial is a well-known aid for helping women

Early detection of breast cancer by mammography screening

Numbers for women aged 50 years and older* who either did or did not participate in mammography screening for approximately 11 years.

1,000 women without screening

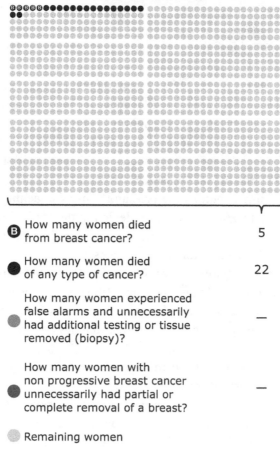

ⓑ How many women died from breast cancer?	5
● How many women died of any type of cancer?	22
● How many women experienced false alarms and unnecessarily had additional testing or tissue removed (biopsy)?	—
● How many women with non progressive breast cancer unnecessarily had partial or complete removal of a breast?	—
● Remaining women	

FIGURE 15.3

Decision aid for mammography.

Adapted from an image courtesy of Harding Center for Risk Literacy; data from P. C. Gøtzsche and K. J. Jørgensen, "Screening for Breast Cancer with Mammography," Cochrane Database of Systematic Reviews 2013, no. 6 (2013): CD001877

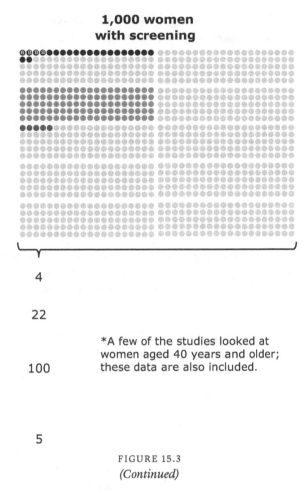

**1,000 women
with screening**

4

22

*A few of the studies looked at
women aged 40 years and older;
these data are also included.

100

5

FIGURE 15.3
(Continued)

think through whether to start mammography at age 40.[9] UpToDate also
has an online decision aid for those considering lung cancer screening.[10]

Several more helpful cancer-screening tools and resources are available online:

- *Making Sense of Screening*, an online brochure published in
  2015 by the organization Sense about Science, is a terrific
  background piece on screening in general, including its
  benefits and harms: https://senseaboutscience.org/wp
  -content/uploads/2016/11/Makingsenseofscreening.pdf.
- "Screening Tests," CDC, last reviewed May 19, 2022, https://
  www.cdc.gov/cancer/dcpc/prevention/screening.htm.

Should I be screened for prostate cancer?

The answer to this question is not the same for everyone. Your doctor can help you decide based on your values and preferences.

The main test used to screen for prostate cancer is a blood test called a "PSA test." Doctors offer screening in the hopes of catching prostate cancer early — before it has a chance to grow, spread, or cause symptoms. But it is not clear if getting screened for prostate cancer can extend a man's life or help him avoid any symptoms or problems.

It might help to ask yourself the following questions when deciding whether or not to be screened:

FIGURE 15.4

Decision aid for PSA screening.

Reproduced with permission from R. M. Hoffman, "Patient Education: Prostate Cancer Screening" (Beyond the Basics), in UpToDate, *edited by T. W. Post (Waltham, MA: UpToDate), accessed Sept. 20, 2022, https://www.uptodate.com /contents/screening-for-prostate-cancer. Copyright © 2022 UpToDate, Inc. and its affiliates and/or licensors. All rights reserved*

- "Cancer Screening Overview (PDQ)—Patient Version," National Cancer Institute, last updated Aug. 18, 2020, https://www.cancer.gov/about-cancer/screening/patient -screening-overview-pdq.
- USPSTF cancer-screening recommendations search results, US Preventive Services Task Force, accessed Feb. 14, 2023, https://www.uspreventiveservicestaskforce.org/uspstf /search_results?searchterm=cancer%20screening.
- For breast cancer specifically: "Weighing the Benefits and Risks of Screening Mammography," Susan G. Komen, updated Nov. 30, 2022, https://www.komen.org/breast -cancer/screening/mammography/benefits-risks/.
- Also for breast cancer: "Mammography for Breast Cancer Screening: Harm/Benefit Analysis," National Breast Cancer Coalition, updated July 2021, https://www.stopbreastcancer .org/information-center/positions-policies/mammography -for-breast-cancer-screening-harm-benefit-analysis/.
- For prostate cancer, "AAFP Updates Its PSA Screening Recommendation," American Academy of Family Physicians, July 20, 2018, https://www.aafp.org/news/health-of -the-public/20180720aafppsarec.html.

- Also for prostate cancer: "Prostate Cancer Screening: Should You Get a PSA Test?," Mayo Clinic, Nov. 3, 2022, https://www .mayoclinic.org/tests-procedures/psa-test/in-depth/prostate -cancer/art-20048087.
- For lung cancer: the University of Michigan's Should I Screen website, last updated October 7, 2021, https://shouldiscreen .com/English/home.

Do these tools help? The bulk of the research suggests they do.[11] Users say they feel more informed, more empowered, and most important, more comfortable with their choices. But the evidence also shows that decision aids are unlikely to have much influence on what a person ultimately chooses to do about screening. One meta-analysis of the research on the impact of decision aids reported, "The two largest studies evaluating choices pertained to breast and prostate screening. The breast screening trial compared a decision aid providing balanced information with usual care in 734 women in Australia, and found no difference in screening rates at one month. The prostate screening trial compared a print-based decision aid, a web-based interactive decision aid, or usual care in 1,879 participants in the US, and also found no significant difference

---

Should I Start Having Mammograms to Screen for Breast Cancer?

Some 40-year-old women start thinking about whether they should attend mammography screening now or wait until they are 50. If you are in this situation, you might find this website helpful.

Researchers from the University of Sydney have compiled the best available evidence regarding mammography screening and created what we call a decision aid. A decision aid is intended to provide you with unbiased information so that you can make a decision after considering the evidence.

The decision aid will take approximately 30 minutes to read and complete. None of your responses are recorded, and at no time do we ask your name or an email address.

If you are interested, click "next" to find out more.

≫ Next

FIGURE 15.5
First page of a mammogram decision aid.
Adapted from "Australian Screening Mammogram Decision Aid Trial," University of Sydney, http://www.mammogram.med.usyd.edu.au

Should I be screened for lung cancer?

The answer to this question is not the same for everyone. Your doctor can help you decide based on your values and preferences. **Quitting smoking** is the most important way to lower your chances of dying from lung cancer. Quitting smoking will improve your health in other ways, too.

The main test used to screen for lung cancer is called a low-dose CT scan (or "CAT scan"). Doctors offer screening to some people in the hopes of catching lung cancer early — before it has a chance to grow, spread, or cause symptoms. If you have cancer, catching and treating it early can improve your chance of being cured and living longer.

It might help to ask yourself the following questions when deciding whether or not to be screened:

FIGURE 15.6

First page of a decision aid for lung cancer screening.
Reproduced with permission from M. E. Deffenbach and L. Humphrey, "Patient Education: Lung Cancer Prevention and Screening" (Beyond the Basics), in UpToDate, edited by T. W. Post (Waltham, MA: UpToDate), accessed Sept. 30, 2022, https://www.uptodate.com/contents/screening-for-lung-cancer. Copyright © 2022 UpToDate, Inc. and its affiliates and/or licensors. All rights reserved

at 13 months."[12] A few studies of online decision aids about PSA testing did show a shift in the choices men expressed.[13] After using online tools like Option Grid (an initiative of the Dartmouth Institute for Health Policy and Clinical Practice, one of the centers behind the overdiagnosis movement), fewer men said they intended to have a PSA test.[14] A study of choices about how to respond to a diagnosis of early stage breast cancer reported "women who used a decision aid were 25% more likely to choose breast-conserving surgery over mastectomy."[15] For the most part, however, while these tools help people work through their decision more carefully and confidently, they seem mostly to help people get to where they were going anyway.

Deciding What to Do about a Diagnosis

Choosing whether to screen for cancer is a far simpler decision than figuring out what to do once you've been diagnosed. The stakes have instantly gone from low to survival itself. The hours and days after the shock of diagnosis are the key period to slow down, not to ignore or deny how you feel but to backpaddle against the emotional whitewater and give yourself more control over your decision making. Decision aids can help here too.

More than aids in deciding whether to screen, tools that help you think through what to do about a diagnosis should be used only in conversation with your physician. If they aren't provided, ask for one. Online decision aids are available for choices about DCIS or low-grade prostate cancer. A word of warning: a review of nearly 40 of them found that they varied in quality. Some are clearly biased toward one particular choice. Some offer information but fail to help the user work through the various emotional aspects of the decision being considered. Many fail to sufficiently encourage the patient and doctor to work together on truly shared decision making.

A good one for deciding what to do about a diagnosis of DCIS is from the researchers conducting the COMET trial (mentioned in chapter 7): "Welcome to the DCIS Decision Support Tool," https://dcisoptions.org /dst.[16] The National Cancer Institute also offers a downloadable booklet on low-risk prostate cancer: *Treatment Choices for Men with Early-Stage Prostate Cancer*, https://www.cancer.gov/publications/patient-education /understanding-prostate-cancer-treatment.[17]

Sadly, as helpful as these valuable decision aids can be, many doctors don't use them. An international survey of physicians in the United States and 10 other developed countries who had been provided with well-tested tools to empower their patients in shared decision making (about a range of health issues, not just cancer) found that only 44% actually used them. The most common explanation doctors gave for not using them with patients was that doing so took too much time, time for which they weren't being compensated.[18] A report from the Commonwealth Fund, a health care foundation, noted, "In spite of the evidence that patients value the tools and learn from them, and in spite of their potential to reduce inappropriate use and control costs, decision aids and shared decision making are not in widespread use." Michael Barry, president of the Informed Medical Decisions Foundation, is quoted as saying, "Given the level of evidence, this may be one of the best-documented but underused interventions in American medicine."[19]

If you want help thinking through the tough choices involved in a diagnosis of a frightening but low-risk type of cancer, ask your doctor for decision aids that might be available. If they don't have one, check with your health insurer. Be alert for bias (the National Comprehensive Cancer Network, a hospital group, has a decision aid on DCIS that mentions nothing about the harms that treatment can cause) and try to find an aid that challenges you to think about how you'd *feel* about certain outcomes. And remember: always use decision aids about treatment in conjunction with your health care provider.

> "Sometimes," Tom recalls, "the waves come back to crash into you again." When we spoke, he had been actively monitoring his cancer with PSA tests, and things looked great. "I took another biopsy one year after the first one, and they did not find any cancer. The doctor said that I probably still have it, but it's clearly not the aggressive sort. It has now been four years since my last biopsy, and my PSA has remained under 4. This is an illness that I'm managing as best as I can, always mindful of the potential resurgence, but I focus my attention to other elements of life's joys."
>
> Tom is also still finding ways to backpaddle against the fear. "I didn't just monitor the cancer. I took action to deal with it. I focused on my diet and took supplements that I found in my research would promote a healthy prostate and boost my immune system." Did a healthier diet help? Almost certainly. Did the supplements help? The evidence is equivocal. But what helped Tom most was the way he fought back against his fears: first, by taking his time, slowing down, backpaddling, and carefully thinking things through rather than going with the first choice that initially felt so right. And second, by finding a way to do what he did as a pilot: "When I was a kid I used to fly airplanes, and what I loved about airplanes was you could see all these dials, and you could figure out what was going on in terms of altitude, windspeed, and I loved having this dashboard of things . . . It gave me a feeling of control. I don't want to be in charge, but I want to know what's going on. Flying a plane, you're never in control of anything, so the illusion about being in control . . . you're really not. I don't want to be naïve. But I want to be aware of what's happening and do what I can do."

That's what combating cancerphobia comes down to: not letting your fear fly your plane. Like a pilot lost in the clouds, our deep fear of this most dreaded of diseases can overwhelm our ability to rely on our instruments—our ability to think about things rationally—and cause us to fly our plane right into the ground. As Katherine Patterson cautioned, "To fear is one thing. To let fear grab you by the tail and swing you around is another." It may feel natural, but it's not likely to lead to the healthiest choices

acknowledgments

Along the long journey of creating this work, I was blessed with an enormous amount of help and support, without which this book would not be in your hands. More important than just the time and ideas these busy people so graciously contributed was their *willingness* to help and their support for the basic idea of this book—that we really need to rethink our fear of cancer—as a valuable contribution to public health. Thank you to everyone who contributed, especially those who challenged my ideas and made me think them though more carefully (or in some instances, toss them out!).

I've done my best to keep track of all those contributors, but almost surely failed, so an apology to those not included and a profound thank-you to everyone who helped, including Dr. Richard Ablin, Sophie Acadie, Janice Audet, Dr. Alexandra Barratt, Dr. Lincoln Berland, Ellen Berlin, Dr. Otis Brawley, Dr. Erica Breslau, Dr. John Brodersen, Dr. Phylis Butow, Dr. Victoria Champion, Dr. Matthew Cooperberg, Dr. Louise Davies, Dr. Karen Emmons, Fahrah Englert, Judy Fortin-Lalone, Dr. Mark Friedberg, Dr. Gird Gigerenzer, Mary Gorden, Dr. Laurel Habel, Dr. Ingrid Hall, Dr. Jimmie Holland, Dr. Mette Kalager, James Kirby, Dr. Daniel Kopans, Dr. Barry Kramer, Dr. Stephen Lam, Dr. Jae-ho Lee, Dr. Robert Mayer, Dr. Diana Miglioretti, Dr. Anthony Miller, Jung Min-Ho, Dr. David Nathan, Dr. Brooke Nickel, Dr. Yuri Nikiforov, Dr. Elissa Ozanne, Dr. Edward Patz, Dr. Ellen Peters, Oscar Poon, Dr. Rinaa Sujata Punglia, Dr. Rita Redberg, Dr. Pooja Saini, David Sampson, Dr. Jacob Sands, Dr. Laura Scherer, Dr. Ya-Chen Tina Shih, Dr. Sudhir Srivastava, Dr. Dawn Stacey, Dr. Peter Ubel, Dr. Robert Volk, Dr. H. Gilbert Welch, Theresa Wickerham, Dr. Renda Soylemez Wiener, Dr. Daniel Wolfson, Dr. Steve Woloshin, Dr. Yousuf Zafar, and Dr. Brian Zikmund-Fisher.

A special thank-you to the several people who reviewed some or all of the book, many of them anonymously. Your suggestions, corrections, and reflections all contributed in important ways. A special thank-you to Professor Steven Pinker, who, when I was wavering about the project, encouraged me to write the book and provided access to critical research resources. My gratitude to eagle-eyed copyeditor Melanie Mallon and to editor Joe Rusko, formerly at Johns Hopkins University Press, for his belief that the challenging premise of this book, which scared so many other publishers away, deserved a voice.

Finally, a deep-hearted thank-you to the hundreds of people who shared their stories with me, sometimes when I asked, but often whenever my research just came up in "What are you up to these days?" conversation. Nearly everyone had a story to tell about how fear of cancer had affected their lives. This book is for them too.

notes

Introduction

1. C. W. Ramers-Verhoeven, G. L. Geipel, and Moira Howie, "New Insights into Public Perceptions of Cancer," *ecancer* 7, art. 349 (2013), https://ecancer.org/en/journal/article/349-new-insights-into-public-perceptions-of-cancer.
2. V. T. DeVita Jr. and E. DeVita-Raeburn, *The Death of Cancer* (New York: Sarah Crichton Books, 2015).
3. M. Roser and H. Ritchie, "Cancer," *Our World in Data*, last updated Nov. 2019, https://ourworldindata.org/cancer.
4. Otis Brawley, "War on Cancer, Year 40: Who's Winning?," TEDMED 2012, video, 9:52, https://www.tedmed.com/talks/show?id=7295.
5. G. Crile Jr., "A Plea against Blind Fear of Cancer," *Life*, Oct. 31, 1955, 127–30; G. Crile Jr., *Cancer and Common Sense* (New York: Viking, 1955).

Chapter 1. The Historical Roots

1. E. J. Odes et al., "Earliest Hominin Cancer: 1.7-Million-Year-Old Osteosarcoma from Swartkrans Cave, South Africa," *South African Journal of Science* 112, no. 7/8 (2016), https://doi.org/10.17159/sajs.2016/20150471.
2. C. Tomasetti, L. Li, and B. Vogelstein, "Stem Cell Divisions, Somatic Mutations, Cancer Etiology, and Cancer Prevention," *Science* 355, no. 6331 (2017): 1330–34.
3. C. Nizamoglu, "Ibn Sina's *The Canon of Medicine*," Muslim Heritage, April 15, 2015, http://www.muslimheritage.com/article/ibn-sinas-canon-medicine.
4. J. Hill, *Cautions against the Immoderate Use of Snuff*, 2nd ed. (London, 1761), National Library of Medicine Digital Collections, https://collections.nlm.nih.gov/bookviewer?PID=nlm:nlmuid-2166041R-bk#page/1/mode/2up.
5. F. Donaldson, "The Practical Application of the Microscope to the Diagnosis of Cancer," *American Journal of the Medical Sciences* 25 (1853): 43–68.
6. "The Purification of the River Thames," *London Evening Standard*, July 5, 1858.
7. "The Dirty Thames," *London City Press*, June 19, 1858.
8. CDC / National Center for Health Statistics, *Leading Causes of Death, 1900–1998*, accessed Jan. 29, 2023, https://www.cdc.gov/nchs/data/dvs/lead1900_98.pdf.

9. J. Burke, *Fear: A Cultural History* (Emeryville, CA: Shoemaker and Hoard, 2005), 298–99.
10. S. H. Adams, *The Great American Fraud* (New York: Collier, 1906).
11. J. Patterson, *The Dread Disease: Cancer and Modern Culture* (Cambridge, MA: Harvard University Press, 1987).
12. Patterson, *Dread Disease.*
13. C. Childe, *The Control of a Scourge: Or, How Cancer Is Curable* (New York: Dutton, 1907).
14. Crile, *Cancer and Common Sense*, 7.
15. H. A. Hare, *Progressive Medicine: A Quarterly Digest of Advances, Discoveries, and Improvements in the Medical and Surgical Sciences*, vol. 2 (Philadelphia: Lea and Febiger, 1921).
16. "Experts Disagree on Treating Cancer: Dr. Ewing Upholds Radium as a Cure, but Thinks an Overdose Killed Bremner," *New York Times*, March 3, 1914.
17. 69 Cong. Rec. 9048–50 (1928).
18. C. Mayo, "Carcinoma of the Right Segment of the Colon," *Annals of Surgery* 83 (1926): 357.
19. Fortune, *Cancer: The Great Darkness* (Garden City, NY: Doubleday, Doran 1937), 4.
20. National Cancer Act of 1937, background and text, National Cancer Institute, posted February 16, 2016, https://www.cancer.gov/about-nci /legislative/history/national-cancer-act-1937.
21. American Society for the Control of Cancer, *Reward of Courage* (New York: Eastern Film Corporation, 1921), NIH National Library of Medicine, 30:39, May 29, 2013, https://www.youtube.com/watch?v=IBlfaHfvXr4.
22. American Cancer Society, *The Traitor Within* (Atlanta, GA: John Sutherland Productions, 1946), NIH National Library of Medicine, 9:45, June 27, 2014, https://www.youtube.com/watch?v=8XoJPoVr7fE.
23. You can listen to the Jimmy broadcast here: "Original Jimmy Fund Radio Broadcast," radio broadcast, May 22, 1948, Dana-Farber Cancer Institute, 8:59, April 17, 2014, https://www.youtube.com/watch?v=eXeYrG-L9L8
24. S. Farber, L. K. Diamond, R. D. Mercer, R. F. Sylvester, and J. A. Wolff, "Temporary Remissions in Acute Leukemia in Children Produced by Folic Acid Antagonist, 4-Aminopteroyl-Glutamic Acid (Aminopterin)," *New England Journal of Medicine*, 238 (1948): 787–93.
25. Patterson, *Dread Disease*, 183.
26. R. Carson, *Silent Spring* (New York: Houghton Mifflin, 1962), 6.
27. Carson, *Silent Spring*, 219–20.
28. P. A. Wingo, C. J. Cardinez, S. H. Landis, R. T. Greenlee, L. A. G. Ries, R. N. Anderson, and M. J. Thun, "Long-Term Trends in Cancer Mortality in the United States, 1930–1998," *Cancer* 97, no. S12 (June 2003): 3133–3275.
29. W. M. Freeman, "Industry Confers to Aid Cigarettes," *New York Times*, Jan. 2, 1954, https://www.nytimes.com/1954/01/02/archives/industry -confers-to-aid-cigarettes-secret-meetings-here-weigh-drive.html.
30. "Expert on Cancer Gives Kindly Nod to Cigarette," *New York Times*, Feb. 24, 1954, https://www.nytimes.com/1954/02/25/archives/expert-on -cancer-gives-kindly-nod-to-cigarette.html.

31. E. C. Hammond and D. Horn, "Smoking and Death Rates—Report on Forty-Four Months of Follow Up of 187,783 Men," *Journal of the American Medical Association* 166, no. 11 (1958): 1294–1308; L. E. Davies, "Cigarettes Found to Raise Death Rate in Men 50 to 70," *New York Times*, June 22, 1954, https://www.nytimes.com/1954/06/22/archives/cigarettes-found-to-raise -death-rate-in-men-50-to-70-death-rate.html.

32. S. Bayne-Jones et al., *Smoking and Health: Report of the Advisory Committee to the Surgeon General of the Public Health Service*, Public Health Service Publication 1103 (Washington, DC: Public Health Service, 1964).

33. From the foreword to *Smoking and Health: Report of the Advisory Committee to the Surgeon General of the Public Health Service* (Public Health Service Publication No. 1103; Washington, DC: Government Printing Office, 1964).

34. Crile, "Plea against Blind Fear of Cancer," 127–30.

35. Crile, *Cancer and Common Sense*, vii, 7–8.

36. S. Sontag, *Illness as Metaphor* (New York: Farrar, Straus, and Giroux, 1988).

37. S. Garb, *Cure for Cancer: A National Goal* (New York: Springer, 1968).

38. S. Mukherjee, *The Emperor of All Maladies* (New York: Scribner, 2010), 146.

39. Mukherjee, *Emperor of All Maladies*, 186–87.

40. J. Paterson, *The Dread Disease* (Cambridge, MA: Harvard University Press, 1987); F. Ingelfinger, editorial, *New England Journal of Medicine* 293 (1975): 1319–20.

41. P. Ehrlich (co-authored by his wife, Anne, who was not credited) *The Population Bomb* (New York: Sierra Club / Ballantine, 1968).

42. Joe Jackson, "Cancer," Eighties Music Channel, Feb. 8, 2013, https:// www.youtube.com/watch?v=WsQyru5ACmA.

43. Paterson, *Dread Disease*, 307.

44. Google NGram search result, March 2023.

45. Google News search result, February 1, 2021.

46. R. Siegel, K. Miller, N.S. Wagle, and A. Jemal, "Cancer Statistics, 2023," *CA: A Cancer Journal for Clinicians*, Jan. 12, 2023, https://acsjournals .onlinelibrary.wiley.com/doi/full/10.3322/caac.21763.

47. V. DeVita Jr. and E. DeVita-Raeburn, *The Death of Cancer* (New York: Farrar, Straus, and Giroux, 2016).

48. M. Finucane, A. Alhakami, P. Slovic, and S. M. Johnson, "The Affect Heuristic in Judgments of Risks and Benefits," *Journal of Behavioral Decision Making* 13 (2000): 1–17.

Chapter 2. The Psychological Roots

1. Crile, *Cancer and Common Sense*, 15–16.

2. H. Ritchie, "How Many People in the World Die from Cancer," *Our World in Data*, Feb. 1, 2018, https://ourworldindata.org/how-many-people-in -the-world-die-from-cancer.

3. T. D. Denberg, T. V. Melhado, and J. F. Steiner, "Patient Treatment Preferences in Localized Prostate Carcinoma: The Influence of Emotion, Misconception, and Anecdote," *Cancer* 107, no. 3 (2006): 620–30.

4. J. E. LeDoux, *The Emotional Brain* (London: Orion Publishing, 2004), 8.

5. Finucane et al., "Affect Heuristic."
6. G. F. Lowenstein, E. U. Weber, C. K. Hsee, and N. Welch, "Risk as Feel-ings," *Psychological Bulletin* 127, no. 2 (2001): 267–86, https://www.cmu.edu/dietrich/sds/docs/loewenstein/RiskAsFeelings.pdf.
7. E. Kaehele, *Living with Cancer* (London: Gollancz, 1953).
8. D. Ropeik, *How Risky Is It, Really? Why Our Fears Don't Always Match the Facts* (New York: McGraw Hill, 2012).
9. J. Chandler, "Life, and Other Plans," *Age* (Melbourne), Aug. 2007, https://www.theage.com.au/technology/life-and-other-plans-20070825-ge5ooz.html.
10. American Society of Clinical Oncology, *ASCO 2018 Cancer Opinions Survey*, October 2018, https://old-prod.asco.org/sites/new-www.asco.org/files/content-files/research-and-progress/documents/2018-NCOS-Results.pdf.
11. C. Balmer, F. Griffiths, and J. Dunn, "A Qualitative Systematic Review Exploring Lay Understanding of Cancer by Adults without a Cancer Diagnosis," *Journal of Advanced Nursing* 70 no. 8 (2014): 1688–1701.
12. D. Colburn, "Cancer: The Word and Its Myths," *Washington Post*, Sept. 30, 1986.
13. "Cancer Army," *Time*, Mar. 22, 1937.
14. Kaehele, *Living with Cancer*.
15. National Cancer Institute, "How much do you agree or disagree with each of the following statements? When I think of cancer, I automatically think of death," Health Information National Trends Survey, Cycle 1, 2017, https://hints.cancer.gov/view-questions-topics/question-details.aspx?PK_Cycle=10&qid=509.
16. A. Jolie, "My Medical Choice," *New York Times*, May 14, 2013, https://www.nytimes.com/2013/05/14/opinion/my-medical-choice.html.
17. K. Robb, A. E. Simon, A. Miles, and J. Wardle, "Public Perceptions of Cancer: A Qualitative Study of the Balance of Positive and Negative Beliefs," *British Medical Journal* 7, no. 4 (2014): e005434, https://bmjopen.bmj.com/content/4/7/e005434.
18. J. Holland and S. Lewis, *The Human Side of Cancer: Living with Hope, Coping with Uncertainty* (New York: Harper Perennial, 2001), 48.
19. Medical historian Robert Aronowitz, *Risky Medicine: Our Quest to Cure Fear and Uncertainty* (Chicago: University of Chicago Press, 2015), 31.
20. Patients quoted in a meta-analysis of several surveys of cancer fears: C. Vrinten, L. M. McGregor, M. Heinrich, C. von Wagner, J. Waller, J. Wardle, and G. B. Black, "What Do People Fear about Cancer? A Systematic Review and Metasynthesis of Cancer Fears in the General Population," *Psycho-oncology* 26, no. 8 (2017): 1070–79.
21. J. Holland and S. Weston, *The Human Side of Cancer: Living with Hope, Coping with Uncertainty* (New York: Harper Perennial, 2001), 48.
22. From a survey of South Asian breast cancer patients living in the UK: G. Karbani, C. E. Chu, J. N. W. Lim, J. Hewison, K. Atkin, K. Horgan, and M. Lansdown, "Culture, Attitude and Knowledge about Breast Cancer and Preventive Measures: A Qualitative Study of South Asian Breast Cancer Patients in the UK," *Asian Pacific Journal of Cancer Prevention* 12 (2011): 1619–26.

23. National Cancer Institute, "Do you think that pesticides or food additives increase a person's chance of getting cancer a lot, a little, or not at all or do you have no opinion?," Health Information National Trends Survey, Cycle 1, 2003, https://hints.cancer.gov/view-questions-topics/question-details .aspx?PK_Cycle=1&qid=488.

24. National Cancer Institute, "Would you say you strongly agree, somewhat agree, somewhat disagree, strongly disagree with the following statements or do you have no opinion? It seems like everything causes cancer," Health Information National Trends Survey, Cycle 3, 2019, https://hints.cancer.gov/view-questions-topics/question-details.aspx ?PK_Cycle=12&qid=500.

25. Tomasetti, Li, and Vogelstein, "Stem Cell Divisions."

26. R. Alleyene, "Cancer Caused by Modern Man as It Was Virtually Non-existent in the Ancient World," *Telegraph* (London), Oct. 14, 2010, https://www.telegraph.co.uk/news/health/news/8064554/Cancer-caused -by-modern-man-as-it-was-virtually-non-existent-in-ancient-world.html.

27. A. R. David and M. R. Zimmerman, "Cancer: An Old Disease, a New Disease or Something in Between?," *Nature Reviews Cancer* 10 (2010): 728–33, https://www.nature.com/articles/nrc2914.

28. K. Arney, "Claims that Cancer Is Only a 'Modern, Man-Made Disease' Are False and Misleading," Cancer Research UK, Oct. 14, 2010, https:// scienceblog.cancerresearchuk.org/2010/10/14/claims-that-cancer-is-only -a-'modern-man-made-disease'-are-false-and-misleading/.

29. American Institute for Cancer Research, *The AICR 2015 Cancer Risk Awareness Survey Report*, 2015, http://www.aicr.org/assets/docs/pdf /education/aicr-awareness-report-2015.pdf.

30. Holland and Weston, *Human Side of Cancer*, 48.

31. Vrinten et al., "What Do People Fear about Cancer?"

32. Vrinten et al., "What Do People Fear about Cancer?"

33. M. Ragland, K. F. Trivers, C. H. A. Andrilla, B. Matthews, J. Miller, D. Lishner, B. Goff, and L. Baldwin, "Physician Nonprofessional Cancer Experience and Ovarian Cancer Screening Practices: Results from a National Survey of Primary Care Physicians," *Journal of Women's Health* 27, no. 11 (2018): 1335–41.

34. Ragland et al., "Physician Nonprofessional Cancer Experience."

35. Vrinten et al., "What Do People Fear about Cancer?"

36. S. M. Banks, P. Salovey, S. Greener, and A. J. Rothman, "The Effects of Message Framing on Mammography Utilization," *Health Psychology* 14, no. 2 (1995): 178–84.

37. J. A. Clark, T. S. Inui, R. A. Silliman, B. G. Bokhour, S. H. Krasnow, R. A. Robinson, M. Spaulding, J. A. Talcott, "Patients' Perceptions of Quality of Life after Treatment for Early Prostate Cancer," *Journal of Clinical Oncology* 21, no. 20 (2003): 3777–84.

38. D. T. Miller and B. R. Taylor, "Counterfactual Thought, Regret, and Superstition: How to Avoid Kicking Yourself," in *Heuristics and Biases: The Psychology of Intuitive Judgment*, ed. T. Gilovich, D. W. Griffin, and D. Kahneman (Cambridge: Cambridge University Press, 2002), 367–76.

39. I. M. Lipkus, G. Samsa, and B. K. Rimer, "General Performance on a Numeracy Scale among Highly Educated Samples," *Medical Decision Making* 21 (2001): 21–37.
40. Karbani et al., "Culture, Attitude and Knowledge."
41. Vrinten et al., "What Do People Fear about Cancer?"
42. C. Vrinten, C. H. M. van Jaarsveld, J. Waller, C. von Wagner, and J. Wardle, "The Structure and Demographic Correlates of Cancer Fear," *BMC Cancer* 14 (2014): 597.

Chapter 3. Overscreening, Overdiagnosis, Overtreatment

1. "Age and Cancer Risk," National Cancer Institute, last updated March 5, 2021, https://www.cancer.gov/about-cancer/causes-prevention/risk/age.
2. H. G. Welch and W. C. Black, "Overdiagnosis in Cancer," *Journal of the National Cancer Institute* 102, no. 9 (2010): 605–13, https://academic.oup.com/jnci/article/102/9/605/894608.
3. "Dr. Barnett Kramer on Over-Diagnosis and Treatment of Cancer," C-Span, video, 37:41, Aug. 8, 2013, https://www.c-span.org/video/?314456-7/dr-barnett-kramer-diagnosis-treatment-cancer.
4. J. Peres, "New PSA Guidelines Discourage Overscreening," *Journal of the National Cancer Institute* 104, no. 1 (2012): 8–9.
5. Phone interview with Dr. Otis Brawley, chief medical officer, American Cancer Society, 2017.
6. L. M. Schwartz, S. Woloshin, F. J. Fowler, and H. G. Welch, "Enthusiasm for Cancer Screening in the United States," *Journal of the American Medical Association* 291, no. 1 (2004): 71–78.
7. D. Petrova, R. Garcia-Retamero, A. Catena, and J. van der Pligt, "To Screen or Not to Screen: What Factors Influence Complex Screening Decisions?" *Journal of Experimental Psychology: Applied* 22, no. 2 (2016): 247–60.
8. L. D. Scherer, K. D. Valentine, N. Patel, S. G. Baker, and A. Fagerlin, "A Bias for Action in Cancer Screening?," *Journal of Experimental Psychology: Applied* 25, no. 2 (2019): 149–61.
9. Scherer et al., "Bias for Action."
10. P. Orenstein, "Our Feel-Good War on Breast Cancer," *New York Times Magazine*, April 25, 2013, https://archive.nytimes.com/www.nytimes.com/2013/04/28/magazine/our-feel-good-war-on-breast-cancer.html.
11. B. Young, L. Bedford, D. Kendrick, K. Vedhara, J. F. R. Robertson, and R. das Nair, "Factors Influencing the Decision to Attend Screening for Cancer in the UK: a Meta-ethnography of Qualitative Research," *Journal of Public Health* 40, no. 2 (2018): 315–39, https://academic.oup.com/jpubhealth/article/40/2/315/3807259.
12. Crile, *Cancer and Common Sense*, 45.
13. "Screening Tests," National Cancer Institute, last updated Nov. 10, 2022, https://www.cancer.gov/about-cancer/screening/screening-tests.
14. "Screening for Various Cancers," World Health Organization, accessed Nov. 1, 2021. http://www.who.int/cancer/detection/variouscancer/en/.
15. A. A. Kotwal, L. C. Walter, S. J. Lee, and W. Dale, "Are We Choosing Wisely? Older Adults' Cancer Screening Intentions and Recalled Discussions with Physicians about Stopping," *Journal of General Internal Medicine*

34 (2019): 1538–45, https://link.springer.com/article/10.1007%2Fs11606
-019-05064-w.

16. T. J. Royce, L. H. Hendrix, and W. A. Stokes, "Cancer Screening Rates in
    Individuals with Different Life Expectancies," *JAMA Internal Medicine*
    174, no. 10 (2014): 1658–65, https://jamanetwork.com/journals
    /jamainternalmedicine/fullarticle/1897549.

17. "Missed Cancer Screenings Not Yet Associated with Increased Cancer Rates
    or Severity," Epic Research, Cosmos Study, news release, Feb. 17, 2023.

18. *Cancer Diagnostics Market Size, Share and Trends Analysis Report*, Grand
    View Research, accessed June 2019, https://www.grandviewresearch
    .com/industry-analysis/cancer-diagnostics-market.

19. *Endoscopy Devices Market Size, Share and Trends Analysis Report*, Grand
    View Research, accessed June 1, 2021, https://www.grandviewresearch
    .com/industry-analysis/endoscopy-devices-market.

20. *Prostate Cancer Diagnostics Market Size, Share and Trends Analysis Report*,
    Grand View Research, accessed June 2020, https://www.grandviewresearch
    .com/industry-analysis/prostate-cancer-diagnostics-market.

21. "North America Breast Cancer Screening Market Forecast to
    2027—COVID-19 Impact and Regional Analysis," *BusinessWire*, https://
    www.businesswire.com/news/home/20201110005704/en/North-America
    -Breast-Cancer-Screening-Market-Forecast-to-2027---COVID-19-Impact
    -and-Regional-Analysis---ResearchAndMarkets.com; "Oncology Market
    Opportunities and Growth Trends," Definitive Healthcare, accessed
    Jan. 20, 2023, https://blog.definitivehc.com/oncology-market-opportunities
    -and-growth-trends.

22. Schwartz et al., "Enthusiasm for Cancer Screening," 6.

23. Crile, *Cancer and Common Sense*, 45.

24. R. Hoffman, "Decision-Making Processes for Breast, Colorectal, and
    Prostate Cancer Screening: Results from the DECISIONS Study," *Medical
    Decision Making* 30, no. S5 (2010): 53S–64S.

25. A. Radhakrishnan, S. A. Nowak, A. M. Parker, K. Visvanathan, and C. E.
    Pollack, "Physician Breast Cancer Screening Recommendations Following
    Guideline Changes: Results of a National Survey," *JAMA Internal Medicine*
    177, no. 6 (2017): 877–88, https://www.ncbi.nlm.nih.gov/pmc/articles
    /PMC5561425/.

26. Welch and Black, "Overdiagnosis in Cancer."

27. O. Brawley and P. Goldberg, *How We Do Harm: A Doctor Breaks Ranks
    about Being Sick in America* (New York: St. Martin's Griffin, 2012).

28. J. W. Mold and H. F. Stein, "The Cascade Effect in the Clinical Care of
    Patients," *New England Journal of Medicine* 314 (1986): 512–14.

29. Crile, *Cancer and Common Sense*, 61.

Chapter 4. Breast Cancer

1. S. Shapiro, P. Strax, and L. Venet, "Periodic Breast Cancer Screening in
   Reducing Mortality from Breast Cancer," *Journal of the American Medical
   Association* 215, no. 11 (1971): 1777–85.

2. B. Lerner, "To See Today with the Eyes of Tomorrow: A History of Screening
   Mammography," background paper for the Institute of Medicine report

Mammography and Beyond: Developing Technologies for the Early Detection of Breast Cancer (Washington, DC: National Academy Press, March 2001).

3. J. Bailar, "Mammography: A Contrary View," *Annals of Internal Medicine* 84, no. 1 (1976): 77–84.
4. Independent UK Panel on Breast Cancer Screening, "The Benefits and Harms of Breast Cancer Screening," *Lancet* 380, no. 9855 (2012): 1778–86.
5. USPSTF, *Final Recommendation Statement, Breast Cancer: Screening,* table 5, Jan. 11, 2016, https://www.uspreventiveservicestaskforce.org/Page /Document/RecommendationStatementFinal/breast-cancer -screening1#tab1.
6. A. B. Miller, C. Wall, C. J. Baines, P. Sun, T. To, and S. A. Narod, "Twenty-Five-Year Follow-Up for Breast Cancer Incidence and Mortality of the Canadian National Breast Screening Study: Randomised Screening Trial," *British Medical Journal* 348, no. 7945 (2014): 348–66, https://www.bmj.com /content/348/bmj.g366.
7. P. C. Gøtzsche and K. Jørgensen, "Screening for Breast Cancer with Mammography," *Cochrane Database of Systematic Reviews,* June 4, 2013, https://www.cochrane.org/CD001877/BREASTCA_screening-for-breast -cancer-with-mammography.
8. P. Autier, M. Boniol, A. Gavin, and L. J. Vatten, "Breast Cancer Mortality in Neighbouring European Countries with Different Levels of Screening but Similar Access to Treatment: Trend Analysis of WHO Mortality Database," *British Medical Journal,* July 28, 2011, https://www.ncbi.nlm.nih .gov/pmc/articles/PMC3145837/.
9. L. A. G. Ries, M. P. Eisner, C. L. Kosary, B. F. Hankey, B. A. Miller, L. Clegg, A. Mariotto, E. J. Feuer, and B. K. Edwards, *Seer Cancer Statistics Review, 1975-2002,* National Cancer Institute, http://seer.cancer.gov/csr/1975_2002/.
10. A. Bleyer and H. G. Welch, "Effect of Three Decades of Screening Mammography on Breast-Cancer Incidence," *New England Journal of Medicine* 367 (2012): 1998–2005, https://www.nejm.org/doi/full/10.1056/NEJMoa1206809.
11. C. Aschwanden, "Cut Back on Mammograms?," *Los Angeles Times,* Aug. 17, 2009.
12. Gøtzsche and Jørgensen, "Screening for Breast Cancer with Mammography."
13. P. C. Gøtzsche, O. J. Hartling, M. Nielsen, and J. Brodersen, *Screening for Breast Cancer with Mammography,* Nordic Cochrane Center, January 2012, https://www.cochrane.dk/sites/cochrane.dk/files/public/uploads/images /mammography/mammography-leaflet.pdf.
14. Canadian Task Force on Preventive Health Care, "Recommendations on Screening for Breast Cancer in Women 40–74 Years of Age Who Are Not at Increased Risk," Breast Cancer Update (2018), https://canadiantaskforce .ca/guidelines/published-guidelines/breast-cancer-update/.
15. USPSTF, *Breast Cancer Screening.*
16. PDQ Screening and Prevention Editorial Board, "Breast Cancer Screening (PDQ)," National Cancer Institute, October 6, 2022, https://www.ncbi.nlm .nih.gov/books/NBK65715/.
17. N. Biller-Andorno and P. Jüni, "Abolishing Mammography Screening Programs? A View from the Swiss Medical Board," *New England Journal of Medicine* 370 (2014): 1965–67.

18. National Breast Cancer Coalition, "NBCC Statement on USPSTF Mammography Screening Recommendations," April 2015.
19. R. E. Hendrick, J. A. Baker, and M. A. Helvie, "Breast Cancer Deaths Averted over 3 Decades," *Cancer*, Feb. 11, 2019, https://onlinelibrary.wiley.com/doi/abs/10.1002/cncr.31954.
20. See the #40not50 home page, accessed Jan. 21, 2023, https://www.40not50.org.
21. "About RadNet," RadNet, accessed Jan. 21, 2023, https://www.radnet.com/about-radnet.
22. L. Tabár et al., "The Incidence of Fatal Breast Cancer Measures the Increased Effectiveness of Therapy in Women Participating in Mammography Screening," *Cancer* 125, no. S1 (2018), https://www.researchgate.net/publication/328830860_The_incidence_of_fatal_breast_cancer_measures_the_increased_effectiveness_of_therapy_in_women_participating_in_mammography_screening.
23. S. R. Drossman, E. R. Port, and E. B. Sonnenblick, "Why the Annual Mammogram Matters," *New York Times*, Oct. 28, 2015, https://www.nytimes.com/2015/10/29/opinion/why-the-annual-mammogram-matters.html.
24. National Breast Cancer Coalition, "Mammography for Breast Cancer Screening: Harm/Benefit Analysis," July 2011, https://www.stopbreastcancer.org/information-center/positions-policies/mammography-for-breast-cancer-screening-harm-benefit-analysis/.
25. N. L. Keating and L. E. Pace, "Breast Cancer Screening in 2018: Time for Shared Decision Making," *Journal of the American Medical Association* 319, no. 17 (2018): 1814–15, https://jamanetwork.com/journals/jama/fullarticle/2679928.
26. N. Patel, M. Lee, and J. L. Marti, "Assessment of Screening Mammography Recommendations by Breast Cancer Centers in the US," *JAMA Internal Medicine*, March 15, 2021, https://jamanetwork.com/journals/jamainternalmedicine/fullarticle/2777520.
27. Radhakrishnan et al., "Physician Breast Cancer Screening Recommendations."
28. Keating and Pace, "Breast Cancer Screening in 2018."
29. US Congress, Protecting Access to Lifesaving Screenings Act of 2019, H.R. 2777, https://www.congress.gov/bill/116th-congress/house-bill/2777?s=1&r=57.
30. Bailar, "Mammography."
31. P. Zahl, J. Maehlen, and H. G. Welch, "The Natural History of Invasive Breast Cancers Detected by Screening Mammography," *Archives of Internal Medicine* 168, no. 21 (2008): 2312–16, https://pss17.files.wordpress.com/2009/01/historianatural_invasivosmama.pdf.
32. "Ductal Carcinoma In Situ (DCIS)," American Cancer Society, Nov. 19, 2021, https://www.cancer.org/cancer/breast-cancer/understanding-a-breast-cancer-diagnosis/types-of-breast-cancer/dcis.html.
33. USPSTF, *Breast Cancer Screening.*
34. S. Narod, J. Iqbal, and V. Giannakeas, "Breast Cancer Mortality after a Diagnosis of Ductal Carcinoma In Situ," *Journal of the American Medical*

Association Oncology 1, no. 7 (2015): 888–96, https://jamanetwork.com
/journals/jamaoncology/fullarticle/2427491.

35. J. Cavallo, "When Is Active Surveillance Appropriate in the Treatment of DCIS?" *ASCO Post*, March 25, 2018, https://ascopost.com/issues/march-25 -2018/when-is-active-surveillance-appropriate-in-the-treatment-of-dcis/.

36. E. Rakovitch, E. Franssen, J. Kim, I. Ackerman, J. Pignol, L. Paszat, K. I. Pritchard, C. Ho, and D. A. Redelmeier, "A Comparison of Risk Perception and Psychological Morbidity in Women with Ductal Carcinoma In Situ and Early Invasive Breast Cancer," *Breast Cancer Research Treatment* 77, no. 3 (2003): 285–93.

37. "Comparison of Operation to Monitoring, with or without Endocrine Therapy (COMET) Trial for Low Risk DCIS," ClinicalTrials.gov, last updated Sept. 21, 2022, https://clinicaltrials.gov/ct2/show/NCT02926911; "Management of Low-Risk DCIS (LORD)," ClinicalTrials.gov, last updated May 26, 2022, https://clinicaltrials.gov/ct2/show/NCT02492607; "LORIS: A Phase III Trial of Surgery versus Active Monitoring for Low Risk Ductal Carcinoma in Situ (DCIS)," Cancer Research UK Clinical Trials Unit, accessed Jan. 21, 2023, https://www.birmingham.ac.uk /research/activity/mds/trials/crctu/trials/loris/index.aspx.

38. Bleyer and Welch, "Effect of Three Decades of Screening Mammography."

39. S. Duffy et al., "Screen Detection of Ductal Carcinoma In Situ and Subsequent Incidence of Invasive Interval Breast Cancers: A Retrospective Population-Based Study," *Lancet Oncology* 17, no. 1 (2015): 109–14, https://www.ncbi.nlm.nih.gov/pubmed/26655422.

40. R. Farber, N. Houssami, S. Wortley, G. Jacklyn, M. L. Marinovich, K. McGeechan, A. Barratt, and K. Bell, "Impact of Full-Field Digital Mammography Versus Film-Screen Mammography in Population Screening: A Meta-Analysis," *Journal of the National Cancer Institute* 113, no. 1 (2021): 16–26, https://www.ncbi.nlm.nih.gov/pmc/articles/PMC7781455/.

41. C. D. Lehman et al., "National Performance Benchmarks for Modern Screening Digital Mammography: Update from the Breast Cancer Surveillance Consortium," *Radiology* 283, no. 1 (2017): 49–58.

42. E. Conant, M. Talley, C. Parghu, B. Sheh, SY. Liang, S Pohlman, A. Rane, Y. Jung, L. Stevens, J. Paulus, and N. Alsheik, "Mammographic Screening in Routine Practice: Multisite Study of Breast Tomosynthesis and Digit Mammography Screenings," *Radiology*, March 14, 2023, https://pubs.rsna .org/doi/10.1148/radiol.221571.

43. I. Ganguli, N. L. Keating, N. Thakore, J. Lii, S. Raza, and L. E. Pace, "Downstream Mammary and Extramammary Cascade Services and Spending Following Screening Breast Magnetic Resonance Imaging vs Mammography among Commercially Insured Women," *JAMA Network Open*, April 13, 2022, https://jamanetwork.com/journals/jamanetworkopen /fullarticle/2791002.

44. D. Hill et al., "Utilization of Breast Cancer Screening with Magnetic Resonance Imaging in Community Practice," *Journal of General Internal Medicine* 33 (2018): 275–83, https://link.springer.com/article/10.1007/s11606-017-4224-6.

45. H. Nelson, E. S. O'Meara, K. Kerlikowske, S. Balch, and D. Miglioretti, "Factors Associated with Rates of False-Positive and False-Negative

Results from Digital Mammography Screening: An Analysis of Registry Data," *Annals of Internal Medicine* 164 (2016): 226–35, https://www.ncbi .nlm.nih.gov/pubmed/26756902.

46. R. A. Hubbard, K. Kerlikowske, C. I. Flowers, B. C. Yankaskas, W. Zhu, and D. Miglioretti, "Cumulative Probability of False-Positive Recall or Biopsy Recommendation after 10 Years of Screening Mammography: A Cohort Study," *Annals of Internal Medicine* 155, no. 8 (2011): 481–92.

47. "Use of Mammography among Women Aged 40 and Over, by Selected Characteristics," table 33, *Health, United States, 2018,* CDC, https://www .cdc.gov/nchs/data/hus/2018/033.pdf.

48. N. T. Brewer, T. Salz, and S. E. Lillie, "Systematic Review: The Long-Term Effects of False-Positive Mammograms," *Database of Abstracts of Reviews of Effects (DARE),* 2007, https://www.ncbi.nlm.nih.gov/books/NBK73699/.

49. A. Bolejko, P. Hagell, C. Wann-Hansson, and S. Zackrisson, "Prevalence, Long-Term Development, and Predictors of Psychosocial Consequences of False-Positive Mammography among Women Attending Population-Based Screening," *Cancer Epidemiology, Biomarkers and Prevention* 24, no. 9 (2015): 1388–97.

50. J. Broderson and V. D. Siersma, "Long-Term Psychosocial Consequences of False-Positive Screening Mammography," *Annals of Family Medicine* 11, no. 2 (2013): 106–15, http://www.annfammed.org/content/11/2/106.full.

51. M. B. El-Tamer, B. M. Ward, T. Schifftner, L. Neumayer, S. Khuri, and W. Henderson, "Morbidity and Mortality Following Breast Cancer Surgery in Women National Benchmarks for Standards of Care," *Annals of Surgery* 245, no. 5 (2007): 665–71, https://www.ncbi.nlm.nih.gov/pmc/articles /PMC1877061/.

52. American Cancer Society, *Cancer Facts and Figures 2017,* https://www .cancer.org/content/dam/cancer-org/research/cancer-facts-and -statistics/annual-cancer-facts-and-figures/2017/cancer-facts-and -figures-2017.pdf.

53. E. S. Hwang, "The Impact of Surgery on Ductal Carcinoma In Situ Outcomes: The Use of Mastectomy," *Journal of the National Cancer Institute* 201, no. 14 (2010): 197–99.

54. A. Shaaban, B. Hilton, K. Clements, E. Provenzano, S. Cheung, M. Wallis, E. Sawyer, J. Thomas, A. Hanby, S. Pinder, and A. Thompson, "Pathological Features of 11,337 Patients with Primary Ductal Carcinoma In Situ (DCIS) and Subsequent Events: Results from the UK Sloane Project," *British Journal of Cancer* 124 (2021): 1009–17, https://www.nature.com /articles/s41416-020-01152-5; P. A. van Luijt, E. A. M. Heijnsdijk, J. Fracheboud, L. I. H. Overbeek, M. J. M. Broeders, J. Wesseling, G. J. den Heeten, and H. J. de Koning, "The Distribution of Ductal Carcinoma In Situ (DCIS) Grade in 4232 Women and Its Impact on Overdiagnosis in Breast Cancer Screening," *Breast Cancer Research* 18, no. (2016): 47, https://www .ncbi.nlm.nih.gov/pmc/articles/PMC4862233/; L. Salvatorelli, L. Puzzo, G. M. Vecchio, R. Caltabiano, V. Virzi, and G. Magro, "Ductal Carcinoma In Situ of the Breast: An Update with Emphasis on Radiological and Morphological Features as Predictive Prognostic Factors," *Cancers* 12, no. 3 (2020): 609, https://www.ncbi.nlm.nih.gov/pmc/articles/PMC7139619/.

55. K. Kummerow, "Nationwide Trends in Mastectomy for Early-Stage Breast Cancer," *Journal of the American Medical Association Surgery* 150, no. 1 (2015): 9–16.

56. This calculation is based on multiple sources, including census data on the female population for those years and data from the CDC, ACS, and several journal articles on the percentage of women undergoing annual mammography.

57. A. Mamtani and M. Morrow, "Why Are There So Many Mastectomies in the United States?" *Annual Review of Medicine* 14, no. 68 (2017): 229–41.

58. Mamtani and Morrow, "Why Are There So Many Mastectomies."

59. D. L. Bloom et al., "Reframing the Conversation about Contralateral Prophylactic Mastectomy: Preparing Women for Postsurgical Realities," *Psycho-Oncology* 8, no. 2 (2019): 394–400.

60. "Post-Mastectomy Pain Syndrome," American Cancer Society, last updated Jan. 3, 2019, https://www.cancer.org/treatment/treatments-and -side-effects/physical-side-effects/pain/post-mastectomy-pain-syndrome .html; "Post-Mastectomy Pain Syndrome," American Chronic Pain Association, accessed Jan. 20, 2023, https://www.theacpa.org/conditions /post-mastectomy-pain-syndrome/; O. J. Viholm, S. Cold, L. Rasmussen, and S. H. Sindrup, "The Postmastectomy Pain Syndrome: An Epidemio-logical Study on the Prevalence of Chronic Pain after Surgery for Breast Cancer," *British Journal of Cancer* 99, no. 4 (2008): 604–10, https://www .ncbi.nlm.nih.gov/pmc/articles/PMC2527825/.

61. O. O. Shiyanbola, B. L. Sprague, J. M. Hampton, K. Dittus, T. A. James, S. Herschorn, R. E. Gangnon, D. L. Weaver, and A. Trentham-Dietz, "Emerg-ing Trends in Surgical and Adjuvant Radiation Therapies among Women Diagnosed with Ductal Carcinoma In Situ," *Cancer* 122, no. 18 (2016): 2810–18.

62. D. J. Indelicato, S. R. Grobmyer, H. Newlin, L. S. Haigh, E. M. Copeland, and N. P. Mendenhall, "Delayed Breast Cellulitis: An Evolving Complica-tion of Breast Conservation," *International Journal of Radiation Oncology, Biology, Physics* 66, no. 5 (2006): 1339–46.

63. H. J. Burstein, K. Polyak, J. S. Wong, S. C. Lester, and C. M. Kaelin, "Ductal Carcinoma In Situ of the Breast," *New England Journal of Medicine* 350 (2004): 1430–41.

64. M. T. King et al., "Patient-Reported Outcomes in Ductal Carcinoma In Situ: A Systematic Review," *European Journal of Cancer* 71 (2017): P95–108.

65. King et al., "Patient-Reported Outcomes."

Chapter 5. Prostate Cancer

1. E. P. DeAntoni, "Eight Years of 'Prostate Cancer Awareness Week': Lessons in Screening and Early Detection," *Cancer* 80, no. 9 (1997): 1845–51.

2. A. B. Mariotto, R. Etzioni, M. Krapcho, and E. Feuer, "Reconstructing PSA Testing Patterns between Black and White Men in the US from Medicare Claims and the National Health Interview Survey," *Cancer* 109, no. 9 (2007): 1877–86.

3. A. L. Potosky, B. A. Miller, P. C. Albertsen, and B. S. Kramer, "The Role of Increasing Detection in the Rising Incidence of Prostate Cancer," *Journal of the American Medical Association* 27, no. 3 (1995): 548–52.

4. "Us Too," Prostate Cancer Foundation, accessed Feb. 1, 2023, https://www
    .pcf.org/ustoo/.
5. R. Ablin and R. Piana, *The Great Prostate Hoax* (New York: St. Martin's
    Press, 2014), 173.
6. Ablin and Piana, *Great Prostate Hoax*, 87.
7. H. G. Welch and P. C. Albertsen, "Reconsidering Prostate Cancer Mortal-
    ity: The Future of PSA Screening," *New England Journal of Medicine* 382
    (2020): 1557–63.
8. R. Martin, et al., "Effect of a Low-Intensity PSA-Based Screening Interven-
    tion on Prostate Cancer Mortality: The CAP Randomized Clinical Trial,"
    Journal of the American Medical Association 3129, no. 9 (2018): 883–95,
    https://jamanetwork.com/journals/jama/article-abstract/2673968.
9. P. F. Pinsky et al., "Extended Mortality Results for Prostate Cancer
    Screening in the PLCO Trial with Median Follow-Up of 15 Years," *Cancer*
    123, no. 4 (2017): 592–99.
10. D. Ilic, M. Djulbegovic, J. Hung Jung, E. Chang Hwang, Q. Zhou, A. Cleves,
    T. Agoritsas, and P. Dahm, "Prostate Cancer Screening with Prostate-Specific
    Antigen (PSA) Test: A Systematic Review and Meta-Analysis," *British Medical
    Journal* 362 (2018), https://www.bmj.com/content/362/bmj.k3519.
11. D. Ilic, M. M. Neuberger, M. Djulbegovic, and P. Dahm, "Screening for
    Prostate Cancer," *Cochrane Database of Systematic Reviews*, Jan. 31, 2013,
    https://www.cochranelibrary.com/cdsr/doi/10.1002/14651858.CD004720
    .pub3/full.
12. S. W. Leslie, T. L. Soon-Sutton, A. R. I, H. Sajjad, and L. E. Siref, "Prostate
    Cancer," *StatPearls*, last updated Nov. 28, 2022, https://www.ncbi.nlm
    .nih.gov/books/NBK470550/.
13. USPSTF, *Final Recommendation Statement: Prostate Cancer Screening*, May 8,
    2018, https://www.uspreventiveservicestaskforce.org/Page/Document
    /RecommendationStatementFinal/prostate-cancer-screening1.
14. R. C. Rabin, "Discuss Prostate Cancer Screening with Your Doctor,
    Experts Now Say," *New York Times*, April 11, 2017, https://www.nytimes.com
    /2017/04/11/well/live/discuss-prostate-screening-with-your-doctor
    -experts-now-say.html.
15. I. J. Hall, S. Hee Rim, G. M. Massetti, C. C. Thomas, J. Li, and L. C.
    Richardson, "Prostate-Specific Antigen Screening: An Update of Physician
    Beliefs and Practices," *Preventive Medicine* 103 (2017): 66–69.
16. K. H. Kensler, C. H. Pernar, B. A. Mahal, P. L. Nguyen, Q. Trinh, A. S. Kibel,
    and T. R. Rebbeck, "Racial and Ethnic Variation in PSA Testing and
    Prostate Cancer Incidence Following the 2012 USPSTF Recommendation,"
    Journal of the National Cancer Institute, Nov. 4, 2020, https://academic.oup
    .com/jnci/article/113/6/719/5955778.
17. National Cancer Institute, "Cancer Stat Facts: Prostate Cancer," Surveil-
    lance, Epidemiology, and End Results Program, accessed June 1, 2021,
    https://seer.cancer.gov/statfacts/html/prost.html.
18. J. Ahmedin et al., "Prostate Cancer Incidence and PSA Testing Patterns in
    Relation to USPSTF Screening Recommendations," *Journal of the American
    Medical Association* 314, no. 19 (2015): 2054–61, https://jamanetwork.com
    /journals/jama/fullarticle/2470446.

19. National Cancer Institute, "Cancer Stat Facts."
20. National Cancer Institute, "Prostate Cancer Screening," Cancer Trends Progress Report, July 2020, https://progressreport.cancer.gov/detection /prostate_cancer.
21. CDC, *Health, United States, 2018.*
22. M. Garnick, "Buffett's Prostate Cancer: Poor Decisions," *Harvard Health Newsletter,* April 23, 2012, https://www.health.harvard.edu/blog/buffetts -prostate-cancer-poor-decisions-201204234621.
23. M. S. Leapman, R. Wang, H. Park, J. B. Yu, P. C. Sprenkle, M. R. Cooperberg, C. P. Gross, and X. Ma, "Changes in Prostate-Specific Antigen Testing Relative to the Revised US Preventive Services Task Force Recommendation on Prostate Cancer Screening," *JAMA Oncology,* Nov. 11, 2021, https:// jamanetwork.com/journals/jamaoncology/article-abstract/2786070.
24. L. B. Squiers, C. M. Bann, S. E. Dolina, J. Tzeng, L. McCormack, and D. Kamerow, "Prostate-Specific Antigen Testing: Men's Responses to 2012 Recommendation against Screening," *American Journal of Preventive Medicine* 45, no. 2 (2013): 182–89.
25. C. Pollack, E. A. Platz, N. A. Bhavsar, G. Noronha, G. E. Green, S. Chen, and H. B. Carter, "Primary Care Providers' Perspectives on Discontinuing Prostate Cancer Screening," *Cancer* 118, no. 22 (2012): 5518–24, https:// onlinelibrary.wiley.com/doi/full/10.1002/cncr.27577.
26. S. Loeb, C. Curnyn, A. Fagerlin, R. S. Braithwaite, M. D. Schwartz, H. Lepor, H. B. Carter, and E. Sedlander, "Qualitative Study on Decision-Making by Prostate Cancer Physicians during Active Surveillance," *British Journal of Urology International* 120, no. 1 (2017): 32–39.
27. J. C. Hunter, A. I. Vines, and V. Carlisle, "African Americans' Perceptions of Prostate-Specific Antigen Prostate Cancer Screening," *Health Education and Behavior* 42, no. 4 (2015): 539–44.
28. E. C. Y. Chan, M. J. Barry, S. W. Vernon, and C. Ahn, "Brief Report: Physicians and Their Personal Prostate Cancer-Screening Practices with Prostate-Specific Antigen: A National Survey," *Journal of General Internal Medicine* 21, no. 3 (2006): 257–59.
29. M. A. Liss, B. Ehdaie, S. Loeb, M. V. Meng, J. D. Raman, V. Spears, and S. P. Stroup, "An Update of the American Urological Association White Paper on the Prevention and Treatment of the More Common Complications Related to Prostate Biopsy," *Journal of Urology* 198, no. 2 (2017): 329–34.
30. USPSTF, "Screening for Prostate Cancer Recommendation Statement," *Journal of the American Medical Association* 19, no. 18 (2018): 1901–13, https://jamanetwork.com/journals/jama/fullarticle/2680553.
31. J. L. Stanford, Z. Feng, A. S. Hamilton, F. D. Gilliland, R. A. Stephenson, J. W. Eley, P. C. Albertsen, L. C. Harlan, and A. L. Potosky, "Urinary and Sexual Function after Radical Prostatectomy for Clinically Localized Prostate Cancer: The Prostate Cancer Outcomes Study," *Journal of the American Medical Association* 283, no. 3 (2000): 354–60, https:// jamanetwork.com/journals/jama/fullarticle/192307.
32. J. J. Fenton, M. S. Weyrich, S. Durbin, Y. Liu, H. Bang, and J. Melnikow, "Prostate-Specific Antigen-Based Screening for Prostate Cancer Evidence Report and Systematic Review for the US Preventive Services Task Force,"

Journal of the American Medical Association 319, no. 18 (2018): 1914–31, https://jamanetwork.com/journals/jama/fullarticle/2680554.
33. Leslie, "Prostate Cancer."
34. M. McNaughton-Collins, F. J. Fowler Jr., J. Caubet, J. Min Lee, A. Hauser, and M. J. Barry, "Psychological Effects of a Suspicious Prostate Cancer Screening Test Followed by a Benign Biopsy Result," *American Journal of Medicine* 17, no. 10 (2004): 719–25.
35. Quoted in A. Shaughnessy, "False-Positive PSA Associated with Increased Worry, Fears," *American Family Physician* 71, no. 10 (2005): 1988.
36. F. Fowler, M. J. Barry, B. Walker-Corkery, J. Caubet, D. W. Bates, J. Min Lee, A. Hauser, and M. McNaughton-Collins, "The Impact of a Suspicious Prostate Biopsy on Patient's Psychological, Socio-Behavioral, and Medical Care Outcomes," *Journal of General Internal Medicine* 21, no. 7 (2006): 715–21.
37. D. A. Katz, D. F. Jarrard, C. A. McHorney, S. L. Hillis, D. A. Wiebe, and D. G. Fryback, "Health Perceptions in Patients Who Undergo Screening and Workup for Prostate Cancer," *Urology* 69, no. 2 (2007): 215–20.
38. J. A. Charnow, "Prostate Cancer Diagnosis Ups Risk of Non-Cancer Hospitalizations," *Renal and Urology News*, Feb. 11, 2016, https://www.renalandurologynews.com/home/news/urology/prostate-cancer/prostate-cancer-diagnosis-ups-risk-of-non-cancer-hospitalizations/.
39. A. D. Raval, S. Madhavan, M. C. Mattes, M. Salkini, and U. Sambamoorthi, "Impact of Prostate Cancer Diagnosis on Non-Cancer Hospitalizations among Elderly Medicare Beneficiaries with Incident Prostate Cancer," *Journal of the National Comprehensive Cancer Network* 14, no. 2 (2016): 185–94, https://www.ncbi.nlm.nih.gov/pmc/articles/PMC4837465/.
40. B. Carter, "Prostate Specific Antigen Revisiting the Evidence," *Journal of the American Medical Association* 319, no. 18 (2018): 1866–68.
41. M. R. Cooperberg and P. R. Carroll, "Trends in Management for Patients with Localized Prostate Cancer, 1990–2013," *Journal of the American Medical Association* 314, no. 1 (2015): 80–82, https://jamanetwork.com/journals/jama/fullarticle/2382968.
42. National Health Service (UK), "PSA Testing," last updated Oct. 18, 2021, https://www.nhs.uk/conditions/prostate-cancer/psa-testing/.
43. National Cancer Institute, "Cancer Stat Facts."
44. M. R. Cooperberg, J. M. Broering, and P. R. Carroll, "Time Trends and Local Variation in Primary Treatment of Localized Prostate Cancer," *Journal of Clinical Oncology* 28, no. 7 (2020): 1117–23.
45. J. Wang, H. H. Xia, Y. Zhang, and L. Zhang, "Trends in Treatments for Prostate Cancer in the United States, 2010–2015," *American Journal of Cancer Research* 11, no. 5 (2021): 2351–68.
46. J. Björklund, Y. Folkvaljon, A. Cole, S. Carlsson, D. Robinson, S. Loeb, P. Stattin, and O. Akre, "Ninety-Day Postoperative Mortality after Robot-Assisted Laparoscopic Prostatectomy and Retropubic Radical Prostatectomy: A Nationwide Population-Based Study," *BJU International* 18, no. 2 (2016): 302–6, https://www.ncbi.nlm.nih.gov/pmc/articles/PMC4942403/.
47. J. Chen, C. Oromendia, J. A. Halpern, and K. V. Ballman, "National Trends in Management of Localized Prostate Cancer: A Population Based Analysis, 2004–2013," *Prostate* 78, no. 7 (2018): 512–20.

48. R. Gulati, A. Tsodikov, R. Etzioni, R. A. Hunter-Merrill, J. L. Gore, A. B. Mariotto, and M. R. Cooperberg, "Expected Population Impacts of Discontinued Prostate-Specific Antigen Screening," *Cancer* 120, no. 22 (2014): 3519–26, https://acsjournals.onlinelibrary.wiley.com/doi/full/10.1002/cncr.28932.
49. F. R. Schroek, T. L. Krupski, L. Sun, D. M. Albala, M. M. Price, T. J. Polascik, C. N. Robertson, A. K. Tewari, and J. W. Moul, "Satisfaction and Regret after Open Retropubic or Robot-Assisted Laparoscopic Radical Prostatectomy," *European Urology* 54, no. 4 (2008): 785–93.
50. D. Ilic, S. M. Evans, C. Allan, J. Jung, D. Murphy, and M. Frydenberg, "Laproscopic and Robot-Assisted versus Open Prostatectomy for the Treatment of Localised Prostate Cancer," *Cochrane Database of Systematic Reviews 2017*, https://www.cochrane.org/CD009625/PROSTATE_laparoscopic-and-robotic-assisted-versus-open-radical-prostatectomy-treatment-localised-prostate.
51. A. R. Mahal et al., "Conservative Management of Low-Risk Prostate Cancer among Young versus Older Men in the United States: Trends and Outcomes from a Novel National Database," *Cancer* 12, no. 21 (2016): 3338–46.
52. J. Wilbur, "Prostate Cancer Screening: The Continuing Controversy," *American Family Physician* 78, no. 12 (2008): 1377–84, https://www.aafp.org/afp/2008/1215/p1377.html.
53. L. Klotz, "Contemporary Approach to Active Surveillance for Favorable Risk Prostate Cancer," *Asian Journal of Urology* 6, no. 2 (2019): 146–52, https://www.ncbi.nlm.nih.gov/pmc/articles/PMC6488691/.
54. F. C. Hamdy et al., "10-Year Outcomes after Monitoring, Surgery, or Radiotherapy for Localized Prostate Cancer," *New England Journal of Medicine* 375 (2016): 1415–24.
55. T. J. Wilt, K. M. Jones, M. J. Barry, G. L. Andriole, D. Culkin, T. Wheeler, W. J. Aronson, and M. K. Brawer, "Follow-Up of Prostatectomy versus Observation for Early Prostate Cancer," *New England Journal of Medicine* 377 (2017): 132–42.
56. K. Marzouk, M. Assel, B. Ehdaie, and A. Vickers, "Long-Term Cancer Specific Anxiety in Men Undergoing Active Surveillance of Prostate Cancer: Findings from a Large Prospective Cohort," *Journal of Urology* 200, no. 6 (2018): 1250–55.
57. R. C. Chen et al., *Active Surveillance for the Management of Localized Prostate Cancer (Cancer Care Ontario Guideline)*, American Society of Clinical Oncology Clinical Practice Guideline Endorsement, eScholarship, https://escholarship.org/uc/item/7rd2v3h6.
58. Loeb et al., "Qualitative Study on Decision-Making," 23.

Chapter 6. Thyroid Cancer

1. Her story comes from a news report by J. Min-ho and J. Sung-eun, "What Caused Jump in Thyroid Cancer Cases?," *Korea Times*, March 27, 2014, http://www.koreatimes.co.kr/www/news/culture/2014/03/319_154183.html.
2. H. S. Ahn, H. J. Kim, and H. G. Welch, "Korea's Thyroid-Cancer 'Epidemic'—Screening and Overdiagnosis," *New England Journal of Medicine* 379, no. 19 (2014): 1765–67, https://www.ecmstudy.com/uploads/3/1/8/8/31885023/nejm-koreas_thyroid-cancer_epidemic-screening_&_overdiagnosis.pdf.

3. J. P. Brito, J. C. Morris, and V. M. Montori, "Thyroid Cancer: Zealous Imaging Has Increased Detection and Treatment of Low Risk Tumours," *British Medical Journal* 347 (2013): 18–21, http://www.bmj.com/bmj /section-pdf/737987?path=/bmj/347/7923/Analysis.full.pdf.
4. Brito, Morris, and Montori, "Thyroid Cancer."
5. "Thyroid Nodules," American Thyroid Association, accessed Jan. 21, 2023, https://www.thyroid.org/thyroid-nodules/.
6. S. Park et al., "Association between Screening and the Thyroid Cancer 'Epidemic' in South Korea: Evidence from a Nationwide Study," *British Medical Journal* 355 (2016): i5745, http://www.bmj.com/content/355/bmj .i5745.
7. B. Aschebrook-Kilfoy et al., "Risk Factors for Decreased Quality of Life in Thyroid Cancer Survivors: Initial Findings from the North American Thyroid Cancer Survivorship Study," *Thyroid* 25, no. 12 (2015): 1313–21.
8. Aschebrook-Kilfoy et al., "Risk Factors for Decreased Quality of Life."
9. K. Ritter, D. Elfenbein, D. Schneider, H. Chen, and R. S. Sippel, "Hypo-parathyroidism after Total Thyroidectomy: Incidence and Resolution," *Journal of Surgical Research* 197, no. 2 (2016): 348–53, https://www.ncbi.nlm .nih.gov/pmc/articles/PMC4466142/.
10. S. L. Lee, "Complications of Radioactive Iodine Treatment of Thyroid Carcinoma," *Journal of the National Comprehensive Cancer Network* 8, no. 1 (2010), https://jnccn.org/view/journals/jnccn/8/11/article -p1277.xml.
11. N. G. Iyer, L. G. T. Morris, R. M. Tuttle, A. R. Shaha, and I. Ganly, "Rising Incidence of Second Cancers in Patients with Low-Risk (T1N0) Thyroid Cancer Who Receive Radioactive Iodine Therapy," *Cancer* 117, no. 19 (2011): 4439–46.
12. N. Bhattacharyya and M. P. Fried, "Assessment of the Morbidity and Complications of Total Thyroidectomy," *JAMA Otolaryngology—Head and Neck Surgery* 128, no. 4 (2002): 389–92, https://jamanetwork.com /journals/jamaotolaryngology/fullarticle/482819.
13. B. C. James, B. Aschebrook-Kilfoy, M. G. White, M. K. Applewhite, S. P. Kaplan, P. Angelos, E. L. Kaplan, and R. H. Grogan, "Quality of Life in Thyroid Cancer—Assessment of Physician Perceptions," *Journal of Surgical Research* 226 (2008): 94–99.
14. H. Kletzien, C. L. Macdonald, J. Orne, D. O. Francis, G. Leverson, E. Wendt, R. S. Sippel, and N. P. Connor, "Comparison between Patient-Perceived Voice Changes and Quantitative Voice Measures in the First Postoperative Year after Thyroidectomy: A Secondary Analysis of a Randomized Clinical Trial," *JAMA Otolaryngology—Head and Neck Surgery* 144, no. 11 (2018): 995–1003.
15. K. H. Yi et al., "The Korean Guideline for Thyroid Cancer Screening," *Journal of the Korean Medical Association* 58, no. 4 (2015): 302–12.
16. International Agency for Research on Cancer, press release no. 246, Aug. 18, 2016, https://www.iarc.fr/en/media-centre/pr/2016/pdfs/pr246_E.pdf.
17. H. S. Ahn and H. G. Welch, "South Korea's Thyroid-Cancer 'Epidemic'— Turning the Tide," *New England Journal of Medicine* 373 (2015): 2389–90.

18. Park et al., "Association between Screening and the Thyroid Cancer 'Epidemic.'"
19. J. Lee and S. W. Shin, "Overdiagnosis and Screening for Thyroid Cancer in Korea," *Lancet* 384, no. 9957 (2014): 1848, https://www.thelancet.com /journals/lancet/article/PIIS0140-6736(14)62242-X/fulltext.
20. Yi et al., "Korean Guideline."
21. *Segye Ilbo*, April 6, 2014.
22. Park et al., "Association between Screening and the Thyroid Cancer 'Epidemic.'"; Lee and Shin, "Overdiagnosis and Screening."
23. S. H. Park, B. Lee, S. Lee, E. Choi, E.-B. Choi, J. Yoo, J. K. Jun, and K. S. Choi, "A Qualitative Study of Women's Views on Overdiagnosis and Screening for Thyroid Cancer in Korea," *BMC Cancer* 15 (2015): 858, https:// bmccancer.biomedcentral.com/articles/10.1186/s12885-015-1877-6.
24. Quoted in Park et al., "Qualitative Study of Women's Views."
25. Park et al., "Qualitative Study of Women's Views."
26. Brito, Morris, and Montori, "Thyroid Cancer."
27. IARC, *Cancer Incidence in Five Continents*, 11 vols. (Lyon: IARC, 2017), http://ci5.iarc.fr/Default.aspx.
28. IARC, *Cancer Incidence*.
29. J. S. Lin, E. J. Aiello Bowles, S. B. Williams, and C. C. Morrison, "Updated Evidence Report and Systematic Review for the US Preventive Services Task Force," *Journal of the American Medical Association* 317, no. 18 (2017): 1888–903, https://jamanetwork.com/journals/jama/fullarticle/2625324.
30. H. Lim, S. S. Devesa, J. A. Sosa, D. Check, and C. M. Kitahara, "Trends in Thyroid Cancer Incidence and Mortality in the United States, 1974–2013," *Journal of the American Medical Association* 317, no. 13 (2017): 1338–1348, https://jamanetwork.com/journals/jama/fullarticle/2613728.
31. Lin et al., "Updated Evidence Report and Systematic Review," 1.
32. L. Davies et al., "American Association of Clinical Endocrinologists and American College of Endocrinology Disease State Clinical Review: The Increasing Incidence of Thyroid Cancer," *Endocrine Practice* 21, no. 6 (2015): 686–96.
33. Davies et al., "American Association of Clinical Endocrinologists."
34. National Cancer Institute, "Cancer Stat Facts: Thyroid Cancer," Surveillance, Epidemiology, and End Results Program, accessed March 16, 2023, https://seer.cancer.gov/statfacts/html/thyro.html.
35. Brito, Morris, and Montori, "Thyroid Cancer."
36. N. Saleh, "Thyroidectomy Still Popular Despite Less Aggressive Treatment Recommendations," *Cancer Network*, April 15, 2019, https://www .cancernetwork.com/view/thyroidectomy-still-popular-despite-less -aggressive-treatment-recommendations.
37. National Cancer Institute, "Cancer Stat Facts: Thyroid Cancer."
38. "Thyroid Cancer: Statistics," Cancer.Net, Jan. 1, 2020, https://www.cancer .net/cancer-types/thyroid-cancer/statistics.
39. B. Haugen et al., "2015 American Thyroid Association Management Guidelines for Adult Patients with Thyroid Nodules and Differentiated Thyroid Cancer," *Thyroid* 26, no. 1 (2016), https://www.liebertpub.com /doi/pdfplus/10.1089/thy.2015.0020.

40. C. Rouvalis, "Yuri Nikiforov: Making Cancer Disappear," *Pitt Chronicle*, Oct. 21, 2016, https://www.chronicle.pitt.edu/story/yuri-nikiforov-making-cancer-disappear.

41. Y. E. Nikiforov et al., "Nomenclature Revision for Encapsulated Follicular Variant of Papillary Thyroid Carcinoma: A Paradigm Shift to Reduce Overtreatment of Indolent Tumors," *JAMA Oncology* 2, no. 8 (2016): 1023–29.

42. B. Nickel, J. P. Brito, A. Barratt, S. Jordan, R. Moynihan, and K. McCaffery, "Clinicians' Views on Management and Terminology for Papillary Thyroid Microcarcinoma: A Qualitative Study," *Thyroid* 27, no. 5 (2017): 661–71.

43. Nickel et al., "Clinicians' Views."

44. Crile, *Cancer and Common Sense*, 27.

45. B. C. James, L. Timsina, R. Graham, P. Angelos, D. A. Haggstrom, "Changes in Total Thyroidectomy versus Thyroid Lobectomy for Papillary Thyroid Cancer during the Past 15 Years," *Surgery* 166, no. 1 (2019): 41–47, https://pubmed.ncbi.nlm.nih.gov/30904172/.

46. L. Caulley et al., "Trends in Diagnosis of Noninvasive Follicular Thyroid Neoplasm with Papillarylike Nuclear Features and Total Thyroidectomies for Patients with Papillary Thyroid Neoplasms," *JAMA Otolaryngology—Head and Neck Surgery* 148, no. 2 (2022): 99–106.

Chapter 7. Lung Cancer
1. "Lung Cancer—Non-Small Cell: Statistics," Cancer.Net, Dec. 2022, https://www.cancer.net/cancer-types/lung-cancer-non-small-cell/statistics.

2. D. R. Aberle et al., "Reduced Lung-Cancer Mortality with Low-Dose Computed Tomographic Screening," *New England Journal of Medicine* 365, no. 5 (2011): 395–409.

3. V. Prasad, J. Lenzer, and D. H. Newman, "Why Cancer Screening Has Never Been Shown to 'Save Lives'—and What We Can Do about It," *British Medical Journal* 352 (2016): h6080.

4. A. Goodman, "NELSON Trial: 'Call to Action' for Lung Cancer CT Screening of High-Risk Individuals," *ASCO Post*, Oct. 25, 2018, https://www.ascopost.com/issues/october-25-2018/nelson-trial/.

5. N. Becker et al., "Lung Cancer Mortality Reduction by LDCT Screening—Results from the Randomized German LUSI Trial," *International Journal of Cancer* 146 (2020): 1503–13.

6. Z. Saghir et al., "CT Screening for Lung Cancer Brings Forward Early Disease. The Randomised Danish Lung Cancer Screening Trial: Status after Five Annual Screening Rounds with Low-Dose CT," *Thorax* 767, no. 4 (2012): 296–301.

7. U. Pastorin et al., "Annual or Biennial CT Screening versus Observation in Heavy Smokers: 5-Year Results of the MILD Trial," *European Journal of Cancer Prevention* 21, no. 3 (2012): 308–15.

8. M. Infante et al., "Long-Term Follow-Up Results of the DANTE Trial, a Randomized Study of Lung Cancer Screening with Spiral Computed Tomography," *American Journal of Respiratory and Critical Care Medicine* 191, no. 10 (2015): 1166–75.

9. L. S. Kinsinger et al., "Implementation of Lung Cancer Screening in the Veterans Health Administration," *Journal of the American Medical Association* 177, no. 3 (2017): 399–406.

10. "Screening for Lung Cancer," Cancer Research UK, last reviewed Sept. 29, 2022, https://www.cancerresearchuk.org/about-cancer/lung-cancer/getting -diagnosed/screening.

11. "Council Updates Its Recommendation to Screen for Cancer," European Council, news release, Dec. 9, 2022, https://www.consilium.europa.eu /en/press/press-releases/2022/12/09/council-updates-its-recommendation -to-screen-for-cancer/.

12. T. B. Richards, V. P. Doria-Rose, A. Soman, C. N. Klabunde, R. S. Cara-ballo, S. C. Gray, K. A. Houston, and M. C. White, "Lung Cancer Screening Inconsistent with U.S. Preventive Services Task Force Recommendations," *American Journal of Preventive Medicine* 56, no. 1 (2019): 66–73, https://www .ncbi.nlm.nih.gov/pmc/articles/PMC6319382/.

13. "Saved by the Scan," American Lung Association, accessed Jan. 24, 2023, https://www.lung.org/our-initiatives/saved-by-the-scan/.

14. L. M. Henderson et al., "Opinions and Practices of Lung Cancer Screening by Physician Specialty," *North Carolina Medical Journal* 80, no. 1 (2019): 19–26, https://ncmedicaljournal.com/article/55155.

15. R. Piana, "Although Evidence Is Clear that Lung Cancer Screening Saves Lives, Adoption Rates Remain Low: A Conversation with Nasser Altorki, MD," *ASCO Post*, March 10, 2019, https://www.ascopost.com/issues /march-10-2019/lung-cancer-screening-evidence-and-adoption/.

16. "Screening for Lung Cancer with Low Dose Computed Tomography (LDCT)," Decision Memo CAG-00439N, Medicare Coverage Database, CMS.gov, Feb. 5, 2015, https://www.cms.gov/medicare-coverage-database /details/nca-decision-memo.aspx?NCAId=274; A. T. Brenner, T. L. Malo, M. Margolis, J. Elston Lafata, S. James, M. B. Vu, and D. S. Reuland, "Evaluating Shared Decision Making for Lung Cancer Screening," *Journal of the American Medical Association* 178, no. 10 (2018): 1311–16, https:// jamanetwork.com/journals/jamainternalmedicine/fullarticle/2696731.

17. Brenner et al., "Evaluating Shared Decision Making."

18. R. F. Redberg, "Failing Grade for Shared Decision Making for Lung Cancer," *Journal of the American Medical Association Internal Medicine* 178, no. 10 (2018): 1295–96.

19. C. Slatore, D. Arenberg, R. Wiener, and M. Sockrider, *Decision Aid for Lung Cancer Screening with Computerized Tomography (CT)*, American Thoracic Society, 2015, https://www.thoracic.org/patients/patient-resources /resources/decision-guide-lcs.pdf.

20. L. Kinsinger, C. Andersen, and J. Kim, "Implementation of Lung Cancer Screening in the Veterans Health Administration," *JAMA Internal Medicine* 177, no. 3 (2017): 399–406.

21. J. Huo, C. Shen, R. J. Volk, and Y. T. Shih, "Use of CT and Chest Radiography for Lung Cancer Screening before and after Publication of Screening Guidelines: Intended and Unintended Uptake," *Journal of the American Medical Association Internal Medicine* 177, no. 3 (2017): 439–41.

22. Richards et al., "Lung Cancer Screening Inconsistent."

23. E. F. Patz et al., "Overdiagnosis in Low-Dose Computed Tomography Screening for Lung Cancer," *Journal of the American Medical Association Internal Medicine* 174, no. 2 (2014): 269–74, https://jamanetwork.com/journals/jamainternalmedicine/fullarticle/1785197.

24. H. J. de Koning et al., "Reduced Lung-Cancer Mortality with Volume CT Screening in a Randomized Trial," *New England Journal of Medicine* 382 (2020): 503–13.

25. B. Heleno, V. Siersma, and J. Brodersen, "Estimation of Overdiagnosis of Lung Cancer in Low-Dose Computed Tomography Screening: A Secondary Analysis of the Danish Lung Cancer Screening Trial," *Journal of the American Medical Association Internal Medicine* 178, no. 10 (2018): 1420–22, https://jamanetwork.com/journals/jamainternalmedicine/article-abstract/2696728.

26. G. Veronesi, P. Maisonneuve, M. Bellomi, C. Rampinelli, I. Durli, R. Bertolotti, and L. Spaggiari, "Estimating Overdiagnosis in Low-Dose Computed Tomography Screening for Lung Cancer: A Cohort Study," *Annals of Internal Medicine* 157, no. 11 (2012): 776–84; Patz et al., "Overdiagnosis."

27. S. Swensen et al., "CT Screening for Lung Cancer: Five-Year Prospective Experience," *Radiology* 235, no. 1 (2005): 259–65.

28. Prasad, Lenzer, and Newman, "Why Cancer Screening."

29. J. Huo, Y. Xu, T. Sheu, R. J. Volk, and Y. T. Shih, "Complication Rates and Downstream Medical Costs Associated with Invasive Diagnostic Procedures for Lung Abnormalities in the Community Setting," *Journal of the American Medical Association Internal Medicine* 179, no. 3 (2019): 324–32.

30. M. R. Freiman, J. A. Clark, C. G. Slatore, M. K. Gould, S. Woloshin, L. M. Schwartz, and R. S. Wiener, "Patients' Knowledge, Beliefs, and Distress Associated with Detection and Evaluation of Incidental Pulmonary Nodules for Cancer: Results from a Multicenter Survey," *Journal of Thoracic Oncology* 11, no. 5 (2016): 700–708, https://www.jto.org/article/S1556-0864(16)00355-5/pdf.

31. D. S. Weiss and C. R. Marmar, "The Impact of Event Scale, Revised," in *Assessing Psychological Trauma and PTSD*, ed. J. P. Wilson, T. M. Keane (New York: Guilford Press, 1997), 399–411.

32. Freiman et al., "Patients' Knowledge."

33. M. Byrne, J. Weissfeld, and M. S. Roberts, "Anxiety, Fear of Cancer, and Perceived Risk of Cancer Following Lung Cancer Screening," *Medical Decision Making* 28, no. 6 (2008): 917–25.

34. C. G. Slatore, R. S. Wiener, S. E. Golden, D. H. Au, and L. Ganzini, "Longitudinal Assessment of Distress among Veterans with Incidental Pulmonary Nodules," *Annals of the American Thoracic Society* 13, no. 11 (2016): 1983–91.

35. H. Zhao, Y. Xu, J. Huo, A. C. Burks, D. E. Ost, and Y. T. Shih, "Updated Analysis of Complication Rates Associated with Invasive Diagnostic Procedures After Lung Cancer Screening," *JAMA Network Open*, Dec. 16, 2020, https://jamanetwork.com/journals/jamanetworkopen/fullarticle/2774245.

36. Zhao et al., "Updated Analysis."

37. M. K. Karmakar and A. M. H. Ho, "Post-thoractomy Pain Syndrome," *Thoracic Surgery Clinics* 14, no. 3 (2004): 345–52.

38. J. Handy, "Hospital Readmission after Pulmonary Resection: Prevalence, Patterns, and Predisposing Characteristics," *Annals of Thoracic Surgery* 7, no. 6 (2001): 1855–60.

39. M. S. Allen et al., "Morbidity and Mortality of Major Pulmonary Resections in Patients with Early-Stage Lung Cancer: Initial Results of the Randomized, Prospective ACOSOG Z0030 Trial," *Annals of Thoracic Surgery* 81, no. 3 (2006): 1013–20.

40. C. D. Wright, H. A. Gaissert, J. D. Grab, S. M. O'Brien, E. D. Peterson, and M. S. Allen, "Predictors of Prolonged Length of Stay after Lobectomy for Lung Cancer: A Society of Thoracic Surgeons General Thoracic Surgery Database Risk-Adjustment Model," *Annals of Thoracic Surgery* 85, no. 6 (2008): 1857–65.

41. M. F. Berry, J. Hanna, B. C. Tong, W. R. Burfeind, D. H. Harpole, T. A. D'Amico, and M. W. Onaitis, "Risk Factors for Morbidity after Lobectomy for Lung Cancer in Elderly Patients," *Annals of Thoracic Surgery* 88, no. 4 (2009): 1093–99.

42. E. Ziarnik and E. L. Grogan, "Post-Lobectomy Early Complications," *Thoracic Surgery Clinics* 25, no. 3 (2015): 355–64.

43. K. Huang, S. Wang, W. Lu, Y. Chang, J. Su, and Y. Lu, "Effects of Low-Dose Computed Tomography on Lung Cancer Screening: A Systematic Review, Meta-analysis, and Trial Sequential Analysis," *BMC Pulmonary Medicine* 19, no. 1 (2019), https://www.ncbi.nlm.nih.gov/pmc/articles/PMC6625016/.

44. Huang et al., "Effects of Low-Dose Computed Tomography."

Chapter 8. Colorectal Cancer

1. American Cancer Society, *Colorectal Cancer Facts and Figures, 2020–2022* (Atlanta, GA: American Cancer Society, 2020), https://www.cancer.org/content/dam/cancer-org/research/cancer-facts-and-statistics/colorectal-cancer-facts-and-figures/colorectal-cancer-facts-and-figures-2020-2022.pdf.

2. P. Cram, A. M. Fendrick, J. Inadomi, M. E. Cowen, D. Carpenter, and S. Vijan, "The Impact of a Celebrity Promotional Campaign on the Use of Colon Cancer Screening: The Katie Couric Effect," *JAMA Internal Medicine* 163, no. 13 (2003): 1601–5.

3. Healthy People 2030, "Increase the Proportion of Adults Who Get Screened for Colorectal Cancer," US Department of Health and Human Services, accessed Jan. 25, 2023, https://health.gov/healthypeople/objectives-and-data/browse-objectives/cancer/increase-proportion-adults-who-get-screened-colorectal-cancer-c-07.

4. Email correspondence with Dr. Ingrid Hall, epidemiologist in the CDC Division of Cancer Prevention and Control's Epidemiology and Applied Research Branch, Sept. 21, 2021; data from the National Health Interview Survey, National Center for Health Statistics, Feb. 24, 2023, https://www.cdc.gov/nchs/nhis/index.htm.

5. Email correspondence with Oscar Poon, business area manager, iData Research, Feb 24, 2023.

6. M. Kalager, P. Wieszczy, I. Lansdorp-Vogelaar, D. A. Corley, M. Bretthauer, and M. F. Kaminski, "Overdiagnosis in Colorectal Cancer Screening: Time to Acknowledge a Blind Spot," *Gastroenterology* 155, no. 3 (2018): 592–595, https://www.gastrojournal.org/article/S0016-5085(18)34825-X /fulltext.

7. M. Arnold, M. S. Sierra, M. Laversanne, I. Soerjomataram, A. Jemal, and F. Bray, "Global Patterns and Trends in Colorectal Cancer Incidence and Mortality," *Gut* 27 no. 4 (2017), https://gut.bmj.com/content/66/4/683.

8. G. Scott, "Waits Are Common for Colonoscopies," *New York Times*, July 9, 2002, https://www.nytimes.com/2002/07/09/health/waits-are-common -for-colonoscopies.html.

9. M. F. Kaminsky and J. Regula, "Adenoma Detection Race at Colonoscopy: The Good and the Bad," *Gastroenterology* 149, no. 2 (2015): 273–74, https://www.gastrojournal.org/article/S0016-5085(15)00878-1/fulltext.

10. M. Adams, D. Leiman, and S. Mathews, "Adenoma Detection Date Removed from MIPS, or Was It?," *GI & Hepatology News*, March 29, 2020, https://www.mdedge.com/gihepnews/article/219752/practice -management/adenoma-detection-rate-removed-2020-mips-or-was-it.

11. O. S. Lin, "Performing Colonoscopy in Elderly and Very Elderly Patients: Risks, Costs and Benefits," *World Journal of Gastrointestinal Endoscopy* 6, no. 6 (2014): 220–26, https://www.ncbi.nlm.nih.gov/pmc/articles /PMC4055990/.

12. T. M. Geiger and R. Ricciardi, "Screening Options for Colorectal Cancer," *Clinics in Colon and Rectal Surgery* 22, no. 4 (2009): 209–17, https://www .ncbi.nlm.nih.gov/pmc/articles/PMC2796104/.

13. P. Wang, T. Xu, S. Ngamruengphong, M. A. Makary, A. Kalloo, and S. Hutfless, "Rates of Infection after Colonoscopy and Osophagogastroduo-denoscopy in Ambulatory Surgery Centres in the USA," *Gut* 67, no. 9 (2018): 1626–36; L. W. Day, A. Kwon, J. M. Inadomi, L. C. Walter, and M. Somsouk, "Adverse Events in Older Patients Undergoing Colonoscopy: A Systematic Review and Meta-analysis," *Gastrointestinal Endoscopy* 74, no. 4 (2011): 885–96, https://www.ncbi.nlm.nih.gov/pmc/articles/PMC3371336/.

14. N. Causada-Calo, K. Bishay, S. Albashir, A. Al Mazroui, and D. Armstrong, "Association between Age and Complications after Outpatient Colonos-copy," *JAMA Open Network* 3, no. 6 (2020), https://jamanetwork.com /journals/jamanetworkopen/fullarticle/2767639.

15. Scott, "Waits Are Common."

16. D. A. Joseph, R. G. S. Meester, A. G. Zauber, D. L. Manninen, L. Winges, F. B. Dong, B. Peaker, and M. van Ballegooijen, "Colorectal Cancer Screen-ing: Estimated Future Colonoscopy Need and Current Volume and Capacity," *Cancer* 122, no. 16 (2016): 2479–86, https://acsjournals .onlinelibrary.wiley.com/doi/full/10.1002/cncr.30070.

17. Joseph et al., "Colorectal Cancer Screening."

18. Poon email correspondence.

19. D. A. Fisher et al., "Complications of Colonoscopy," *Gastrointestinal Endoscopy* 74, no. 4 (2011), https://www.asge.org/docs/default-source /education/practice_guidelines/doc-56321364-c4d8-4742-8158 -55b6bef2a568.pdf.

Chapter 9. Underscreening

1. J. Reece, E. F. G. Neal, P. Nguyen, J. McIntosh, and J. D. Emery, "Delayed or Failure to Follow-up Abnormal Breast Cancer Screening Mammograms in Primary Care: A Systematic Review," *BMC Cancer* 21, article 373 (2021). https://bmccancer.biomedcentral.com/articles/10.1186/s12885-021 -08100-3.
2. M. R. Andersen, R. Smith, H. Meischke, D. Bowen, and N. Urban, "Breast Cancer Worry and Mammography Use by Women with and without a Family History in a Population-Based Sample," *Cancer Epidemiology, Biomarkers, and Prevention* 12, no. 4 (2003): 314–20, https://cebp .aacrjournals.org/content/12/4/314.
3. Andersen et al., "Breast Cancer Worry."
4. K. M. Kash, J. C. Holland, M. S. Halper, and D. G. Miller, "Psychological Distress and Surveillance Behaviors of Women with a Family History of Breast Cancer," *Journal of the National Cancer Institute* 84, no. 1 (1992): 24–30.
5. N. S. Consedine, C. Magai, Y. S. Krivoshekova, L. Ryzewicz, and A. I. Neugut, "Fear, Anxiety, Worry, and Breast Cancer Screening Behavior: A Critical Review," *Cancer Epidemiology, Biomarkers, and Prevention* 13 (2004): 1–10, https://cebp.aacrjournals.org/content/13/4/501.
6. L. Clemow, M. E. Costanza, W. P. Haddad, R. Luckmann, M. J. White, D. Klaus, and A. M. Stoddard, "Underutilizers of Mammography Screening Today: Characteristics of Women Planning, Undecided about, and Not Planning a Mammogram," *Annals of Behavioral Medicine* 22, no. 1 (2000): 80–88; C. S. Skinner, C. L. Arfken, and R. K. Sykes, "Knowledge, Perceptions, and Mammography Stage of Adoption among Older Urban Women," *American Journal of Preventive Medicine* 14, no. 1 (1998): 54–63.
7. J. L. Hay, T. R. Buckley, and J. S. Ostroff, "The Role of Cancer Worry in Cancer Screening: A Theoretical and Empirical Review of the Literature," *Psycho-oncology* 14, no. 7 (2005): 517–34.
8. R. M. Jones, K. J. Devers, A. J. Kuzel, and S. H. Woolf, "Patient-Reported Barriers to Colorectal Cancer Screening: A Mixed-Methods Analysis," *American Journal of Preventive Medicine* 38, no. 5 (2010): 508–16.
9. R. C. Rabin, "Why People Aren't Screened for Colon Cancer," *New York Times*, Jan. 20, 2011, https://well.blogs.nytimes.com/2011/01/20/why -people-arent-screened-for-colon-cancer/.
10. National Cancer Institute, "I'd rather not know my chance of getting cancer," Health Information National Trends Survey (HINTS), https:// hints.cancer.gov/view-questions/question-detail.aspx?qid=1419.
11. National Cancer Institute, "You are afraid of finding colon cancer if you were checked," HINTS 1 (2003), https://hints.cancer.gov/view-questions -topics/question-details.aspx?PK_Cycle=1&qid=1041.
12. National Cancer Institute, HINTS 2 (2005), https://hints.cancer.gov/view -questions-topics/question-details.aspx?PK_Cycle=2&qid=473.
13. S. L. Quaife, C. Vrinten, M. Ruparel, S. M. Janes, R. J. Beeken, J. Waller, and Andy McEwen, "Smokers' Interest in a Lung Cancer Screening Programme: A National Survey in England," *BMC Cancer* 18, no. 1 (2018): 497.

14. Prostate Cancer Foundation, *Public Perceptions of Prostate Cancer*, PCF 3P Report 2018, https://www.pcf.org/wp-content/uploads/2018/08/PublicPerception_PCF.pdf.
15. A. A. Kotwal, P. Schumm, S. G. Mohile, and W. Dale, "The Influences of Stress, Depression, and Anxiety on PSA Screening Rates in a Nationally Representative Sample," *Medical Care* 50, no. 12 (2012): 1037–44.
16. O. Bratt, J. Damber, M. Emanuelsson, U. Kristoffersson, R. Lundgren, H. Olsson, and H. Grönberg, "Risk Perception, Screening Practice and Interest in Genetic Testing among Unaffected Men in Families with Hereditary Prostate Cancer," *European Journal of Cancer* 36, no. 2 (2000): 235–41.
17. M. G. Oscarsson, B. E. Wijma, and E. G. Benzein, "'I Do Not Need to . . . I Do Not Want to . . . I Do Not Give It Priority . . .'—Why Women Choose Not to Attend Cervical Cancer Screening," *Health Expectations* 11, no. 1 (2008): 26–34.
18. S. L. Pruitt, M. J. Shim, P. D. Mullen, S. W. Vernon, and B. C. Amick III, "Association of Area Socioeconomic Status and Breast, Cervical, and Colorectal Cancer Screening: A Systematic Review," *Cancer Epidemiology, Biomarkers and Prevention* 18, no. 10 (2009): 2579–99, https://cebp.aacrjournals.org/content/18/10/2579.
19. C. von Wagner, A. Good, K. L. Whitaker, and J. Wardle, "Psychosocial Determinants of Socioeconomic Inequalities in Cancer Screening Participation: A Conceptual Framework," *Epidemiologic Reviews* 33, no. 1 (2011): 135–47, https://academic.oup.com/epirev/article/33/1/135/478690.
20. Von Wagner et al., "Psychosocial Determinants."
21. S. Assari, P. Khoshpouri, and H. Chalian, "Combined Effects of Race and Socioeconomic Status on Cancer Beliefs, Cognitions, and Emotions," *Healthcare* (Basel) 7, no. 1 (2019): 17, https://www.ncbi.nlm.nih.gov/pmc/articles/PMC6473681/.
22. J. Wardle, K. McCaffery, M. Nadel, and W. Atkin, "Socioeconomic Differences in Cancer Screening Participation: Comparing Cognitive and Psychosocial Explanations," *Social Science and Medicine* 59, no. 2 (2004): 249–61.
23. S. G. Smith, L. M. McGregor, R. Raine, J. Wardle, C. Wagner, and K. A. Robb, "Inequalities in Cancer Screening Participation: Examining Differences in Perceived Benefits and Barriers," *Psycho-oncology* 25, no. 10 (2016): 1168–74.
24. C. Lerman, M. Daly, C. Sands, and A. Balshem, "Mammography Adherence and Psychological Distress Among Women at Risk for Breast Cancer," *Journal of the National Cancer Institute* 85, no. 13 (1993): 1074–80.
25. Z. A. Rivera-Ramos and L. P. Buki, "I Will No Longer Be a Man! Manliness and Prostate Cancer Screenings among Latino Men," *Psychology of Men and Masculinity* 12, no. 1 (2011): 13–25.
26. Rivera-Ramos and Buki, "I Will No Longer Be a Man!"
27. R. F. Bakemeier, L. U. Krebs, J. R. Murphy, Z. Shen, and T. Ryals, "Attitudes of Colorado Health Professionals toward Breast and Cervical Cancer Screening in Hispanic Women," *Journal of the National Cancer Institute Monographs* 18 (1995): 95–110.

28. L. T. Austin, F. Ahmad, M. McNally, and D. E. Stewart, "Breast and Cervical Cancer Screening in Hispanic Women: A Literature Review Using the Health Belief Model," *Women's Health Issues* 2, no. 3 (2002): 122–28.

29. L. P. Buki, E. A. Borrayo, B. M. Feigal, and I. Y. Carillo, "Are All Latinas the Same? Perceived Breast Cancer Screening Barriers and Facilitative Conditions," *Psychology of Women Quarterly* 28, no. 4 (2004): 400–411.

30. Buki et al., "Are All Latinas the Same?"

31. Austin et al., "Breast and Cervical Cancer Screening in Hispanic Women."

32. "How Do Breast Cancer Screening Rates Compare among Different Groups in the U.S.?," Susan G. Komen, last updated Jan. 24, 2023, https://www.komen.org/breast-cancer/screening/screening-disparities/.

33. M. E. Peek, J. V. Sayad, and R. Markwardt, "Fear, Fatalism and Breast Cancer Screening in Low-Income African-American Women: The Role of Clinicians and the Health Care System," *Journal of General Internal Medicine* 23, no. 11 (2008): 1847–53, https://www.ncbi.nlm.nih.gov/pmc/articles/PMC2585682/.

34. J. C. Jernigan, J. M. Trauth, D. Neal-Ferguson, and C. Cartier-Ulrich, "Factors that Influence Cancer Screening in Older African American Men and Women: Focus Group Findings," *Family Community Health* 24, no. 3 (2001): 27–33.

35. L. K. Christman, A. D. Abernethy, R. L. Gorsuch, and A. Brown, "Intrinsic Religiousness as a Mediator Between Fatalism and Cancer-Specific Fear: Clarifying the Role of Fear in Prostate Cancer Screening," *Journal of Religions and Health* 53, no. 3 (2014): 760–72.

36. C. L. Melvin, M. S. Jefferson, L. J. Rice, K. B. Cartmell, and C. H. Halbert, "Predictors of Participation in Mammography Screening among Non-Hispanic Black, Non-Hispanic White, and Hispanic Women," *Frontiers in Public Health*, Sept. 6, 2016, https://www.frontiersin.org/articles/10.3389/fpubh.2016.00188/full.

37. E. L. Cohen, "Naming and Claiming Cancer among African American Women: An Application of Problematic Integration Theory," *Journal of Applied Communication Research* 37, no. 4 (2009): 397–417, https://www.ncbi.nlm.nih.gov/pmc/articles/PMC2760846/.

Chapter 10. **Delayed Diagnosis**

1. G. Garg, N. Bansal, P. Dixit, and A. Sharma, "Auto-Amputation of Penis due to Advanced Carcinoma Penis," *BMJ Case Reports* 2018 (2018), https://casereports.bmj.com/content/2018/bcr-2018-226505.

2. E. Skeppner, S. Andersson, J. Johansson, and T. Windahl, "Initial Symptoms and Delay in Patients with Penile Carcinoma," *Scandinavian Journal of Urology and Nephrology* 46, no. 5 (2012): 319–25, https://www.researchgate.net/publication/230878272_Initial_symptoms_and_delay_in_patients_with_penile_carcinoma.

3. V. Devita Jr. and E. Devita-Raeburn, *The Death of Cancer* (New York: Sarah Crichton Books, 2015).

4. U. Macleod, E. D. Mitchell, C. Burgess, S. Macdonald, and A. J. Ramirez, "Risk Factors for Delayed Presentation and Referral of Symptomatic Cancer: Evidence for Common Cancers," *British Journal of Cancer* 101,

no. 101 (2009): S92–S101, https://www.ncbi.nlm.nih.gov/pmc/articles /PMC2790698/.

5.   E. Mitchell, S. Macdonald, N. C. Campbell, D. Weller, and U. Macleod, "Influences on Pre-hospital Delay in the Diagnosis of Colorectal Cancer: A Systematic Review," *British Journal of Cancer* 98, no. 1 (2008): 60–70, https://www.ncbi.nlm.nih.gov/pmc/articles/PMC2359711/.

6.   A. Almuammar, C. Dryden, and J. A. Burr, "Factors Associated with Late Presentation of Cancer: A Limited Literature Review," *Journal of Radiotherapy in Practice* 9, no. 2 (2010): 117–23.

7.   A. E. Simon, J. Waller, K. Robb, and J. Wardle, "Patient Delay in Presentation of Possible Cancer Symptoms: The Contribution of Knowledge and Attitudes in a Population Sample from the United Kingdom," *Cancer Epidemiology, Biomarkers, and Prevention* 19, no. 9 (2010): 2272–77, https:// cebp.aacrjournals.org/content/19/9/2272.

8.   A. Bish, A. Ramirez, C. Burgess, and M. Hunter, "Understanding Why Women Delay in Seeking Help for Breast Cancer Symptoms," *British Journal of Cancer* 58, no. 4 (2005): 321–26.

9.   J. A. Fish, I. Prichard, K. Ettridge, E. A. Grunfeld, and C. Wilson, "Psychosocial Factors That Influence Men's Help-Seeking for Cancer Symptoms: A Systematic Synthesis of Mixed Methods Research," *Psycho-oncology* 24, no. 10 (2015): 1222–32, https://onlinelibrary.wiley.com/doi/full/10.1002 /pon.3912.

10. L. K. Smith, C. Pope, and J. L. Botha, "Patients' Help-Seeking Experiences and Delay in Cancer Presentation: A Qualitative Synthesis," *Lancet* 366 (2005): 825–31.

11. C. Burgess, M. S. Hunter, and A. J. Ramirez, "A Qualitative Study of Delay among Women Reporting Symptoms of Breast Cancer," *British Journal of General Practice* 51, no. 473 (2001): 967–71.

12. A. Peroskie, R. A. Ferrer, and W. M. P. Klein, "Association of Cancer Worry and Perceived Risk with Doctor Avoidance: An Analysis of Information Avoidance in a Representative US Sample," *Journal of Behavioral Medicine* 37 (2014): 977–87.

13. Populus Research/Strategy, cancer polling, June 2018, https://yonder consulting.com/poll-archive/cancer-polling-survey.pdf.

14. R. J. Beeken, A. E. Simon, C. von Wagner, K. L. Whitaker, and J. Wardle, "Cancer Fatalism: Deterring Early Presentation and Increasing Social Inequalities?," *Cancer Epidemiology, Biomarkers, and Prevention* 20, no. 10 (2011): 2127–31, https://www.ncbi.nlm.nih.gov/pmc/articles/PMC3189396 /pdf/ukmss-36356.pdf.

15. G. Lyratzopoulos, M. Pang-Hsiang Liu, G. A. Abel, J. Wardle, and N. L. Keating, "The Association between Fatalistic Beliefs and Late Stage at Diagnosis of Lung and Colorectal Cancer," *Cancer Epidemiology, Biomarkers, and Prevention* 24, no. 4 (2015): 720–26.

16. Buki et al., "Are All Latinas the Same?"

17. N. C. Facione, M. J. Dodd, W. Holzemer, and A. I. Meleis, "Helpseeking for Self-Discovered Breast Symptoms: Implications for Early Detection," *Cancer Practice* 5, no. 4 (1996): 220–27.

18. Sharon, "I Was the Worst Daughter They Ever Saw," *Ex-Christian Scientist*, Jan. 17, 2016, https://exchristianscience.com/2016/01/17/i-was-the -worst-daughter-they-ever-saw/.

19. A. Iskandarsyah, C. D. Klerk, D. R. Suardi, M. P. Soemitro, S. S. Sadarjoen, and J. Passchier, "Psychosocial and Cultural Reasons for Delay in Seeking Help and Nonadherence to Treatment in Indonesian Women with Breast Cancer: A Qualitative Study," *Health Psychology* 33, no. 3 (2014): 214–21.

20. M. M. Gullatte, O. Brawley, A. Kinney, B. Powe, and K. Mooney, "Religiosity, Spirituality, and Cancer Fatalism Beliefs on Delay in Breast Cancer Diagnosis in African American Women," *Journal of Religion and Health* 49, no. 1 (2010): 62–72.

21. P. G. Moorman et al., "Effect of Cultural, Folk, and Religious Beliefs and Practices on Delays in Diagnosis of Ovarian Cancer in African American Women," *Journal of Women's Health* 28, no. 4 (2019): 444–52.

22. B. N. Polite, T. M. Cipriano-Steffens, F. J. Hlubocky, P. Jean-Pierre, Y. Cheng, K. C. Brewer, G. H. Rauscher, and G. A. Fitchett, "Association of Externalizing Religious and Spiritual Beliefs on Stage of Colon Cancer Diagnosis among Black and White Multicenter Urban Patient Populations," *Cancer* 124, no. 12 (2018): 2578–87, https://acsjournals.onlinelibrary.wiley .com/doi/full/10.1002/cncr.31351; K. A. Wallston, V. L. Malcarne, L. Flores, I. Hansdottir, C. A. Smith, M. J. Stein, M. H. Weisman, and P. J. Clements, "Does God Determine Your Health? The God Locus of Health Control Scale," *Cognitive Therapy and Research* 2, no. 2 (1999): 131–42.

23. R. Neal et al., "Is Increased Time to Diagnosis and Treatment in Symptomatic Cancer Associated with Poorer Outcomes? Systematic Review," *British Journal of Cancer* 112 (2015): S92–S107, https://www.nature.com /articles/bjc201548.

24. M. A. Richards, "The Size of the Prize for Earlier Diagnosis of Cancer in England," *British Journal of Cancer* 101 (2009): S125–S129.

Chapter 11. The Stunning Economic Cost of Our Sometimes Excessive Fear of Cancer

1. X. Ma et al., "The Cost Implications of Prostate Cancer Screening in the Medicare Population," *Cancer* 120 (2014): 96–102, https://acsjournals .onlinelibrary.wiley.com/doi/pdf/10.1002/cncr.28373.

2. J. G. Trogdon, A. D. Falchook, R. Basak, W. R. Carpenter, and R. C. Chen, "Total Medicare Costs Associated with Diagnosis and Treatment of Prostate Cancer in Elderly Men," *JAMA Oncology* 5, no. 1 (2019): 60–66, https://pubmed.ncbi.nlm.nih.gov/30242397/.

3. Ong, Mei-Sing, et al., "National Expenditure for False-Positive Mammograms and Breast Cancer Overdiagnoses Estimated at $4 Billion a Year," *Health Affairs* 34, no. 4 (2015), https://www.healthaffairs.org/doi/full/10 .1377/hlthaff.2014.1087.

4. C. P. Gross et al., "The Cost of Breast Cancer Screening in the Medicare Population," *JAMA Internal Medicine* 173, no. 3 (2013): 220–26, https:// jamanetwork.com/journals/jamainternalmedicine/fullarticle/1555815.

5. E. Lopez, T. Neuman, G. Jacobson, and L. Levitt, "How Much More than Medicare Do Private Insurers Pay? A Review of the Literature," Kaiser

Family Foundation, April 15, 2020, https://www.kff.org/medicare/issue
-brief/how-much-more-than-medicare-do-private-insurers-pay-a-review
-of-the-literature/. The 85% estimate was deemed reasonable and reliable
by Larry Levitt, executive vice president for health policy at the Kaiser
Family Foundation and senior author of Lopez et al., "How Much More
than Medicare," in a video conversation, October 7, 2020.

6. A. Vlahiotis, B. Griffin, A. T. Stavros, and J. Margolis, "Analysis of Utiliza-
    tion Patterns and Associated Costs of the Breast Imaging and Diagnostic
    Procedures after Screening Mammography," *ClinicoEconomics and
    Outcomes Research* 2018, no. 10 (2018): 157–67.

7. Hwang, "Impact of Surgery on Ductal Carcinoma In Situ Outcomes."

8. H. Blumen, K. Fitch, and V. Polkus, "Comparison of Treatment Costs for
    Breast Cancer, by Tumor Stage and Type of Service," *American Health
    Drug Benefits* 9, no. 1 (2016): 23–32, https://www.ncbi.nlm.nih.gov/pmc
    /articles/PMC4822976/.

9. P. A. Cronin, C. Olcese, S. Patil, M. Morrow, K. J. Van Zee, "Impact of Age
    on Risk of Recurrence of DCIS: Outcomes of 2996 Women Treated with
    Breast-Conserving Surgery over 30 Years," *Annals of Surgical Oncology* 23,
    no. 9 (2016): 2816–24, https://www.ncbi.nlm.nih.gov/pmc/articles
    /PMC4995886/.

10. H. Panchal and E. Matros, "Current Trends in Post-Mastectomy Breast
    Reconstruction," *Plastic Reconstructive Surgery* 140, no. 5 (2017): 7S–13S,
    https://www.ncbi.nlm.nih.gov/pmc/articles/PMC5722225/.

11. A. M. Miller, C. A. Steiner, M. L. Barrett, K. R. Fingar, and A. Elixhauser,
    "Breast Reconstruction Surgery for Mastectomy in Hospital Inpatient
    Ambulatory Settings, 2009–2014," *Healthcare Cost and Utilization
    Project*, Agency of Health Quality Research Statistical Brief 228, Oct. 2017,
    https://www.hcup-us.ahrq.gov/reports/statbriefs/sb228-Breast
    -Reconstruction-For-Mastectomy.pdf.

12. S. N. Razdan et al., "Cost-Effectiveness Analysis of Breast Reconstruc-
    tion Options in the Setting of Postmastectomy Radiotherapy Using the
    BREAST-Q," *Plastic and Reconstructive Surgery* 137, no. 3 (2017): 510e–517e,
    https://www.ncbi.nlm.nih.gov/pmc/articles/PMC4986994/; N. L. Berlin,
    K. C. Chung, E. Matros, J. Chen, A. O. Momoh, "The Costs of Breast
    Reconstruction and Implications for Episode-Based Bundled Payment
    Models," *Plastic and Reconstructive Surgery* 146, no. 6 (2020): 721e–730e;
    J. I. Billig, A. Duncan, L. Zhong, O. Aliu, E. D. Sears, K. C. Chung, and A. O.
    Momoh, "The Cost of Contralateral Prophylactic Mastectomy in Women
    with Unilateral Breast Cancer," *Plastic and Reconstructive Surgery* 141,
    no. 5 (2018): 1094–1102, https://pubmed.ncbi.nlm.nih.gov/29659447/;
    J. I. Billig, Y. Lu, A. O. Momoh, and K. C. Chung, "A Nationwide Analysis
    of Cost Variation for Autologous Free Flap Breast Reconstruction," *JAMA
    Surgery* 152, no. 11 (2017): 1039–47, https://pubmed.ncbi.nlm.nih.gov
    /28724133/; A. M. Fitzpatrick et al., "Cost and Outcome Analysis of
    Breast Reconstruction Paradigm Shift," *Annals of Plastic Surgery* 73, no. 2
    (2014): 141–49; Y. Cai, S. R. Boas, L. Summerville, and A. Kumar, "National
    Trends in Hospitalization Charges for Autologous Free Flap Breast Recon-
    struction," *Annals of Plastic Surgery* 85, no. S1 (2020): S135–S140; N. M.

Krishnan, J. P. Fischer, M. N. Basta, and M. Y. Nahabedian, "Is Single-Stage Prosthetic Reconstruction Cost Effective? A Cost-Utility Analysis for the Use of Direct-to-Implant Breast Reconstruction Relative to Expander-Implant Reconstruction in Postmastectomy Patients," *Plastic and Reconstructive Surgery* 138, no. 3 (2016): 537–47; C. A. Steiner, A. J. Weiss, M. L. Barrett, K. R. Fingar, and P. H. Davis, "Trends in Bilateral and Unilateral Mastectomies in Hospital Inpatient and Ambulatory Settings, 2005–2013," *Healthcare Cost and Utilization Project*, AHRQ Statistical Brief 201, March 2016, https://www.hcup-us.ahrq.gov/reports/statbriefs/sb201 -Mastectomies-Inpatient-Outpatient.jsp.

13. T. L. Mills, "Six Payment Opportunities You May Have Missed," *Family Practice Medicine* 15, no. 9 (2008): 27–32, https://www.aafp.org/fpm/2008 /1100/p27.html.

14. A. B. Weiner et al., "The Cost of Prostate Biopsies and Their Complications: A Summary of Data on All Medicare Fee-for-Service Patients over 2 Years," *Urology Practice* 7, no. 2 (2020), https://www.auajournals.org/doi /abs/10.1097/UPJ.0000000000000072.

15. Number of tests per urologist: J. A. Halpern et al., "National Trends in Prostate Biopsy and Radical Prostatectomy Volumes Following the US Preventive Services Task Force Guidelines against Prostate-Specific Antigen Screening," *JAMA Surgery* 152, no. 2 (2017): 192–98, https://jamanetwork .com/journals/jamasurgery/fullarticle/2571537. Number of urologists: American Urological Association, accessed March 23, 2023, https://www .auanet.org.

16. M. D. Gross, M. N. Alshak, J. E. Shoag, A. A. Laviana, M. A. Gorin, A. Sedrakyan, and J. C. Hu, "Healthcare Costs of Post-Prostate Biopsy Sepsis," *Urology*, 133 (2019): 11–15, https://www.sciencedirect.com /science/article/abs/pii/S0090429519305503.

17. R. P. Werntz and S. E. Eggener, "Use of Active Surveillance or Watchful Waiting for Low-Risk Prostate Cancer and Management Trends across Risk Groups in the United States, 2010–2015," *Journal of the American Medical Association* 321, no. 7 (2019): 704–6.

18. V. Sharma, K. M. Wymer, B. J. Borah, D. A. Barocas, R. H. Thompson, R. J. Karnes, and S. A. Boorjian, "Cost-Effectiveness of Active Surveillance, Radical Prostatectomy and External Beam Radiotherapy for Localized Prostate Cancer: An Analysis of the ProtecT Trial," *Journal of Urology* 202, no. 5 (2019): 964–72. F. C. Hamdy et al., "10-Year Outcomes after Monitoring, Surgery, or Radiotherapy for Localized Prostate Cancer," *New England Journal of Medicine* 375 (2016): 1415–24, https://www.nejm.org/doi/full/10 .1056/nejmoa1606220.

19. T. Walsh, "Cost of Penile Implants and Insurance Coverage for ED Treatments," EDCURE.org, accessed January 25, 2023, https://www .edcure.org/articles/insurance-coverage-for-penile-implants-cost-should -not-be-a-barrier-to-erectile-restoration/.

20. M. M. Boltz, C. S. Hollenbeak, E. Schaefer, D. Goldenberg, B. D. Saunders, "Attributable Costs of Differentiated Thyroid Cancer in the Elderly Medicare Population," *Surgery* 154, no. 6 (2013): 1363–70.

21. C. C. Lubitz, C. Y. Kong, P. M. McMahon, G. H. Daniels, Y. Chen, K. P. Economopoulos, S. Gazelle, and M. C. Weinstein, "Annual Financial Impact of Well-Differentiated Thyroid Cancer Care in the United States," *Cancer* 123, no. 9 (2014): 1345–52.
22. A. Hauch, Z. Al-Qurayshi, G. Randolph, and E. Kandil, "Total Thyroidectomy Is Associated with Increased Risk of Complications for Low- and High-Volume Surgeons," *Annals of Surgical Oncology* 21 (2014): 3844–52.
23. T. B. Richards, V. P. Doria-Rose, A. Soman, C. N. Klabunde, R. S. Caraballo, S. C. Gray, K. A. Houston, and M. C. White, "Lung Cancer Screening Inconsistent with U.S. Preventive Services Task Force Recommendations," *American Journal of Preventive Medicine* 56, no. 1 (2019): 66–73, https://www.ncbi.nlm.nih.gov/pmc/articles/PMC6319382/.
24. S. A. Fedewa et al., "State Variation in Low-Dose Computed Tomography Scanning for Lung Cancer Screening in the United States," *Journal of the National Cancer Institute*, Nov. 12, 2020, https://academic.oup.com/jnci/advance-article/doi/10.1093/jnci/djaa170/5970481.
25. "Medicare Reimbursement for Lung Cancer Screening Using Low-Dose CT," Healthcare Administrative Partners, Feb. 12, 2016, https://info.hapusa.com/blog-0/medicare-reimbursement-for-lung-cancer-screening-using-low-dose-ct.
26. B. H. L. Goulart, M. E. Bensink, D. G. Mummy, and S. D. Ramsey, "Lung Cancer Screening with Low-Dose Computed Tomography: Costs, National Expenditures, and Cost-Effectiveness," *Journal of the National Comprehensive Cancer Network* 10, no. 2 (2012): 267–70.
27. Richards et al., "Lung Cancer Screening Inconsistent."
28. Patz et al., "Overdiagnosis in Low-Dose Computed Tomography Screening."
29. Goulart et al., "Lung Cancer Screening."
30. E. Ziarnik and E. L. Grogan, "Post-Lobectomy Early Complications," *Thoracic Surgery Clinics* 25, no. 3 (2015): 355–64.
31. Goulart et al., "Lung Cancer Screening."
32. Goulart et al., "Lung Cancer Screening."
33. A. Shaukat, J. Holub, I. M. Pike, M. Pochapin, D. Greenwald, C. Schmitt, and G. Eisen, "Benchmarking Adenoma Detection Rates for Colonoscopy: Results from a US-Based Registry," Brief Communication, *American Journal of Gastroenterology* 16, no. 9 (2021): 1946–49, https://journals.lww.com/ajg/Abstract/2021/09000/Benchmarking_Adenoma_Detection_Rates_for.26.aspx.
34. Lieberman et al., "Utilization of Colonoscopy."
35. Phone conversation with Brad Conway, VP public policy, American College of Gastroenterology, Feb. 2, 2021.
36. American College of Radiology, "Updated USPSTF Lung Cancer Screening Guidelines Would Help Save Lives," July 7, 2020, https://www.acr.org/Media-Center/ACR-News-Releases/2020/Updated-USPSTF-Lung-Cancer-Screening-Guidelines-Would-Help-Save-Lives.
37. USPSTF, *Final Recommendation Statement, Colorectal Cancer: Screening*, May 18, 2021, https://www.uspreventiveservicestaskforce.org/uspstf/recommendation/colorectal-cancer-screening.

38. USPSTF, *Breast Cancer: Screening*.
39. R. Jagsi et al., "Treatment Decisions and the Employment of Breast Cancer Patients: Results of a Population-Based Survey," *Cancer* 123, no. 4 (2017): 4791–99, https://www.ncbi.nlm.nih.gov/pmc/articles/PMC5716845/.
40. "Prostatectomy: What to Expect during Surgery and Recovery," Johns Hopkins Medicine, accessed March 23, 2023, https://www.hopkinsmedicine.org/health/conditions-and-diseases/prostate-cancer/prostatectomy-what-to-expect-during-surgery-and-recovery.
41. "What to Expect Before and After Thyroid Surgery," Penn Medicine, accessed March 23, 2023, https://www.pennmedicine.org/for-patients-and-visitors/find-a-program-or-service/surgery/thyroid-surgery/what-to-expect-at-penn.
42. US Bureau of Labor Statistics, "Employer Costs for Employee Compensation Summary," news release, Dec. 15, 2022, https://www.bls.gov/news.release/ecec.nro.htm.

Chapter 12. Environmentalism's Contribution to Our Fear of Cancer

1. R. Carson, *Silent Spring* (New York: Houghton Mifflin, 1962).
2. Google Books NGram viewer, carcinogens, 1800–2019, https://books.google.com/ngrams/graph?content=carcinogens&year_start=1800&year_end=2019.
3. B. Israel, "How Many Cancers Are Caused by the Environment?," *Scientific American*, May 21, 2010, https://www.scientificamerican.com/article/how-many-cancers-are-caused-by-the-environment/.
4. National Cancer Institute, "Would you say you strongly agree, somewhat agree, somewhat disagree, strongly disagree with the following statements or do you have no opinion: It seems like everything causes cancer," HINTS 5, cycle 2, 2018, https://hints.cancer.gov/view-questions-topics/question-details.aspx?PK_Cycle=11&qid=500.
5. "Environmental Hazards and Health Effects: Cancer Clusters," CDC, accessed March 24, 2023, https://www.cdc.gov/nceh/clusters/fallon/ddtfaq.htm.
6. A. Ferriman, "Attempts to Ban DDT Have Increased Deaths," *BMJ* 322, no. 7297 (2001): 1270, https://www.ncbi.nlm.nih.gov/pmc/articles/PMC1173321/.
7. L. McLaren, S. Patterson, S. Thawer, P. Faris, D. McNeil, M. Potestio, and L. Shwart, "Measuring the Short-Term Impact of Fluoridation Cessation on Dental Caries in Grade 2 Children Using Tooth Surface Indices," *Community Dentistry and Oral Epidemiology* 44, no. 3 (2016): 274–82, https://onlinelibrary.wiley.com/doi/full/10.1111/cdoe.12215.
8. J. Meyer, V. Margaritis, and A. Mendelsohn, "Consequences of Community Water Fluoridation Cessation for Medicaid-Eligible Children and Adolescents in Juneau, Alaska," *BMC Oral Health* 18, art. 215 (2018), https://bmcoralhealth.biomedcentral.com/articles/10.1186/s12903-018-0684-2.
9. J. R. Bucher, M. R. Hejtmancik, J. D. Toft II, R. L. Persing, S. L. Eustis, J. K. Haseman, "Results and Conclusions of the National Toxicology Program's

Rodent Carcinogenicity Studies with Sodium Fluoride," *International Journal of Cancer* 18, no. 5 (1991): 733–37, https://onlinelibrary.wiley.com /doi/abs/10.1002/ijc.2910480517.

10. "2018 Fluoridation Statistics," CDC, last reviewed Sept. 8, 2020, https://www.cdc.gov/fluoridation/statistics/2018stats.htm.

11. H. Ritchie, "What Was the Death Toll from Chernobyl and Fukushima?," Our World in Data, updated Dec. 1, 2021, https://ourworldindata.org/what -was-the-death-toll-from-chernobyl-and-fukushima.

12. *Health Risk Assessment from the Nuclear Accident after the 2011 Great East Japan Earthquake and Tsunami,* World Health Organization, 2013, https:// apps.who.int/iris/bitstream/handle/10665/78218/9789241505130_eng .pdf;jsessionid=3B34.

13. E. Marcus, "No Evidence Reactor Leak Caused Cancer," *Washington Post*, Sept. 1, 1990, https://www.washingtonpost.com/wp-srv/national /longterm/tmi/stories/study090190.htm.

14. "Life Span Study (LSS)," Radiation Effects Research Institute, accessed Jan. 25, 2023, https://www.rerf.or.jp/en/programs/research_activities_e /outline_e/proglss-en/.

15. Congressional Research Service, *U.S. Nuclear Plant Shutdowns, State Interventions, and Policy Concerns,* June 10, 2021, https://crsreports .congress.gov/product/pdf/R/R46820/3.

16. Public comment in a Municipal Light Plant meeting to discuss the smart meter program proposed for Concord, MA, Nov. 22, 2021.

17. "Cell Phone Towers," American Cancer Society, last revised June 1, 2020, https://www.cancer.org/cancer/cancer-causes/radiation-exposure /cellular-phone-towers.html.

18. T. B. Wheeler, "Angelos Joins Lawsuit on Cell Phone Injuries," *Baltimore Sun*, Jan. 17, 2001, https://www.baltimoresun.com/news/bs-xpm-2001 -01-17-0101170078-story.html.

19. "Cell Phones and Cancer Risk," National Cancer Institute, March 10, 2022, https://www.cancer.gov/about-cancer/causes-prevention/risk/radiation /cell-phones-fact-sheet.

20. A. J. Schutt, "The Power Line Dilemma: Compensation for Diminished Property Value Caused by Fear of Electromagnetic Fields," *Florida State University Law Review* 24, no. 1, art. 5 (1996), https://ir.law.fsu.edu/cgi /viewcontent.cgi?article=1427&context=lr.

21. J. Smith, "GMOS and Cancer," Institute for Responsible Technology, Sept. 21, 2021, https://www.responsibletechnology.org/gmos-and-cancer/; K. Loria, "Most Plastic Products Contain Potentially Toxic Substances," *Consumer Reports*, last updated Oct. 2, 2019, https://www.consumerreports .org/toxic-chemicals-substances/most-plastic-products-contain -potentially-toxic-chemicals/; "Disinfection Byproducts," Environmental Working Group, April 2020, https://www.ewg.org/tapwater/reviewed -disinfection-byproducts.php; S. Kobylewski and M. F. Jacobson, *Food Dyes: A Rainbow of Risks*, Center for Science in the Public Interest, June 2010, https://cspinet.org/sites/default/files/attachment/food-dyes -rainbow-of-risks.pdf; L. Suhaila, "High Fructose Corn Syrup and Pancreatic Cancer," *Natural Medicine Journal* 4, no. 10 (2012), https://www

.naturalmedicinejournal.com/journal/2012-10/high-fructose-corn-syrup
-and-pancreatic-cancer.

22. "The Pollution in People: Cancer-Causing Chemicals in Americans'
Bodies," Environmental Working Group, June 14, 2016, https://www.ewg
.org/research/pollution-people.

23. C. Tomasetti and B. Vogelstein, "Variation in Cancer Risk among Tissues Can
Be Explained by the Number of Stem Cell Divisions," *Science* 347, no. 6217
(2015): 78–81, https://www.ncbi.nlm.nih.gov/pmc/articles/PMC4446723/.

24. Tomasetti and Vogelstein, "Variation in Cancer Risk"; A. Kasprak, "Cancer,
Juries, and Scientific Uncertainty: The Monsanto Roundup Ruling Explained," Snopes, Aug. 17, 2018, https://www.snopes.com/news/2018/08/17
/cancer-juries-scientific-certainty-monsanto-roundup-ruling-explained/.

Chapter 13. Other Societal Impacts of Our Fear of Cancer

1. M. Gavidia, "Overall US Cancer Mortality Rate Reaches 26-Year Decline,
but Obesity-Related Cancer Deaths Rise," *American Journal of Managed
Care*, Jan. 8, 2020, https://www.ajmc.com/view/overall-us-cancer-mortality
-rate-reaches-26year-decline-but-obesityrelated-cancer-deaths-rise.

2. S. Simon, "Facts and Figures 2020 Reports Largest One-Year Drop in
Cancer Mortality," American Cancer Society, Jan. 8, 2020, https://www
.cancer.org/latest-news/facts-and-figures-2020.html.

3. Gavidia, "Overall US Cancer Mortality Rate."

4. A. L. Goodkind, C. W. Tessum, J. S. Coggins, J. D. Hill, and J. D. Marshall,
"Fine-Scale Damage Estimates of Particulate Matter Air Pollution Reveal
Opportunities for Location-Specific Mitigation of Emissions," *Proceedings
of the National Academy of Sciences* 116, no. 18 (2019), https://www.pnas
.org/content/pnas/116/18/8775.full.pdf.

5. Consumer Defense Grp. v. Rental Housing Indus. Members, 137 Cal. App.
4th 1185, 1208 (2006).

6. J. Rosenblatt, "Bayer Wins Court Ruling Blocking California's Roundup
Warning," *Bloomberg Business*, June 22, 2020, https://www.bloomberg.com
/news/articles/2020-06-22/bayer-wins-court-ruling-blocking-california-s
-roundup-warning.

7. A. Kasprak, "Cancer, Juries, and Scientific Certainty: The Monsanto
Roundup Ruling Explained," Snopes, Aug. 17, 2018.

8. Schutt, "Power Line Dilemma."

9. Norfolk and Western Railway Company v. Ayers, 58 U.S. 135 (2003),
https://www.oyez.org/cases/2002/01-963.

10. B. E. Sirovich, S. Woloshin, and L. M. Schwartz, "Too Little? Too Much?
Primary Care Physicians' Views on US Health Care: A Brief Report,"
Archives of Internal Medicine 171, no. 17 (2011): 1582–85, https://pubmed
.ncbi.nlm.nih.gov/21949169/.

11. R. Hanscom, M. Small, and A. Lambrecht, *Diagnostic Accuracy: Room for
Improvement*, Coverys, accessed Jan. 29, 2023, https://coverys.com/PDFs
/Coverys_Diagnostic_Accuracy_Report.aspx.

12. P. Legant, "Oncologists and Medical Malpractice," *Journal of Oncological
Practice* 2, no. 4 (2006): 164–69, https://www.ncbi.nlm.nih.gov/pmc
/articles/PMC2793617/.

13. G. S. Regev and A. M. Ser, "Breast Cancer Medical Malpractice Litigation in New York: The Past 10 Years," *Breast* 46 (2019): 1–3.
14. J. G. Elmore et al., "Does Litigation Influence Medical Practice? The Influence of Community Radiologists' Medical Malpractice Perceptions and Experience on Screening Mammography," *Radiology* 236, no. 1 (2005): 37–46, https://www.ncbi.nlm.nih.gov/pmc/articles/PMC3143020/.
15. S. D. Kamath, S. M. Kircher, and A. B. Benson III, "Comparison of Cancer Burden and Nonprofit Organization Funding Reveals Disparities in Funding across Cancer Types," *Journal of the National Comprehensive Cancer Network* 17, no. 7 (2019), https://jnccn.org/view/journals/jnccn/17/7/article-p849.xml.
16. "Financial Reports," Susan G. Komen, accessed Jan. 29, 2023, https://www.komen.org/about-komen/financials/.
17. M. Carter, "Backlash against 'Pinkwashing' of Breast Cancer Awareness Campaigns," *British Medical Journal* 351 (2015): h5339.
18. "About Think Before You Pink," Breast Cancer Action, accessed Jan. 29, 2023, https://www.bcaction.org/about-think-before-you-pink/.
19. G. A. Sulik, *Pink Ribbon Blues: How Breast Cancer Culture Undermines Women's Health* (New York: Oxford University Press, 2012), 186.
20. "Organic Purchasing," Organic Trade Association, accessed Jan. 29, 2023, https://ota.com/organic-market-overview/organic-purchasing.
21. Pew Research Center, "Americans' Views about and Consumption of Organic Foods," in *The New Food Fights: US Public Divides over Food Science*, Dec. 1, 2016, https://www.pewresearch.org/science/2016/12/01/americans-views-about-and-consumption-of-organic-foods/.
22. UK Food Standards Agency, "The Food Standards Agency's Current Stance: Organic Food," Aug. 2006, https://web.archive.org/web/20100331234955/http://extras.timesonline.co.uk/organicfood2.pdf.
23. M. C. R. Alavanja and M. R. Bonner, "Occupational Pesticide Exposures and Cancer Risk: A Review," *Journal of Toxicology and Environmental Health, Part B: Critical Review* 15, no. 4 (2018): 238–63, https://www.ncbi.nlm.nih.gov/pmc/articles/PMC6276799/. See also "Organic Foods and Cancer Risk: Separating Myth from Fact," American Institute for Cancer Research, Feb. 5, 2019, https://www.aicr.org/resources/blog/organic-foods-and-cancer-risk-separating-myth-from-fact/.
24. "Dietary Supplement Use Reaches All Time High," Council for Responsible Nutrition, news release, Sept. 30, 2019, https://www.crnusa.org/newsroom/dietary-supplement-use-reaches-all-time-high.
25. E. Guallar, S. Stranges, C. Mulrow, L. J. Appel, and E. R. Miller, "Stop Wasting Money on Vitamin and Mineral Supplements," *Annals of Internal Medicine* 159 (2013): 850.
26. S. P. Fortmann, B. U. Burda, C. A. Senger, J. S. Lin, and E. P. Whitlock, "Vitamin and Mineral Supplements in the Primary Prevention of Cardiovascular Disease and Cancer: An Updated Systematic Evidence Review for the U.S. Preventive Services Task Force," *Annals of Internal Medicine* 159, no. 12 (2013): 824–34.
27. "Do Not Use Supplements for Cancer Prevention," World Cancer Research Fund International, accessed March 13, 2023, https://www.wcrf.org/dietandcancer/recommendations/dont-rely-supplements.

28. "Do Not Use Supplements for Cancer Prevention."
29. M. E. Martinez, E. T. Jacobs, J. A. Baron, J. R. Marshall, and T. Byers, "Dietary Supplements and Cancer Prevention: Balancing Potential Benefits against Proven Harms," *Journal of the National Cancer Institute* 104, no. 10 (2012): 732–39, https://www.ncbi.nlm.nih.gov/pmc/articles/PMC3352833/.
30. "Cancer Costs Projected to Reach at Least $158 Billion in 2020," National Institutes of Health, Jan. 12, 2011, https://www.nih.gov/news-events/news-releases/cancer-costs-projected-reach-least-158-billion-2020.
31. J. Park and K. A. Look, "Health Care Expenditure Burden of Cancer Care in the United States," *Inquiry* 56 (2019), https://www.ncbi.nlm.nih.gov/pmc/articles/PMC6778988/.
32. "Cancer Care: The Deceptive Marketing of Hope," Truth in Advertising, Oct. 22, 2018, https://www.truthinadvertising.org/cancer-care-the-deceptive-marketing-of-hope/.
33. Quoted in "Cancer Care: The Deceptive Marketing of Hope," Truth in Advertising, Oct. 22, 2018, https://truthinadvertising.org/articles/cancer-care-the-deceptive-marketing-of-hope/.
34. L. B. Vater, J. M. Donohue, R. Arnold, D. B. White, E. Chu, and Y. Schenker, "What Are Cancer Centers Advertising to the Public? A Content Analysis," *Annals of Internal Medicine* 160, no. 12 (2014): 813–20, https://www.ncbi.nlm.nih.gov/pmc/articles/PMC4356527/.
35. "Companies that Purport to Successfully Treat Cancer Agree to Settle FTC Charges over Their Claims," Federal Trade Commission, March 13, 1996, https://www.ftc.gov/news-events/press-releases/1996/03/companies-purport-successfully-treat-cancer-agree-settle-ftc.
36. Grand View Research, *Cancer Diagnostics.*
37. Grand View Research, *Endoscopy Devices.*
38. Global Market Insights, *In-Vitro Colorectal Cancer Screening Tests Market Size by Test Type*, Feb. 2019, updated in 2021, https://www.gminsights.com/industry-analysis/in-vitro-colorectal-cancer-screening-tests-market-report.
39. "North America Breast Cancer Screening Market Forecast to 2027—COVID-19 Impact and Regional Analysis, ResearchAndMarkets.com," *Business Wire*, Nov. 10, 2020, https://www.businesswire.com/news/home/20201110005704/en; T. Morris, "Oncology Market Opportunities and Growth Trends," Definitive Healthcare, March 18, 2020, https://blog.definitivehc.com/oncology-market-opportunities-and-growth-trends.
40. Grand View Research, *Prostate Cancer Diagnostics.*
41. Market Research Future, *Lung Cancer Therapeutics Market Research Report*, July 2019, https://www.marketresearchfuture.com/reports/lung-cancer-market-1185.
42. Research and Markets, "United States $15.39 Billion Solid Tumor Testing Markets: Analysis 2019–2020 and Forecast to 2030," *PRNewswire*, Oct. 27, 2020, https://www.prnewswire.com/news-releases/united-states-15-39-billion-solid-tumor-testing-markets-analysis-2019-2020--forecast-to-2030--301160647.html.
43. P. Castle, "Screening for many Cancers with One Test: Uncertainty Abounds," National Cancer Institute, April 21, 2022, https://www.cancer.gov/news-events/cancer-currents-blog/2022/finding-cancer-early-mced-tests.

44. "3D Mammogram," Mayo Clinic, Sept. 16, 2022, https://www.mayoclinic
    .org/tests-procedures/3d-mammogram/about/pac-20438708; S. Hofvind,
    A. S. Holen, H. S. Aase, N. Houssami, S. Sebuødegård, T. A. Moger, R. S.
    Haldorsen, and L. A. Akslen, "Two-View Digital Breast Tomosynthesis
    versus Digital Mammography in a Population-Based Breast Cancer Screen-
    ing Programme (To-Be): A Randomised, Controlled Trial," *Lancet* 20, no. 6
    (2019): 795–805, https://www.thelancet.com/pdfs/journals/lanonc/PIIS1470
    -2045(19)301615.pdf.
45. US Preventive Services Task Force, "Breast Cancer: Screening," Final
    Recommendation Statement, Jan. 11, 2016, https://www.uspreventiveservice
    staskforce.org/uspstf/recommendation/breast-cancer-screening.
46. "TMIST: Study Comparing Digital Mammograms (2-D) with Tomosynthe-
    sis Mammograms (3-D)," National Cancer Institute, updated Nov. 8, 2022,
    https://www.cancer.gov/about-cancer/treatment/clinical-trials/nci
    -supported/tmist#trial.
47. GE HealthCare, *2019 Reimbursement for Information for Mammography,
    CAD and Digital Breast Tomosynthesis*, April 2019, https://www
    .gehealthcare.com/-/jssmedia/f4d636930a51452ea80d207da4bd8bao
    .pdf?la=en-us.
48. L. Szabo, "A Million-Dollar Juggernaut Pushes 3D Mammograms," *Kaiser
    Health News*, Oct. 22, 2019, https://khn.org/news/a-million-dollar-marketing
    -juggernaut-pushes-3d-mammograms/.

Chapter 14. **Combating Cancerphobia**
1. J. Ryle, "The Twenty-First Maudsley Lecture," *British Journal of Psychiatry*
   94, no. 394 (1948): 1–17.
2. Ryle, "Twenty-First Maudsley Lecture."
3. Crile, *Cancer and Common Sense*, vii; Crile, "Plea against Blind Fear of
   Cancer."
4. F. Hamdy, J. Donovan, J. Athene Lane, C. Metcalfe, M. Davis, E. Turner, R.
   Martin, G. Young, E. Walsh, R. Bryant, P. Bollina, and A. Doble, "Fifteen-
   Year Outcomes after Monitoring, Surgery, or Radiotherapy for Prostate
   Cancer," *New England Journal of Medicine,* March 11, 2023.
5. M. G. Sanda et al., "Clinically Localized Prostate Cancer: AUA/ASTRO/
   SUO Guideline (2017)," *Journal of Urology*, Dec. 15, 2017.
6. R. Choo et al., "Feasibility Study: Watchful Waiting for Localized Low to
   Intermediate Grade Prostate Carcinoma with Selective Delayed Intervention Based on Prostate Specific Antigen, Histological and/or Clinical
   Progression," *Journal of Urology* 167, no. 4 (2002): 1664–69, https://www
   .auajournals.org/doi/abs/10.1016/S0022-5347%2805%2965174-9.
7. J. J. Tosoian, H. Ballentine Carter, A. Lepor, and S. Loeb, "Active Surveillance for Prostate Cancer: Current Evidence and Contemporary State of
   Practice," *Nature Reviews Urology* 13, no. 4 (2016): 205–15.
8. R. R. Parikh, S. Kim, M. N. Stein, B. G. Haffty, I. Y. Kim, and S. Goyal,
   "Trends in Active Surveillance for Very Low-Risk Prostate Cancer:
   Do Guidelines Influence Modern Practice?," *Cancer Medicine* 6,
   no. 10 (2017): 2410–18, https://www.ncbi.nlm.nih.gov/pmc/articles
   /PMC5633554/.

9.   A. Miyauchi, "Clinical Trials of Active Surveillance of Papillary Microcarcinoma of the Thyroid," *World Journal of Surgery* 40 (2016): 516–22, https://dx.doi.org/10.1007/s00268-015-3392-y.

10. P. Harrison, "Patients Accept Watchful Waiting for Low-Risk Thyroid Cancer," *Medscape Medical News*, Oct. 29, 2019, https://www.medscape.com/viewarticle/920509#vp_2.

11. N. A. Melville, "Active Surveillance for Low-Risk Thyroid Cancer: Lessons from Japan," *Medscape Medical News*, May 23, 2018, https://www.medscape.com/viewarticle/897114.

12. L. Davies, B. R. Roman, M. Fukushima, Y. Ito, and A. Miyauchi, "Patient Experience of Thyroid Cancer: Active Surveillance in Japan," *JAMA Otolaryngology—Head and Neck Surgery* 145, no. 4 (2019): 363–70.

13. J. Cavallo, "When Is Active Surveillance Appropriate in the Treatment of DCIS?." *ASCO Post*, March 25, 2018, https://ascopost.com/issues/march-25-2018/when-is-active-surveillance-appropriate-in-the-treatment-of-dcis/.

14. Welch and Black, "Overdiagnosis in Cancer."

15. L. Esserman et al., "Addressing Overdiagnosis and Overtreatment in Cancer: A Prescription for Change," *Lancet Oncology* 15, no. 6 (2014): e234–e242, https://pubmed.ncbi.nlm.nih.gov/24807866/.

16. D. J. Grignon, "The Current Classification of Urothelial Neoplasms," *Modern Pathology* 22 (2009): S60–S69, https://doi.org/10.1038/modpathol.2008.235.

17. Nikiforov et al., "Nomenclature Revision."

18. P. R. Dixon, G. Tomlinson, J. D. Pasternak, O. Mete, C. M. Bell, A. M. Sawka, D. P. Goldstein, and D. R. Urbach, "The Role of Disease Label in Patient Perceptions and Treatment Decisions in the Setting of Low-Risk Malignant Neoplasms," *JAMA Oncology* 5, no. 6 (2019): 817–23, https://jamanetwork.com/journals/jamaoncology/fullarticle/2728810.

19. "Role of Active Surveillance in the Management of Men with Localized Prostate Cancer," NIH State-of-the-Science Conference, Dec. 5–7, 2011, Bethesda, MD, https://consensus.nih.gov/2011/prostatefinalstatement.htm.

20. S. E. Eggener, A. Berlin, A. J. Vickers, G. P. Paner, H. Wolinsky, M. R. Cooperberg, "Low-Grade Prostate Cancer: Time to Stop Calling It Cancer," *Journal of Clinical Oncology*, April 18, 2022, https://ascopubs.org/doi/full/10.1200/JCO.22.00123.

21. "Diagnosis and Management of Ductal Carcinoma in Situ (DCIS)," NIH State-of-the-Science Conference, Sept. 22–24, 2009, Bethesda, MD, https://consensus.nih.gov/2009/dcisstatement.htm.

22. Z. B. Omer, E. S. Hwang, L. J. Esserman, R. Howe, and E. M. Ozanne, "Impact of Ductal Carcinoma In Situ Terminology on Patient Treatment Preferences," *JAMA Internal Medicine* 173, no. 19 (2013): 1830–31, https://jamanetwork.com/journals/jamainternalmedicine/fullarticle/1731962.

23. K. McCaffery, B. Nickel, R. Moynihan, J. Hersch, A. Teixeira-Pinto, L. Irwig, and A. Barratt, "How Different Terminology for Ductal Carcinoma In Situ Impacts Women's Concern and Treatment Preferences: A Randomised Comparison within a National Community Survey," *BMJ Open* 5, no. 11 (2015): e008094, https://bmjopen.bmj.com/content/bmjopen/5/11/e008094.full.pdf.

24. H. Adami, M. Kalager, U. Valdimarsdottir, M. Bretthauer, and J. P. A. Ioannidis, "Time to Abandon Early Detection Cancer Screening," *European Journal of Clinical Investigation* 49, no. 3 (2018), https://onlinelibrary.wiley .com/doi/abs/10.1111/eci.13062.
25. Adami et al., "Time to Abandon."
26. Adami et al., "Time to Abandon."
27. Y. Shieh, M. Eklund, G. F. Sawaya, W. C. Black, B. S. Kramer, and L. J. Esserman, "Population-Based Screening for Cancer: Hope and Hype," *National Review of Clinical Oncology* 13, no. 9 (2016): 550–65, https://www .ncbi.nlm.nih.gov/pmc/articles/PMC6585415/.
28. N. Biller-Andorno and P. Jüni, "Abolishing Mammography Screening Programs? A View from the Swiss Medical Board," *New England Journal of Medicine* 370 (2014): 1965–67, https://www.nejm.org/doi/full/10.1056 /NEJMp1401875.
29. M. G. Marmot, D. G. Altman, D. A. Cameron, J. A. Dewar, S. G. Thompson, and M. Wilcox, "The Benefits and Harms of Breast Cancer Screening: An Independent Review," *British Journal of Cancer* 108 (2013): 2205–40, https://www.nature.com/articles/bjc2013177.
30. S. Srivastava, S. Ghosh, J. Kagan, and R. Mazurchuk, "The Making of a Pre-Cancer Atlas: Promises, Challenges, and Opportunities," *Trends in Cancer* 4, no. 8 (2018): 523–36.
31. National Comprehensive Cancer Network, *Breast Cancer Screening and Diagnosis,* 2022, NCCN, June 2, 2022, https://www.nccn.org/patientresources /patient-resources/guidelines-for-patients/guidelines-for-patients-details ?patientGuidelineId=66.
32. E. S. Koh, A. Y. J. Lee, B. Ehdaie, and J. L. Marti, "Comparison of US Cancer Center Recommendations for Prostate Cancer Screening with Evidence-Based Guidelines," *JAMA Internal Medicine* 182, no. 5 (2022): 555–56.
33. "22 Myths and Truths," National Breast Cancer Coalition, accessed Feb. 12, 2023, https://www.stopbreastcancer.org/information-center/myths -truths/.
34. "Weighing the Benefits and Risks of Screening Mammography," Susan G. Komwn, last updated November 30, 2022, https://www.komen .org/breast-cancer/screening/mammography/benefits-risks/.
35. "Limitations of Mammograms," American Cancer Society, last revised Jan. 14, 2022, https://www.cancer.org/cancer/breast-cancer/screening-tests -and-early-detection/mammograms/limitations-of-mammograms.html.
36. "Prostate Cancer Early Detection, Diagnosis, and Staging," American Cancer Society, last revised Aug. 1, 2019, https://www.cancer.org/content /dam/CRC/PDF/Public/8795.00.pdf.
37. "Should I Be Screened?," Prostate Cancer Foundation, accessed March 16, 2023, https://www.pcf.org/about-prostate-cancer/what-is-prostate -cancer/the-psa-test/should-i-be-screened/.
38. "Don't Recommend Screening for Breast, Colorectal, Prostate, or Lung Cancers without Considering Life Expectancy and the Risks of Testing, Overdiagnosis, and Overtreatment," American Academy of Family Physicians, accessed Feb. 12, 2023, https://www.aafp.org/pubs/afp /collections/choosing-wisely/189.html.

39. "Breast Cancer Risk Assessment and Screening in Average-Risk Women," *ACOG Practice Bulletin* 170 (2017), https://www.acog.org/clinical/clinical -guidance/practice-bulletin/articles/2017/07/breast-cancer-risk -assessment-and-screening-in-average-risk-women.

40. "Early Detection of Prostate Cancer, AUA Guideline," *Journal of Urology*, Aug. 1, 2013, https://www.auajournals.org/doi/10.1016/j.juro.2013.04.119.

41. "To Screen or Not to Screen? The Benefits and Harms of Screening Tests," *NIH News in Health*, March 2017, https://newsinhealth.nih.gov/2017/03 /screen-or-not-screen.

42. Tribune Content Agency, "Prostate Cancer Screening Is No Longer Automatic: That's Turned Out to Be a Sensible Change," *Greater Milwaukee Today*, Dec. 18, 2020, https://www.gmtoday.com/health/prostate -cancer-screening-is-no-longer-automatic-thats-turned-out-to-be-a -sensible-change/article_25178aa0-4151-11eb-ba02-a3c51088611a.html; J. E. Brody, "Debating the Value of PSA Prostate Screening," *New York Times*, Feb. 24, 2020, https://www.nytimes.com/2020/02/24/well/live /prostate-testing-PSA-cancer-screening.html; L. Rapaport, "More Doctors Say Men Should Think Twice about Prostate Cancer Screening," *Reuters Health*, Sept. 25, 2018, https://www.reuters.com/article/us-health -cancer-prostate-screening-idUSKCN1M52XL; S. Begley, "Mammograms More Likely to Cause Unneeded Treatment than to Save Lives," *STAT News*, Oct. 12, 2016, https://www.statnews.com/2016/10/12/mammogram -overdiagnose-breast-cancer/; A. Park, "The Case for Annual Mammograms Is More Complicated than Ever," *Time*, Jan. 9, 2017, https://time .com/4629245/who-needs-a-mammogram-for-breast-cancer-guidelines /; "Breast Cancer Screening Programme 'Does More Harm than Good,'" *BBC News*, May 5, 2018, https://www.bbc.com/news/health-44016206; D. Grady, "Quandary with Mammograms: Get a Screening, or Just Skip It?," *New York Times*, Nov. 2, 2009, https://www.nytimes.com/2009/11/03 /health/03second.html; "Screening for Lung Cancer Is a Controversial Idea," *Economist*, April 27, 2019, https://www.economist.com/science-and -technology/2019/04/27/screening-for-lung-cancer-is-a-controversial -idea; S. Reinberg, "Colonoscopies Can Cause Greater Infection Risk," *HealthDay News*, June 6, 2018, https://www.webmd.com/colorectal-cancer /news/20180606/colonoscopies-can-cause-greater-infection-risk#1; "Are We Now Doing Too Much Cancer Screening?," 1200 WOAI, Dec. 26, 2017, https://woai.iheart.com/content/2017-12-26-are-we-now-doing-too-much -cancer-screening/.

43. L. Davenport, "'Overdiagnosis' in about 20% of Common Cancers," *Medscape Medical News*, Jan. 30, 2020, https://www.medscape.com /viewarticle/924550; A. E. Cha, "Breast Cancer and Mammograms: Study Suggests 'Widespread Overdiagnosis,'" *Washington Post*, July 6, 2015, https://www.washingtonpost.com/news/to-your-health/wp/2015/07 /06/breast-cancer-and-mammograms-study-suggests-widespread -overdiagnosis/; L. Lagnado, "Debate over Early-Stage Cancer: To Treat or Not to Treat?," *Wall Street Journal*, Oct. 19, 2015, https://www.wsj.com /articles/debate-over-early-stage-cancer-to-treat-or-not-to-treat -1445276596; J. Belluz, "We Really Need to Rethink How We Diagnose

and Treat Breast Cancer," *Vox*, Aug. 21, 2015, https://www.vox.com/2015/8/21/9185739/breast-cancer-treatment-mastectomy; G. Kolata, "Doubt Is Raised over Value of Surgery for Breast Lesion at Earliest Stage," *New York Times*, Aug. 20, 2015, https://www.nytimes.com/2015/08/21/health/breast-cancer-ductal-carcinoma-in-situ-study.html; "Thousands of Australians Undergo Chemo after Being 'Overdiagnosed' with Cancer Each Year," *Sunrise*, 7News.com.au, Jan. 26, 2020, https://7news.com.au/sunrise/on-the-show/thousands-of-australians-overdiagnosed-with-cancer-each-year-c-666254; S. McCaffery, "What Is DCIS and Is This Type of Breast Cancer Overtreated?," *Atlanta Journal-Constitution*, May 9, 2019, https://www.ajc.com/lifestyles/health/stage-zero-can-less-more/W45VkpeKI1U86joqqszSzL/; P. Neighmond and R. Knox, "When Treating Abnormal Breast Cells, Sometimes Less Is More," NPR, Aug. 5, 2013, https://www.npr.org/sections/health-shots/2013/08/05/208239545/when-treating-abnormal-breast-cells-sometimes-less-is-more; L. Abraham, "The Danger of DCIS, the Breast 'Cancer' That's Often Not," *ELLE*, June 8, 2015, https://www.elle.com/culture/news/a28636/a-radical-idea/.

44. T. Mathias, "Doctors Debate Whether to Stop Calling Low-Risk Tumors 'Cancer,'" Reuters, Feb. 6, 2019, https://www.reuters.com/article/us-health-cancer-labels/doctors-debate-whether-to-stop-calling-low-risk-tumors-cancer-idUSKCN1PV2ED; G. Kolata, "'Cancer' or 'Weird Cells': Which Sounds Deadlier?," *New York Times*, Nov. 21, 2011, https://www.nytimes.com/2011/11/22/health/cancer-by-any-other-name-would-not-be-as-terrifying.html; A. Thompson, "Doctors Should Stop Using the Word Cancer: Low-Risk Tumours Should Be Renamed 'Indolent' Because the C-word Traumatises Patients, Leading Expert Says," *Daily Mail* (London), Jan. 23, 2019, https://www.dailymail.co.uk/health/article-6624081/Low-risk-cancers-renamed-indolent-oncologist-urges.html.

45. R. H. Nagler, E. Franklin Fowler, N. Marino, K. M. Mentzer, and S. E. Gollust, "The Evolution of Mammography Controversy in the News Media: A Content Analysis of Four Publicized Screening Recommendations, 2009–2016," *Women's Health Issues* 29, no. 1 (2019): 87–95, https://www.ncbi.nlm.nih.gov/pmc/articles/PMC6295242/.

46. A. B. Miller, "Basic Issues in Populations Screening for Cancer," in *Screening in Cancer*, ed. A. B. Miller (Technical Report Series 40; Geneva: UICC, 1978).

47. W. C. Black and H. G. Welch, "Advances in Diagnostic Imaging and Overestimation of Disease Prevalence and the Benefits of Therapy," *New England Journal of Medicine* 328, no. 17 (1993): 1237–43, https://www.nejm.org/doi/full/10.1056/nejm199304293281706.

48. A. E. Raffle, A. Mackie, and J. A. Muir Gray, *Screening: Evidence and Practice* (Oxford: Oxford University Press, 2007).

49. W. C. Black, "Overdiagnosis: An Underrecognized Cause of Confusion and Harm in Cancer Screening," *Journal of the National Cancer Institute* 92, no. 16 (2000): 1280–82, https://academic.oup.com/jnci/article/92/16/1280/2905911; Welch and Black, "Overdiagnosis in Cancer."

50. S. Brownlee, *Overtreated: Why Too Much Medicine Is Making Us Sicker and Poorer* (New York: Bloomsbury, 2008).

51. Welch, Schwartz, and Woloshin, *Overdiagnosed*; Brawley, *How We Do Harm*; Sulik, *Pink Ribbon Blues*; A. H. Horan, *How to Avoid the Over-Diagnosis and Over-Treatment of Prostate Cancer* (Broomfield, CO: On the Write Path, 2012).

52. R. J. Albin and R. Piana, *The Great Prostate Hoax: How Big Medicine Hijacked the PSA Test and Caused a Public Health Disaster* (New York: St. Martin's Press, 2014).

53. R. Pellerin, *Conspiracy of Hope: The Truth about Breast Cancer Screening* (Fredericton, NB: Goose Lane, 2018).

Chapter 15. Combating Cancerphobia in Yourself

1. D. Kahneman, *Thinking, Fast and Slow* (New York: Farrar, Straus, and Giroux, 2013).

2. Breast Cancer Surveillance Consortium Risk Calculator, last modified Jan. 31, 2016, https://tools.bcsc-scc.org/BC5yearRisk/.

3. Prostate Cancer Prevention Trial Risk Calculator Version 2.0, last updated 2018, https://riskcalc.org/PCPTRC/.

4. M. J. Barry and S. Edgman-Levitan, "Shared Decision Making—The Pinnacle of Patient-Centered Care," *New England Journal of Medicine* 366, no. 9 (2012): 780–81.

5. A. O'Connor, H. Llewellyn-Thomas, and D. Stacey, *IPDAS Background Document*, International Patient Decision Aids Standards Collaboration, Dec. 17, 2005, http://ipdas.ohri.ca/IPDAS_Background.pdf.

6. T. J. Caverly, R. A. Hayward, E. Reamer, B. J. Zikmund-Fisher, D. Connochie, M. Heisler, and A. Fagerlin, "Presentation of Benefits and Harms in US Cancer Screening and Prevention Guidelines: Systematic Review," *Journal of the National Cancer Institute* 108, no. 6 (2016): djv436, https://academic.oup.com/jnci/article/108/6/djv436/2412660.

7. A. J. Housten et al., "A Review of the Presentation of Overdiagnosis in Cancer Screening Patient Decisions Aids," *MDM Policy and Practice* 4, no. 2 (2019), https://journals.sagepub.com/doi/10.1177/2381468319881447.

8. "Should I Be Screened for Prostate Cancer?," UpToDate, 2021, https://www.uptodate.com/contents/image?imageKey=ONC%2F110294&topicKey=PI%2F883.

9. "Australian Screening Mammography Decision Aid Trial," University of Sydney, accessed Feb. 1, 2023, http://www.mammogram.med.usyd.edu.au.

10. "Should I Be Screened for Lung Cancer?," UpToDate, 2021, accessed Feb. 1, 2023, https://www.uptodate.com/contents/image?imageKey=ONC%2F110643.

11. D. Stacey et al., "Decision Aids for People Facing Health Treatment or Screening Decisions," *Cochrane Database of Systematic Reviews* 28, no. 1 (2014): CD001431, https://pubmed.ncbi.nlm.nih.gov/24470076/.

12. T. A. Trikalinos, L. S. Wieland, G. Phyfe Adam, A. Zgodic, and E. Ntzani, *Decision Aids for Cancer Screening and Treatment*, Comparative Effectiveness Reviews no. 145, Agency for Healthcare Research and Quality, Dec. 2014, https://www.ncbi.nlm.nih.gov/books/NBK269409/.

13. R. Evans et al., "Supporting Informed Decision Making for Prostate Specific Antigen (PSA) Testing on the Web: An Online Randomized Controlled Trial," *Journal of Medical Internet Research* 12, no. 3 (2010): e27; P. Scalia, G. Elwyn, J. Kremer, M. Faber, and M. Durand, "Assessing Preference Shift and Effects on Patient Knowledge and Decisional Conflict: Cross-Sectional Study of an Interactive Prostate-Specific Antigen Test Patient Decision Aid," *Journal of Medical Internet Research* 4, no. 2 (2018): e11102.

14. G. Elwyn, J. Adams, Z. Berger, B. Dropkin, E. Hyams, D. Frosch, S. Stewart, and M. Durand, eds., "Prostate Specific Antigen: Yes or No?," Option Grid decision aid, accessed March 16, 2023, https://www.mahealthcare.com /pdf/mahp/PSA_Decision_Grid.pdf.

15. J. Waljee, M. Rogers, and A. Alderman, "Decision Aids and Breast Cancer: Do They Influence Choice for Surgery and Knowledge of Treatment Options?" *Journal of Clinical Oncology* 25, no. 9 (2007): 1067–73, https:// www.ncbi.nlm.nih.gov/books/NBK73450/.

16. S. Hwang, A. Thompson, and A. Partridge, "Welcome to the DCIS Decision Support Tool," accessed Feb. 1, 2023, https://dcisoptions.org/dst.

17. *Treatment Choices for Men with Early-Stage Prostate Cancer*, National Cancer Institute, last updated Jan. 2011, https://www.cancer.gov/publications /patient-education/understanding-prostate-cancer-treatment.

18. D. Stacey, V. Suwalska, L. Boland, K. B. Lewis, J. Presseau, and R. Thomson, "Are Patient Decision Aids Used in Clinical Practice after Rigorous Evaluation? A Survey of Trial Authors," *Medical Decision Making* 39, no. 7 (2019): 805–15.

19. M. Hostetter and S. Klein, "Helping Patients Make Better Choices with Decision Aids," *Improving Health Care Quality*, Oct.–Nov. 2012, Commonwealth Fund, https://www.commonwealthfund.org/publications/newsletter -article/helping-patients-make-better-treatment-choices-decision-aids ?redirect_source=/publications/newsletters/quality-matters/2012/october -november/in-focus.

index

Page numbers in *italic* refer to figures; those in **bold** refer to tables.